Kevin J. McWilliams

12 - 5 - 2014

Purchased by

Corinne McGoran

Protein Power

BY THE SAME AUTHORS

Michael R. Eades, M.D.
Thin So Fast

Mary Dan Eades, M.D.
If It Runs in Your Family: Breast Cancer
If It Runs in Your Family: Arthritis
Freeing Someone You Love from Eating Disorders
The Doctor's Complete Guide to Vitamins and Minerals

Protein Power

Michael R. Eades, M.D.
& Mary Dan Eades, M.D.

BANTAM BOOKS
New York · Toronto · London · Sydney · Auckland

The diet plan presented here is not intended for anyone with kidney problems or for pregnant women or women trying to get pregnant. Readers who are on medication to control cholesterol, blood pressure, fluid retention, or blood sugar or who have an abnormal heart rhythm or have had a heart attack within the last six months must not under any circumstances begin this diet plan without a physician's guidance and close supervision. Even other readers, however, should consult a physician regarding their individual needs before starting any diet or fitness program.

PROTEIN POWER
A Bantam Book / February 1996

All rights reserved.
Copyright © 1996 by Creative Paradox, LLC

Figure 6.1 is modified and used with permission of Dr. Barry Sears.

Book design by Irving Perkins Associates

Illustrations by Roberto Osti

Library of Congress Cataloging-in-Publication Data
Eades, Michael R.
    Protein power : the metabolic breakthrough / Michael R. Eades and
Mary Dan Eades.
        p.   cm.
    Includes index.
    ISBN 0-553-10183-8
    1. Low-carbohydrate diet. 2. Insulin resistance.   I. Eades, Mary
Dan.   II. Title.
RM237.73E23 1996
613.2'8—dc20   95-32738
                                                         CIP

Published simultaneously in the United States and Canada

Bantam Books are published by Bantam Books, a division of Bantam Doubleday Dell Publishing Group, Inc. Its trademark, consisting of the words "Bantam Books" and the portrayal of a rooster, is Registered in U.S. Patent and Trademark Office and in other countries. Marca Registrada. Bantam Books, 1540 Broadway, New York, New York 10036.

PRINTED IN THE UNITED STATES OF AMERICA

BVG   30 29 28 27 26 25 24

To British physician John Yudkin, M.D., Ph.D., who was fighting the good fight before we were born.

And to our sons, Ted, Daniel, and Scott Eades, who will continue to fight it after we're gone.

There was an old man of Tobago,
Who lived on rice, gruel, and sago;
Till, much to his bliss,
His physician said this—
To a leg, sir, of mutton you may go.

JOHN MARSHALL, 1822

Contents

Acknowledgments

We would like to thank the many people who were instrumental in helping us bring this book to you. It's been a long and sometimes difficult process through which we had the unfailing support of our agent and friend Channa Taub, who consoled and cajoled us through some stressful times and was always willing to sharpen her editorial pencil when needed. Channa brought us to Carol Mann, who gets many thanks for bringing our work to the wonderful group at Bantam Books. Thanks to Fran McCullough, our editor, for her interest in and understanding of this project and for all the work she did to streamline and improve the manuscript. And to everyone at Bantam—especially Irwyn Applebaum, Nita Taublib, Allen Goodman, Amanda Mecke, Barb Burg, and Lauren Janis.

To our sons, Ted, Dan, and Scott, who put up with erratic family schedules and cranky parents during the writing of this book, we love you.

Our faithful staff at the clinic, who fielded calls, juggled schedules, and held down the fort while we wrote, deserve special mention—thanks to Rhonda Mallison, Mary Clendaniel, Linda Tullos, Valerie Wilkins, Michelle Denton, and Deya Devorak.

Thanks to Barbara Witt, who contributed most of the recipes.

We are grateful for the support, help, criticism, and advice from our many professional and scientific colleagues who read and commented on this manuscript during its writing. Special thanks to Barry Sears, Ph.D., who has helped us refine our thinking by engaging us in hundreds of hours of how-many-angels-can-dance-on-the-head-of-a-pin-type arguments on the merits of our respective dietary philosophies. And to Allen Hill, M.D., whose suggestions and support have been invaluable, we give heartfelt thanks. Not only has he taken much time from his busy practice to read and help improve our manuscript, he has also graciously taken over the care of our patients innumerable times, often at a moment's notice, during the many absences this project required of us.

And finally, thanks to Cathy Hemming, our erstwhile agent and always our friend, who believed in the merits of this book and this paradigm before anyone else.

Introduction

You may be wondering how a couple of physicians who specialize in weight loss in a relatively small city in Middle America devised a nutritional program that works as well as this one does, while most of the scientists in the major universities are headed off in the opposite direction, puzzling over why their success with low-fat diet plans has been so minimal. In a nutshell, we lucked out. We lucked out because that's how science works. Science progresses because people continue to question why. Researchers propose hypotheses based on their understanding of the natural world and then test them—and most of the time these theories blow up in their faces. The lucky ones stumble onto the hypotheses that turn out to be valid. But of course there's more than luck involved, because as Louis Pasteur said, "Chance favors the prepared mind," and in our case our minds were prepared by many years of clinical practice with patients suffering all the illnesses that are heir to disordered insulin metabolism as well as by our unique combination of medical interests. Mike is a collector of diet books and old medical texts and has a strong interest in paleopathology and biochemistry; Mary Dan is interested in anthropology and has published a book on eating disorders and the deranged metabolic status of eating-disordered patients.

We have a copy of the earliest diet book ever to sweep the nation, *Banting's Letter on Corpulence,* first printed in the middle 1800s. This restricted-carbohydrate diet worked like a charm for Banting and, if sales were any indication, many others. It has always intrigued us because it completely flies in the face of today's low-fat paradigm. At about the same time we ran across Banting we began attending paleopathology conferences and studying anthropology, where we learned what paleopathologists and anthropologists have known for years: the agricultural revolution and the increased consumption of carbohydrates it brought along with it played havoc with the health of early man. Mary Dan's extensive study of eating disorders and metabolic hormonal derangements combined with Mike's interest in biochemistry rounded out the "preparation" of our minds. We looked at Banting's success with carbohydrate restriction along with the paleopathological/anthropological data showing a decline in health accompanying an increase in carbohydrate intake and concluded that maybe the intake of large amounts of carbohydrates wasn't necessarily a good thing. That became our first mini-hypothesis: excess carbohydrate consumption isn't good. But why not?

We knew, as does every doctor, that the immediate effect of carbohydrate consumption is increased blood glucose, then an increased insulin level. We thought that perhaps the increased insulin levels might be to blame for part of the problem. As we studied the medical literature, we found that researchers the world over were finding elevated insulin levels associated with obesity, heart disease, high blood pressure, and diabetes—the common diseases of modern man. We also found that the same researchers were for the most part trying to treat these patients by giving them more of the same thing we were beginning to believe may have caused the problem in the first place: the high-carbohydrate, low-fat diet. It made more sense to us that if excess insulin indeed *causes* these disorders, or at the very least makes them worse, as the increasing mountain of research indicated, perhaps patients would be better off *reducing* their carbohydrate intake, not increasing it.

We took then as our working hypothesis that excess carbohydrate leads to excess insulin, which leads to obesity, high blood pressure, and all the rest. It fit with the anthropological and paleopathological data and, at least as far as obesity was concerned, with Banting's dietary theory. We then began to examine this hypothesis from a basic biochemical perspective and found that it worked beautifully. From all perspectives our hypothesis looked good on paper, so we began to test it carefully, first on ourselves, then on patients in our practice. We found that the results were rapid, dramatic, and pretty much uniform—just what we expected based on the underlying science. As we worked with our patients, we continued to refine our techniques, expand our range of dietary choices, and in general collect those little tips and tricks that make the practice of medicine an art as well as a science. We are still learning and refining every day, and, as with any technique that works, more and more practitioners are beginning to use a restricted-carbohydrate diet for their patients and are adding their own unique refinements to the rapidly growing body of data.

This book is arranged in basically the sequence of our own development and refinement of our hypothesis. The first chapters give an overview and an explanation from a historical, anthropological, and biochemical perspective, which should give you the information and explanations you need to become comfortable with these seemingly radical ideas. If you don't care about the "why" of all this, just read "The Bottom Line," the summaries at the end of each chapter. The latter part of the book is a nuts-and-bolts primer on how to implement these nutritional strategies in your own health-preserving and rejuvenation program. (On the other hand, if you'd like to read more, please write to us in care of our publisher, and we'll send you a bibliography.)

You'll find the program in a nutshell on page 155, but please read all of Chapter 10, all about exercise in Chapter 12, and the essential list of vitamins at the end of Chapter 8, in addition to the Bottom Line Summaries.

Will this program work for you? In good conscience, we can only say probably. The reason we hedge a little is because of biochemical individuality—we are all as different biochemically as we are in appearance. Every doctor has encountered patients in whom medicines seem to work in an opposite fashion to that intended, patients who are kept awake by sleeping pills and pass out on stimulants. These and similar experiences keep practiced physicians from ever making blanket this-will-work-in-all-circumstances statements. All we can tell you is that in the almost ten years we have been treating patients with this program we have *never* had a negative outcome. If you're like the vast majority of our patients, you will find the results as striking and life changing as we have and will adopt this program, modified to your own unique lifestyle and tastes, for the rest of your life.

Little Rock
June 1995

Protein Power

Chapter I

A New Nutritional Perspective

Every man is the creature of the age in which he lives; very few are able to raise themselves above the ideas of the time.

VOLTAIRE

We have a medical book published in 1822 passed down to Michael from his great-grandfather, a country doctor from the Ozark Mountains. A long section deals with yellow fever—in the 1800s no one knew what caused it or how it spread. Now, of course, we understand that the mosquito is the carrier of the virus that causes yellow fever, but then the cause eluded the best minds in medical science. Read what this standard 1822 medical textbook says about yellow fever:

> . . . it rises from the exposure of putrid animal and vegetable substances on the public wharfs . . . it always begins in the lowest part of a populous mercantile town near the water, and continues here without much affecting the higher parts. It rages most where large quantities of new ground have been made by banking out the rivers for the purpose of constructing wharfs. . . . the yellow fever is generated by the impure air or vapour which issues from the new-made earth or ground raised on the muddy and filthy bottom of rivers. . . .

From our contemporary vantage point we want to reach back and tell them, "Look, it's a mosquito; why can't you see the big picture?"

The medical problems that confound us today will probably amaze scientists in the twenty-first century as they puzzle over why we medical pioneers of today were unable to reach out and grasp the obvious, why we were so advanced in certain areas of medical treatment yet so abysmally deficient in others. Why, they may ask, could our surgeons perform open-heart surgery so skillfully as to make it a routine operation while at the same time our nutritional experts couldn't determine the optimal diet for preventing most of the problems necessitating that procedure? Why spend so much time and effort developing complex surgical techniques and other wondrous medical procedures that prolong the life of a diseased body for a few months or, at best, a few years instead of focusing on nutritional changes capable of prolonging healthy life for decades? Why can't *we* see the big picture?

The Failure of the Low-Fat, High-Carbohydrate Diet

Yes, doctors today are aware that diet plays a significant role in the development and progression of the major diseases afflicting modern man—heart disease, diabetes, obesity, high blood pressure, and many kinds of cancers. As a consequence dietitians, nutritionists, and physicians constantly exhort us to eat properly to avoid these disorders. By their definition, eating properly means rooting out fat from our diets and replacing it with complex carbohydrate.

Ever since the surgeon general recommended in 1988 that Americans severely reduce their consumption of fat, especially saturated fat, the race to zero fat products has been on. Eggs, red meat, and other superior protein sources have been virtually drummed out of the American kitchen. Reduce fat intake to almost nothing, we are told by battalions of nutritional experts, and good-bye obesity, heart disease, diabetes, and all the rest. Sounds great in theory, but—and here's why physicians a hundred years from now will be shaking their heads—it doesn't work.

The low-fat, high-complex-carbohydrate approach has proven a failure. It doesn't reduce cholesterol levels to any great degree unless followed to an almost ridiculous extreme, in which case it can actually cause other equally sinister problems, as you will soon discover. It gives diabetes sufferers endless grief in trying to regulate their blood sugar levels. It doesn't reduce high blood pressure unless it brings about significant weight loss. Its success rate for weight loss is almost nonexistent. (You may be surprised to learn that we've treated many people who have *gained* weight on the low-fat diet.) The result of the current no-fat mania has been a fatter and less healthy America, thanks in part to the zeal of food manufacturers who have given us an endless variety of fat-free high-carbohydrate junk to replace the fat-filled junk we were eating before.

In the face of this dismal record, what do we as medical professionals do? Do we write off the low-fat diet as something that sounded good on paper but didn't work in practice, abandon it and begin searching for something better, as we would a new drug that had failed? No. Instead we say, "Bring on more of the same. Let's try harder, let's try longer, let's be more diligent." We tell our patients that it must be *their* fault if their condition doesn't improve on a low-fat diet; they must not be following it correctly. But such thinking flies in the face of metabolic reality because *dietary fat alone is not the problem.* The problem lies in the biochemical structure of the low-fat diet and the mixed signals it gives to the body's essential metabolic processes. Ironically, not only does the low-fat diet fail to solve the health problems it addresses; it actually makes them even worse.

The program we outline in this book triumphs where the high-complex-carbohydrate, low-fat diet fails. It reduces cholesterol rapidly *without* increasing other risk factors; it reverses, or at least significantly improves, adult-onset (type II) diabetes; it drops elevated blood pressure like a rock; it offers a long-term solution for the problem of excess weight—all without asking you to count fat grams or worry about fat percentages. It does all this simply by selecting foods that work *with* your body's metabolic biochemistry instead of against it.

The human body is a remarkably resilient, reactive, regenerative piece of biochemical machinery. Like any piece of complex equipment, it functions best when treated properly. The proponents of low-fat dieting believe the best way to treat the body is by restricting the amount of fat, particularly saturated fat, the body takes in and replacing it with complex carbohydrate. Their flawed thinking goes like this: too much fat accumulation in the arteries causes heart disease and other problems, too much fat accumulation in the fat cells causes obesity, and too much fat intake exacerbates diabetes, so if we reduce fat intake, we'll solve all these problems. Although it seems logical, it doesn't work because it doesn't take into account the body's biochemistry and the ways our metabolic hormones cause us to store fat. When we understand and control these potent body chemicals, we can achieve our health goals by controlling fat from within rather than trying to eliminate it from without. To begin to understand how this works, let's first examine food from a biochemical perspective.

What Is This Thing Called Food?

All food, from pancakes to sushi, is composed of macronutrients, micronutrients, and water. Aside from water, which makes up the lion's share of everything, food is made primarily of the macronutrients protein, fat, and carbohydrate. These three macronutrients are the only food components that provide energy—measured as calories—to maintain life. The micronutrients—vitamins, minerals, and trace elements—provide no caloric energy but are nevertheless essential for life. They perform a multitude of cellular functions, many of which involve the efficient use and disposal of the macronutrients. Without macronutrients we would suffer malnutrition, starvation, and death; without the micronutrients we would suffer deficiency diseases, a precipitous health decline, and death. The nutrients from both groups are necessary for life.

BALANCING THE BIG THREE

Since the entire caloric content of food comes from the three macronutrients, it is obvious that decreasing any one macronutrient—fat, for instance—requires increasing another (carbohydrate or protein or both) to maintain any given caloric level. If your metabolic needs for a day require 2,000 calories, and, in accordance with the recommendations of the nutritional establishment, you reduce your fat intake, what happens? You increase your intake of carbohydrate and protein to make up for the calories lost by removing the fat, right? Actually, it's a little more complicated than that. You don't go to the grocery store and buy three scoops of protein, five scoops of carbohydrate, and two scoops of fat; you buy meat, eggs, vegetables, fruits, dairy products. Some foods, meat and eggs, for instance, contain only protein and fat, while others such as apples and grapes are practically all carbohydrate with only a trace of protein. You can trim the visible fat from cuts of meat to reduce fat content, but otherwise it's difficult to extract just one macronutrient from a particular food item. So the only way to change the ratios of fat, protein, and carbohydrate is to change the types of foods eaten. If you want to decrease your fat intake, you simply eat less meat, eggs, and dairy products and replace them with fruits and vegetables. Sounds reasonable, but is it?

Not really, and here's why. Humans don't require equal amounts of the three macronutrients for optimal health. The average person requires at least 70 to 100 grams of protein per day, or about 300 calories' worth, and at least 6 to 10 grams of linoleic acid (a type of fat that is essential to health), about 75 calories' worth. What about carbohydrate? The actual amount of carbohydrate *required* by humans for health is *zero*.[1] We haven't made these figures up; they represent the consensus of scientific wisdom today. Now, this doesn't mean that as long as you get 75 grams of protein and 6 grams of fat you'll do fine. You need more calories to provide energy for your bodily functions. It does mean that if you got

---

[1] As you will discover in a later chapter, your body has all the biochemical machinery necessary to make all the blood sugar you need to nourish the tissues that require it—red blood cells, some parts of the eye, brain, and kidney.

enough energy from either protein or fat and maintained your minimum intake of each, you would do fine. Eskimos eat very little carbohydrate, in fact no carbohydrate during the winter, and survive nicely to a ripe old age. Although their traditional diet is composed of a large quantity of protein and an enormous amount of fat, Eskimos suffer very little heart disease, diabetes, obesity (despite the cartoons), high blood pressure, and all the other diseases we associate with a more civilized lifestyle. Furthermore, Eskimos don't have metabolic systems from an alien planet; they have the exact same biochemistry and physiology that we do. Yes, *you* could eat the same diet and tolerate it nicely.[2]

Bearing in mind that protein and fat are essential to health and carbohydrate isn't, what happens when we cut back our fat as the nutritional establishment recommends? Since we can't for the most part remove the fat from the food, we end up replacing foods that contain fat with those that don't. Since most sources of good-quality protein—meat, eggs, and dairy products—contain a fair amount of fat, to cut back on fat we end up cutting back on protein as well and replacing them both with carbohydrate. Most vegetable sources of protein—beans and grains—are incomplete unless combined carefully and contain far more carbohydrate than protein. In the end if we strictly follow the low-fat prescription we can end up deficient in protein (it's difficult to be deficient in fat because the only essential fat is linoleic acid, which is found in vegetable oils).

But possibly the worst news of all is that eating more carbohydrates stimulates your body's fat storage. In attempting to reduce fat intake, you wind up actually getting fatter, because some macronutrients stimulate profound metabolic hormonal changes. Surprisingly, fat doesn't do much. If you were to swill down a dish of lard while hooked up to a laboratory device to measure the levels of your metabolic hormones—chiefly insulin and glucagon—you wouldn't see much activity, because fat is essentially metabolically inert. Carbohydrate, however, would set off a Mad Hatter's tea party of metabolic activity. Eating a handful of grapes

---

[2] We know this because of the famous study done in 1929 and 1930 using the explorers Vilhjalmur Stefansson and Karsten Anderson. These men returned from the Arctic reporting that Eskimos were able to live on nothing but caribou meat all winter while performing arduous work, expending great amounts of energy without consequence. To prove that not only Eskimos had this capability, both explorers volunteered to be studied while hospitalized in Bellevue Hospital in New York City for one year. During this time they ate a meat diet composed of more than 2,500 calories a day, which was 75 percent fat. At the end of the year both had lost about 6 pounds of weight, their cholesterol levels and other blood chemistry values were normal, and neither experienced any adverse effects.

while hooked to the same device would initiate a wild swinging of gauge needles indicating a rapid increase in insulin and a decrease in its opposing hormone glucagon, all perfectly normal metabolic responses kindled by the consumption of carbohydrate. It follows logically that the constant consumption of large quantities of carbohydrate would then produce large quantities of insulin, which indeed it does.

Even complex carbohydrates stimulate the response because *all* carbohydrates are basically sugar. Various sugar molecules—primarily glucose—hooked together chemically compose the entire family of carbohydrates. Your body has digestive enzymes that break these chemical bonds and release the sugar molecules into the blood, where they stimulate insulin and the other metabolic hormones. This means that if you follow a 2,200-calorie diet that is 60 percent carbohydrate—the very one most nutritionists recommend—your body will end up having to contend metabolically with *almost 2 cups of pure sugar per day.*

What's Insulin Got to Do with It?

So, what does insulin have to do with anything other than diabetes? And if you don't have diabetes, why should you care about insulin at all? Because it's important to your health.

Insulin, a hormone produced and released into the blood by the pancreas, affects virtually every cell in the body. Insulin occupies a chapter or two in every medical biochemistry and physiology textbook, entire sections in endocrinology texts, and even two pages of tiny print in our fifteen-year-old *Encyclopaedia Britannica.* Whole textbooks are devoted to its myriad activities. Insulin regulates blood sugar, yes, but it does much more. It controls the storage of fat, it directs the flow of amino acids, fatty acids, and carbohydrate to the tissues, it regulates the liver's synthesis of cholesterol, it functions as a growth hormone, it is involved in appetite control, it drives the kidneys to retain fluid, and much, much more. This master hormone of metabolism is a substance absolutely essential to life; without it, you would perish—quickly.

But insulin is also a monster hormone; it has a dark side. In the proper amount it is life sustaining; too much of it causes enormous health problems. Reams of scientific studies, with more added to the stack daily, implicate excess insulin as a *primary* cause of or significant risk factor for high blood pressure, heart disease, obesity, elevated cholesterol and other blood fats, and diabetes (yes, insulin itself can *cause* diabetes, a concept we will explore at length later in this book).

If you don't have diabetes now, that doesn't mean you won't develop it in the future, especially if it runs in your family. The same goes for heart disease, high blood pressure, and all the rest. Insulin problems have a strong genetic basis, so a good way to determine if you are at risk for any of the insulin-related disorders is to examine your family tree closely. If your parents or grandparents had or have any of the following, you are at risk:

- heart disease,
- high blood pressure,
- accumulation of fat around the waistline,
- elevated cholesterol,
- elevated triglycerides and other blood fats,
- type II diabetes,
- excess fluid retention (swelling of ankles).

As you consider the health profiles of your family members, be aware that the more of these disorders you identify, the more at risk you are for developing them. If you are at risk, you have a pressing reason to care about insulin, because controlling it can literally save your life; if you have already been afflicted with one (or more) of these disorders, controlling your insulin can restore your health.

Taming the Monster: Controlling Insulin Through Diet

How do you go about controlling it? With our nutritional regimen—a carbohydrate-restricted, moderate-fat, adequate-protein diet that modulates the body's metabolic hormones, including insulin. Diet is what makes insulin levels go haywire in the first place, so it stands to reason that dietary changes should be able to reverse the problem. Diet is, in fact, the *only* way to solve this problem.

The foods we eat exert a profound influence on what happens within our bodies hormonally—both for good and for bad. By eating the correct balance of foods we can almost medicinally alter what goes on inside us in a healthful way; by eating the wrong foods we can precipitate health disasters. We can more easily dig our graves with a fork and spoon than with a shovel.

Our plan uses food as a tool to reverse, or at the very least markedly improve, disorders engendered by a metabolic system out of whack. Our easy-to-follow dietary regimen is tasty, filling, nutritionally complete, and even allows for the consumption of alcoholic beverages—in moderation. It works. And best of all it works quickly.

How quickly? In terms of feeling better and more energetic, within a week or less; for cholesterol reduction, substantial reductions in blood levels by three weeks, maybe sooner (we say maybe sooner because we've never checked anyone before three weeks). Victims of high blood pressure—a condition that is usually insulin related—typically achieve a greatly lowered, or normal, blood pressure within a week or two. Those with diabetes and related problems generally find their blood sugar levels normalized or at least greatly improved within just a few weeks—sometimes only days. High blood pressure, elevated cholesterol, type II diabetes—this program corrects or greatly improves them all in short order by normalizing the body's disrupted metabolic hormonal status, which causes all these problems in the first place.

Obesity, the other major health problem rooted in a disturbed insulin metabolism, doesn't disappear as quickly, of course. Although our nutritional program opens all the metabolic pathways to allow an efficient burning of body fat for energy, the body fat still has to be burned—and depending on how much there is to burn, that can take some time. The good news is, however, that long before our patients lose much weight on the program the medical problems afflicting most of them—high blood pressure, elevated cholesterol, diabetes, gout, and a host of others—improve dramatically or even vanish. Now, granted, on the typical low-calorie, low-fat, high-complex-carbohydrate weight-reduction diet these medical disorders will sometimes *gradually* improve as body weight falls, but on our diet these improvements are almost immediate due to the rapid metabolic changes effected.

Of course we don't have all the answers; but we do have a nutritional program that we've tested on ourselves, our three sons, thousands of our patients, and countless people nationwide, without a single adverse reaction.[3]

Our approach is scientifically valid, historically valid, and can be explained using not a few obscure scientific articles but standard medical textbooks. This is important because it means that we've based our conclusions on scientific fact, not theory. Medical scientists doing cutting-edge research publish their findings in medical/scientific journals, initiating a firestorm of debate and a flurry of activity in other laboratories the world over. Many scientists then repeat the experiments, sometimes obtaining the same results, sometimes not. Before any particular piece of scientific knowledge is generally considered valid, it must be confirmed by multiple long-term tests, performed in many different labs, all

---

[3] In 1989 Michael wrote a book, *Thin So Fast,* published by Warner Books that described our nutritional regimen as applied solely to weight loss. Since then we've received countless letters from readers all over the world, recounting their successes after years of failure on more conventional diets.

with the same result. Only then does it enter the medical literature as fact, and only then is it published in medical textbooks. Not only can *all* the concepts underlying our program be found in every basic medical textbook, but studies confirming our approach are beginning to appear throughout the medical journals (again, write to us in care of our publisher for a bibliography).

Could anyone have seen this big picture earlier?

Interestingly enough, the answer is a qualified yes. The history of dieting begins in 1825, when the Frenchman Jean-Anthelme Brillat-Savarin published an essay entitled "Preventative or Curative Treatment of Obesity" in his gastronomic classic *The Physiology of Taste* in which he stated: "Now, an antifat diet is based on the commonest and most active cause of obesity, since, as it has already been clearly shown, it is only because of grains and starches that fatty congestion can occur, as much in a man as in the animals; this effect . . . plays a large part in the commerce of fattened beasts for our markets, and it can be deduced, as an exact consequence, that a more or less rigid abstinence from everything that is starchy or floury will lead to the lessening of weight." Brillat-Savarin had obviously empirically stumbled onto the virtues of a restricted-carbohydrate diet and published his findings. In 1862 William Banting, an upscale London undertaker, found himself so obese that he could not tie his shoes and had to walk downstairs backward. He tried all the fashionable cures of the day without success until his physician put him on a diet free of starchy and sugary foods. Banting followed this diet to the letter and lost a pound a week until he reached a normal weight and restored his health and his ability to walk down the stairs face first. He was so overjoyed with his success that, at his own expense, he published and distributed 2,500 copies of his *Letter on Corpulence,* describing his treatment and his own modifications of the plan. Demand was so great for this pamphlet that it rapidly went through many editions on both sides of the Atlantic before his death in 1878 at eighty-one years of age. His diet was so well known that his name became synonymous with dieting; people weren't dieting; they were banting. In America, Banting's lean-meat diet led to the development of the American Salisbury steak, a staple of life in the late 1800s.

The next popular weight loss and health book was *Eat and Grow Thin* by Vance Thompson, husband of actress Lillian Spencer and founder of *M'lle New York* magazine. This slim book touting the virtues of a restricted-carbohydrate diet (allegedly written by the Asian sage Mahdah) was an enormous best-seller that went through its 112th printing in 1931.

These early diet books all have in common the fact that their authors were untrained as physicians or scientists (Brillat-Savarin was a lawyer) and basically promoted and adhered to these diets simply because they worked, as testified to by the hundreds of thousands of "patients" who followed them. In the late 1920s mainstream medical scientists observed and reported on the efficacy of the restricted-carbohydrate diet when the Arctic explorer Vilhjalmur Stefansson and a colleague submitted themselves to a meat-only diet for a year (see footnote 2).

In England in more recent times T. L. Cleave, the surgeon-captain of the Royal Navy, and John Yudkin, M.D., Ph.D., professor of nutrition at Queen Elizabeth College, London University, have studied and written extensively on the merits of the restricted-carbohydrate diet. Dr. Yudkin has published papers on restricted-carbohydrate dieting from both a scientific and a natural history perspective in most of the prestigious medical journals during a career spanning six decades. At eighty-five, he continues to write and publish. His books, *This Slimming Business* and *A–Z of Slimming*, are classics on the subject.

The three most popular diet books in America in recent years were all written by physicians detailing their own versions of the restricted-carbohydrate diet. Dr. Irwin Stillman published his *Quick Weight Loss Diet* in 1967, describing how he overcame middle-aged obesity and a heart attack by cutting carbohydrates and drinking large quantities of water. Dr. Robert Atkins wrote *Dr. Atkins' Diet Revolution*, another multimillion-copy best-seller, in 1972, detailing his own experiences as well as those of his many patients with low-carbohydrate dieting. In 1979 Dr. Herman Tarnower explained his approach to low-carbohydrate dieting with his cardiology and internal medicine patients in *The Complete Scarsdale Medical Diet*. These books in hardcover and paperback have sold over 20 million copies (amazingly, the last two are still in print twenty years later), and there is probably not a dieter alive who hasn't at least heard of one of these books, if not all. Why are they so popular? Because they work.

None of the authors of any of these popular diet books wrote about the underlying science involved; they just found carbohydrate restriction to be an effective means to bring about weight loss and health improvement in an easy-to-follow diet. In essence these authors "discovered" by trial and error the same thing that Brillat-Savarin, Banting, and the others found the same way. There has been no doubt that these diets work. The only question has been: why? In the chapters to come, you will learn the biochemistry and physiology of the why. And in learning how carbohydrate restriction works through insulin reduction, you will be able to use our techniques to expand on the restricted programs of those who came before us.

First let's look at the most extensive study of the high-complex-carbohydrate, low-fat nutritional approach ever undertaken—the civilization of ancient Egypt. You can draw your own conclusions from the pages of history.

The Bottom Line

At the end of each chapter you'll find a succinct summary of everything you need to remember. If you want to race through the book and get to the program itself as soon as possible, read these Bottom Line boxes (they're listed in the Index) and then proceed to Chapter 10.

Chapter 2

Curse of the Mummies

Historical pathology gives descriptions of diseases in all ages that can be exactly applied to diseases of today....

C. G. CUMSTON, medical historian

From time immemorial the fertile valley along the Nile River has produced an abundance of plant life. The river itself teemed with fish in ancient times and provided food and cover for birds, while the lush floodplain provided rich grazing for every sort of wild animal. Out of this flourishing, verdant landscape the early inhabitants, the ancient Egyptians, carved the beginnings of one of the greatest civilizations of all time—pharaonic Egypt.

During the almost 3,000 years from 2500 B.C. to A.D. 395, the Egyptians refined the art of mummification and extended its practice through all social strata. The number of mummies from that period has been estimated by some experts to equal the population of Egypt today. Medical scientists have analyzed many of these mummified remains in such detail that they have been able to determine not only blood type and body size and shape but the presence of specific bacterial or parasitic infections and other diseases and the cause of death. In effect this legion of mummies provides us with a thirty-century-long study of health and disease.

In addition, we have the written history the Egyptians left us. Archaeologists have unearthed tens of thousands of papyrus fragments describing all aspects of life along the Nile in dynastic times. From translations of their meticulous and voluminous records we know how they lived and in what kinds of houses, where and how they worked, how much they were paid, and, most important for our purposes, what they ate.

What the Mummies Ate

The diet of the average Egyptian consisted primarily of carbohydrates. Their staple crops, wheat and barley, supplied a coarse stone-ground whole-wheat flour, which they baked into a flat bread and consumed in great quantity. In fact, during the later periods, the Egyptian army rationed each of its soldiers about five pounds of bread per day, a quantity so impressive that the Greeks of the time called these soldiers *artophagoi*, "the bread eaters."

Egyptian farmers cultivated a wide variety of fruits, such as grapes, dates, jujube, melons, peaches, olives, pears, pomegranates, carob, apples, and nuts, and several varieties of vegetables—mainly garlic, onions, lettuce, cucumbers, peas, lentils, and papyrus. They sweetened their food with honey (since sugar didn't arrive on the scene until about A.D. 1000) and used olive, safflower, linseed, and sesame oils for cooking and medicinal purposes.

The papyrus records tell us that the early Egyptians sat down to dine on a diet consisting primarily of bread, cereals, fresh fruit and vegetables, some fish and poultry, almost no red meat, olive oil instead of lard, and goat's milk for drinking and to make into cheese—a veritable nutritionist's nirvana. Except for papyrus, the Egyptians could have obtained their entire diet from the shelves of any health food store in America.

With such a bounty available, rich in all the foods believed to promote health and almost devoid of saturated fat and cholesterol, it would seem that the ancient Egyptians should have lived forever or at least should have lived long, healthy lives and died of old age in their beds. But did they? Let's look at the archaeological evidence.

What Ailed the Egyptians

We have two ways of estimating the health of these ancient people: searching the surviving papyrus writings of the time for any mention of diseases and examining the actual mummified remains of the ancient Egyptians. Through the science of paleopathology—the application of modern techniques of pathology and other scientific disciplines to the remains of early man, from bone fragments to entire preserved bodies—scientists can determine not only the state of health at the time of death but also the almost indiscernible responses of the flesh to the rigors of primitive life. Obviously the more complete the specimen, the more reliable the analysis. And when scientists can study many fairly intact remains, such as the enormous number of Egyptian mummies available, all from a particular time and place, they can spot disease trends and can speculate with a good deal of certainty about the health status of the population.

Certainly we would expect to find evidence of bacterial and parasitic infections, because at that time there were no antibiotic or antiparasitic medications—those were not developed until the twentieth century. And indeed we do find evidence of widespread infections and infestations. The ancient Egyptians suffered pneumonia, tuberculosis, probably leprosy, and many other less exotic bacterial infections, along with parasites that occur from drinking and bathing in contaminated water.

With no refined sugar in the diet, we would expect that the ancient Egyptians would have perfect teeth, right? Absolutely wrong. Mummies from all socioeconomic strata suffered terrible dental problems. Their teeth were worn down to such an extensive degree that both enamel and dentin were gone, exposing the soft pulp. Without this protective outer surface, the living tissue within the tooth dies, and the empty canal (the area dentists fill when they do a root canal) becomes a source of chronic infection, often leading to abscess formation. The incidence of actual tooth *decay* was not particularly high because the teeth were worn down to the nub before decay could set in.

The Egyptians also had severe gum disease, which most experts believe was caused by two factors—diet and poor dental hygiene. We know little of the oral hygiene habits of the ancient Egyptians, but we can suppose that they wouldn't be any worse than their primitive hunting-gathering ancestors, who weren't particularly afflicted with gum disease, which scientists always find with increasing frequency in societies ascending the ladder of civilization. It stands to reason that the "civilized" diet plays some role in its promotion.

Subsisting as they did on a diet of fresh fruits and vegetables and coarse whole-grain bread, at least we would not expect to find fat Egyptians. After all, the basic Egyptian diet is the very one most experts prescribe for weight loss today. But here is yet another health problem that doesn't correlate with our "healthy diet" paradigm: obesity. Many ancient Egyptians, based on examination of their mummified remains, weren't just a little overweight, but were actually fat. Paleopathologists have described huge folds of excess skin of a type and distribution that indicate the presence of severe obesity. People in that early age probably viewed excess fat much as we do today—not as a thing of beauty. But just as we find the pages of our magazines covered with pictures of slender models, so the ancient Egyptians painted and carved idealized pictures showing their citizens as slender, svelte in their form-fitting pleated linen garments. In view of this discrepancy between the actual and the idealized, it seems unlikely that the Egyptians actively worked to *become* obese—instead, as it does today, it probably just happened to them.

Finally, in view of the low-fat content of the diet, we would anticipate very little, if any, evidence of heart disease, but again, the low-fat, high-complex-carbohydrate paradigm fails the test. The evidence of heart and vascular disease found in the mummy and papyrus chronicles proves that cardiovascular disease occurred extensively throughout ancient Egypt.

When paleopathologists dissected the arteries of the Egyptian mummies, they did not find smooth, supple arterial walls but rather arteries choked with greasy, cholesterol-laden deposits that were often calcified, exhibiting an advanced stage of atherosclerotic disease. Many subjects had arteries that were scarred and thickened, indicating the presence of high blood pressure. Pathologists today find the same diseased changes when examining tissue from a victim of a heart attack, stroke, diabetes, or other disease found in conjunction with late-stage heart disease. In fact it appears that cardiovascular disease was as prevalent in ancient Egypt as it is in America today.

We have further proof that the ancient Egyptians suffered from heart disease. Among the enormous number of papyrus documents that have been discovered are several that were apparently medical textbooks of the time. One in particular, the papyrus *Ebers*, written in about 1500 B.C., describes the pain from heart disease:

> If thou examinest a man for illness in his cardia, and he has pains in his arms, in his breasts, and in one side of his cardia . . . it is death threatening him.

This account perfectly describes the ominous signs of an impending heart attack: pain in the left side of the chest radiating down the arms. Keep in mind that the average Egyptian enjoyed a much shorter life span than we do, and therefore the vast amount of arterial disease found in the mummified remains gives us a fair indication that "illnesses in their cardia" must have threatened death at a relatively early age.

So a picture begins to emerge of an Egyptian populace rife with disabling dental problems, fat bellies, and crippling heart disease. From the evidence, we know atherosclerotic cholesterol plaque and the effects of high blood pressure narrowed their arteries at a young age. Sounds a lot like the afflictions of millions of people in America today, doesn't it? The Egyptians didn't eat much fat, had no refined carbohydrates as we know them today, and ate almost nothing but whole grains, fresh fruits and vegetables, and fish and fowl, yet were beset with all the same diseases that afflict modern man. Modern man, who is exhorted to eat loads of whole grains, fresh fruits, and vegetables to prevent or reverse these diseases.

In the words of Aidan Cockburn (in *Mummies, Disease and Ancient Cultures*), founder of the Paleopathology Association and the first to bring together an interdisciplinary team of scientists to examine mummies with all the sophisticated equipment available today:

> Atheromatous disease of the arteries is . . . a common finding in mummies. Nowadays, a great deal of emphasis is placed on the stress of modern life or on modern diet as factors in the high incidence of this disorder in our present-day industrialized civilization, but the etiological influences were certainly there in the ancient world, and this fact should be taken into account in any theorizing regarding causation.[1]

What does all this mean in the great scheme of things? We think it means that there are some real problems with the low-fat, high-carbohydrate diet. Perhaps, you might argue, it simply indicates that the ancient Egyptians, maybe for genetic reasons, had difficulty dealing with a high-carbohydrate diet physiologically and the same disorders wouldn't occur in other groups of ancient people on a similar diet. In fact, they do. Throughout history, when man has turned away from the traditional "prehistoric" diet that evolution designed him to eat to an agrarian (grain-based) one, this decline in health has recurred. We think you will find the following data comparing these two kinds of diets startling as well as fascinating.

The Diet We Were Meant to Eat

Most experts agree that game-hunting was the primary means of sustenance for our ancestors 700,000 years ago. From that time until the beginnings of agriculture (about 8,000 to 10,000 years ago), man lived on a diet composed predominantly of meat of one sort or another. In fact scientists estimate that from 60 to 90 percent of the calories these early people consumed were in the form of large and small game animals, birds, eggs, reptiles, and insects. The forces of natural selection acting over some 7,000 centuries shaped and molded our physiology to function optimally on a diet consisting predominantly of meat supplemented with roots, shoots, berries, seeds, and nuts. Only within the last 100 centuries have we reversed the order to become mainly carbohydrate eaters

---

[1] Interestingly, cancer was virtually nonexistent in ancient populations of both hunter-gatherers and agriculturalists, so diet may not be a major factor in cancer development. But remember that both protein and fat are crucial for a strong immune system—your first defense against cancer. There's a stronger case for heavy metal toxins as a cancer cause; the tissues of modern man have 10 times more lead than is found in ancient tissues, for instance.

with meat as the supplement. This dietary reversal—from a diet providing, on average, about 75 percent of its calories from some sort of meat with the remainder coming from plants to one in which only 25 percent of calories come from meat, the rest from other sources—has taken place in approximately 400 to 500 generations, far short of the 1,000 to 10,000 generations deemed necessary by geneticists to allow any substantial genetic changes to take place. We may yet adapt to the high-carbohydrate agricultural diet, but history tells us it will probably take another 10,000 years.

Farming Away Fitness

The change to the agricultural diet created many health problems for early man. The fossil remains tell us that in preagricultural times human health was excellent. People were tall, lean, had well-developed, strong, dense bones, sound teeth with minimal, if any, decay, and little evidence of severe disease. After the advent of agriculture and a change in diet this picture of robust health began to deteriorate. Postagricultural man was shorter, had more brittle bones, extensive tooth decay, and a high incidence of malnutrition and chronic disease—a health picture similar to that of the Egyptians.

The remarkable thing about this generalized decline in health is that it occurred throughout the world. From the eastern Mediterranean to Peru, whenever people changed from a high-protein to a high-carbohydrate diet they became less healthy. In fact archaeologists consider this health disparity so predictable that when they unearth the skeletal remains of a prehistoric society they classify the people as hunters or farmers by the state of their bones and teeth. If the teeth are excellent and nondecayed and the bones strong, dense, and long, the people were hunter-gatherers; if the teeth are decayed and the bones frail and deformed, scientists know the remains are those of agriculturists.

THE DECLINE OF THE HARDIN VILLAGERS

A study by Claire M. Cassidy, Ph.D., an anthropologist with the University of Maryland and the Smithsonian Institution, compares two groups of people arising from the same genetic pool, living in the same area and in roughly the same size community—two similar groups of people separated only by time and diet. Her paper, published in 1980, documents the health differences between hunter-gatherers and agriculturists (or farmers) as a function of diet. Dr. Cassidy's subjects were the skeletal remains of a group of farmers who inhabited an area identified as Hardin Village, in what is now Kentucky, from approximately 1500 to 1675 and a comparison group of hunter-gatherers who occupied a location called Indian Knoll centuries earlier, around 3000 B.C.

These two groups of people were similar in virtually all respects except diet: they lived in the same part of the country, had the same climate to deal with, and had the same types of wild plants and animals available. Both lived in about the same-size population group and were sedentary or semisedentary, removing the variable of degree of exercise. The farmers ate primarily "corn, beans, and squash. Wild plants and animals (especially deer, elk, small mammals, wild turkey, box turtle) provided supplements to a largely agricultural diet." The hunters, on the other hand, consumed "very large quantities of river mussels and snails. . . . Other meat was provided by deer, small mammals, wild turkey, box turtle, and fish; dog was sometimes eaten ceremonially." Dr. Cassidy sums up the differences: "The Hardin Village [farmers'] diet was high in carbohydrates, while that at Indian Knoll [hunters'] was high in protein."

She evaluated the skeletal remains of these two groups for bone and tooth changes indicative of iron-deficiency anemia, growth arrest from disease or malnutrition, and decay, and was able to determine the effects of the different diets on these otherwise similar peoples. She found the life expectancies for all ages lower and infant mortality higher among the farmers. Iron-deficiency anemia was nonexistent among the hunters but identified in 8.2 percent of the farmers. Growth arrests among the hunters were periodic and of short duration, possibly due to regularly occurring food shortages at certain times of the year, while growth arrests among the farmers were random and of much longer duration, indicating chronic malnutrition. More children suffered infection in the farmer population, with evidence of infection in the long bones thirteen times more common in farmers than hunters. Tooth decay, widespread among the farmers, rarely occurred among the hunters.[2] In Dr. Cassidy's words, "the agricultural Hardin Villagers were clearly less healthy than the Indian Knollers, who lived by hunting and gathering." She attributes this disparity in health to the difference in diet: "The health data provide convincing evidence that the diet of the agriculturists was the inferior of the two. The archaeological dietary data support this conclusion."

Dr. Cassidy is not alone in reporting this phenomenon. Many scientific

---

[2] The farmers had an average of 6.74 decayed teeth, while the hunters had only 0.73. Interestingly, no hunter children had tooth decay, whereas some farmer children had developed cavities by the second year of life.

papers have been written on this subject, and they present even the most passionate believer in the superiority of the high-carbohydrate diet with some food for thought. As Dr. Kathleen Gordon, like Dr. Cassidy an anthropologist at the Smithsonian Institution, writes in one such paper: "Not only was the agricultural 'revolution' not really so revolutionary at its inception, it has also come to represent something of a nutritional 'devolution' for much of mankind."

The Thrifty Gene: Store That Fat!

The anthropological record provides plenty of evidence that the change to a high-carbohydrate diet caused a general decline in health of people designed to eat a high-protein, carbohydrate-restricted diet. Why? What is there about a high-carbohydrate diet that causes the trouble?

There has been discussion in the scientific community for years about the so-called "thrifty gene." First used with reference to diabetes, this phrase has come to mean the genetic material that has been passed along to us by our prehistoric ancestors that allows us to better survive hunger and privation. Since periodic famines, brought on by game scarcity, heavy winters, droughts, or other natural disasters, were a part of prehistoric life, it makes sense that the people best suited to survive these deprivations would live to reproduce. Obviously this happened. Natural selection culled the weak and left a population that had the biochemistry and physiology necessary to squeeze every possible calorie from the food at hand and store it efficiently. This energy efficiency or biological thriftiness was precisely what we needed to survive in prehistoric times—but what about now?

When we eat a meal, we know that we are going to eat again in a few hours, but our enzymes and hormones don't. When the food comes in and is broken down into its components by our prehistoric digestive enzymes, it is absorbed into the blood and attacked by our primordial digestive hormones. Each calorie is put to work to meet the body's immediate demands with the remainder being stored as fat to be called on as needed. When the next meal comes along in four hours instead of four days, this whole process repeats. Since we eat meals regularly, we end up storing too much fat, which creates a new set of problems probably never experienced by prehistoric man.

The primary hormone involved in this entire process is insulin. Insulin is our main anabolic, or bodybuilding, hormone and is called into action each time we eat—especially if we eat or drink a food containing carbohydrates. Insulin increases the storage of fat, drives the sugar from the blood into the cells, and in general performs all the energy-conserving functions that allowed our ancestors to survive. Unfortunately, in our plentiful time of high-carbohydrate intake insulin works to our detriment. When levels of insulin become too high, as they do on our modern diet, this hormone causes us to retain sodium (and with it excess fluid), leading to high blood pressure; it causes our bodies to increase the production of cholesterol; it causes some damage to the arteries; it makes us store fat in a particularly unhealthy way; and it even can start the entire process leading to atherosclerosis and heart disease. All this treachery from a hormone that allowed us to survive prehistoric times.

In the following chapters we'll look at the hard scientific facts that inescapably point to the critical role of insulin excess in causing this host of "modern" ills that you now have seen are not so modern. You'll understand the body's metabolism and what drives it, how insulin works, and why it causes both the good and bad effects it does. Once you have this background, you'll clearly see why the high-carbohydrate, low-fat diet recommended by today's nutritionists—and our government itself—promotes an outpouring of excess insulin and why adhering to such a diet will ultimately lead us to the same end that it did the ancient Egyptians.

The Bottom Line

Modern nutritional wisdom would predict that the diet of the ancient Egyptians—high in complex carbohydrates, low in fat, no refined sugar, almost no red meat—should have brought health, fitness, and longevity to the Egyptians of old. But it didn't.

Translations of the ancient Egyptian papyrus writings and modern examination of their mummified remains by pathologists tell us quite a different tale. The evidence speaks of a people afflicted with rotten teeth and severe atherosclerosis, suffering from elevated blood pressure and dying in their thirties with heart attacks. And contrary to the paintings of the willowy svelte figures in pleated linen that adorned their tomb walls, the large skin folds of the mummies tell us that their ancient low-fat, high-carbohydrate diet left them obese as well.

The Egyptians are not the only ancient people whose health suffered because of a diet consisting mainly of complex carbohydrates. An anthropologist examining skeletal remains of early man can tell immediately whether the bones and teeth belonged to a hunter-gatherer (mainly protein eater) or a farmer (mainly carbohydrate eater) simply by their condition. The hunters grew tall, with strong, well-formed bones and sound teeth, and the remains of the farmers usually show skeletal signs of malnutrition, stunted growth, and tooth decay.

For 700,000 years humans ate a diet of mainly meat, fat, nuts, and berries. Eight thousand years ago we learned to farm, and as our consumption of grains increased, our health declined. Genetic evolutionary changes take a minimum of 1,000 generations—or another 8,000 to 10,000 years to adapt.

Our metabolic machinery was designed to cope with an unpredictable food supply. We had to store food away for the lean times ahead. The hormone insulin did this for us. Unfortunately, a diet heavy in carbohydrate also sends our insulin levels soaring, and our body interprets this as a need to store calories, to make cholesterol, and to conserve water—all important to our survival way back then. Some of us inherit this conservation ability—a *thrifty gene*—in great measure. People who have this trait gain weight easily and have a more difficult time losing their excess, and the current nutritional low-fat, high-carbohydrate prescription leads to overweight and weight-related health problems even more quickly among them.

Chapter 3

The Symptom Treatment Trap

All great truths begin as blasphemies.

GEORGE BERNARD SHAW

"You want me to eat *what?*"

The middle-aged lady sitting across the desk from us was incredulous and becoming more so by the second as we explained to her the changes she needed to make in her diet—changes necessary to reduce the dangerously elevated level of fat in her blood. She didn't have a serious weight problem; she had come to us seeking advice on the treatment of her cholesterol problem, but she was having difficulty accepting that advice.

"But if I eat all these foods you're telling me to eat, won't my cholesterol just go higher? I can't see how I can eat an egg or red meat in my condition. Are you sure this is going to work?"

We explained how her physiology worked and why her cholesterol was high. Her metabolism would change as she followed our nutritional plan, and these changes would result in a dramatic reduction in her cholesterol levels. We told her that once she got started on the proper diet she would see major results within just a few weeks instead of the months it usually takes for diets to work—if they do at all. Then she could judge for herself whether or not she was on the right track. She may not have been convinced by the scientific explanations of her problem and its solution, but she brightened at the thought of seeing results so quickly.

"Six weeks!? Do you really think I will have improved much by then?" she asked.

"You will be pleasantly surprised."

"I hope so. I don't know if I can go through another experience like the last time. I worked so hard with my previous doctor. I faithfully followed the diet he prescribed, and for what? Practically nothing. I don't mean to be such a whiner, but you've got to understand that I'm at my wit's end with this. If I don't get this cholesterol under control and start feeling better, I'm going to be a basket case."

We certainly understood. Although her problem is more serious than most, Jayne Bledsoe[1] is fairly typical of the patients we treat in our metabolic practice. We have heard variations of her history from countless other patients who have gotten stuck on the cholesterol treadmill.

Treating the Symptom, Missing the Problem

Jayne had been unaware that she even had a problem until she went for a routine physical examination. Her doctor checked her over, told her she appeared to be in good health, drew some blood, and told her he would call her when the results came back from the lab. He called the next day and dropped the bombshell: her blood fats were dangerously elevated. Her serum cholesterol was 750 mg/dl (milligrams/deciliter)—normal is anything below 200 and her triglycerides (another blood fat usually measured in the 100-to-250-mg/dl range) were a whopping 3,000 mg/dl! Most physicians get excited over a cholesterol of 300 mg/dl, let alone 750, and become outright alarmed at such a triglyceride level. So it's no surprise that her doctor—following standard medical protocol—completely bypassed Step One and immediately started her on the National Cholesterol Awareness Program Step-Two Diet *and* two potent cholesterol-lowering medications.[2]

Jayne faithfully followed her doctor's orders for six months, although not without difficulty. The medications nauseated her, and the diet kept her constantly hungry. Her condition was the talk of her friends and relatives, one of whom actually remarked to her, "I didn't know a person

---

[1] Most of the case histories in this book are, like this one, actual patients whose names have been changed. Occasionally a composite patient history is used to illustrate a particular point.

[2] From the "Report of the National Cholesterol Education Program Expert Panel on Detection, Evaluation, and Treatment of High Blood Cholesterol in Adults," *Archives of Internal Medicine* 148:36–69, January 1988. Under these guidelines physicians treat patients with elevated cholesterol in a stepwise fashion starting with dietary modification that limits fat to 30 percent and protein to 10 to 20 percent of calories and encourages the consumption of large amounts of carbohydrate. This is called the Step-One Diet. If the blood cholesterol level refuses to fall or doesn't fall far enough on the Step-One Diet, a more stringent one that further reduces fat intake—the Step-Two Diet—follows. In those cases in which diet alone fails, most physicians turn to one or more of the many cholesterol-lowering drugs.

could still be alive with a cholesterol of 750!" By the time Jayne returned for her recheck, she was desperate for improvement. And she had improved some, but not nearly enough. Her cholesterol had dropped from 750 mg/dl to 475 mg/dl and her triglycerides from 3,000 mg/dl to 2,000 mg/dl—an improvement to be sure, but still cause for great concern to both Jayne and her physician. They discussed her treatment options. Her doctor suggested either increasing the dosage of her cholesterol-lowering medications or adding yet another medicine to her regimen. Jayne wanted to think about it before she decided which option to take. She decided to do neither until she got a second opinion from another physician, so she came to our clinic.

After listening to her history, we drew another blood sample and found that indeed she did have extraordinarily elevated levels of cholesterol and triglycerides in her blood—495 mg/dl and 1,900 mg/dl, respectively. In addition, her blood sugar was elevated to 155 mg/dl (normal is below 115 mg/dl), an ominous sign of impending diabetes.

We instructed Jayne to stop taking both of her cholesterol-lowering medications and to change her diet drastically. Her new nutritional regimen allowed meat (even red meat), eggs, cheese, and many other foods that most people view as *causing* cholesterol problems, not solving them. We told her to call in three weeks to check in and to come back to have her blood checked in six weeks.

She called at her appointed time and reported that she "felt grand" and that her nausea and hunger had vanished. The results of her blood work astounded her. Jayne's cholesterol level had fallen to 186 mg/dl and her triglycerides to 86 mg/dl. Her blood sugar had dropped to 90 mg/dl; everything was back in the normal range. As you might imagine, she was ecstatic.

How could this happen? How can a diet virtually everyone believes should raise cholesterol actually lower it—and in a person who doesn't have just a slight cholesterol elevation but a major one? We know Jayne Bledsoe's case is not a freak happenstance or an aberration because we've tried variations of the same regimen on countless other patients—all with the same results. The results make perfect sense, because Jayne's problem, her illness, is not the elevated cholesterol level—that's merely a sign of the underlying problem. Her problem is *hyperinsulinemia,* a chronic elevation of serum insulin.

When Jayne first came to our office, her insulin level was almost 20 mU/ml (milliUnits/milliliter), about double what we consider normal, which is anything below 10 mU/ml. After six weeks on a diet designed to lower her insulin level, Jayne's lab work showed that she had dropped hers to 12 mU/ml, almost normal. By treating her real problem—excess

insulin—we were able to solve her secondary problems of elevated cholesterol, triglycerides, and blood sugar. Standard medical therapies treat
the symptoms of excess insulin—elevated cholesterol, triglycerides, blood
sugar, blood pressure, and obesity—instead of treating the excess insulin
itself. Unfortunately, the standard treatment of the symptoms may even
raise the insulin levels and worsen the underlying problem. Let's look at
what happens when we treat symptoms instead of causes with a common
scenario of conventional medical wisdom at work.

Suppose your father were to develop high blood pressure. At first the
readings are not alarming, and his doctor prescribes a mild medication to
lower the pressure and tells him to cut down on salt. Months pass, and
when he visits his doctor again for a checkup his blood pressure is indeed
better. But he learns that now his cholesterol is up a bit, and he has begun to put on a little weight. So his doctor recommends a low-calorie,
low-fat diet and warns that if his cholesterol remains too high, he will add
another medication to lower it. Time marches on, and perhaps years later
he visits the doctor and learns that now his blood sugar has begun to rise;
he is developing diabetes. He receives more low-fat, high-complex-
carbohydrate dietary instruction and perhaps yet another pill for his sugar
problem. It seems that the more the physician treats your dad's problems, the more problems he develops.

Excess Insulin: The Real Culprit

A substance that fundamentally influences every cell in the body, insulin
is the master controller of the metabolic system without which all metabolic processes would be rudderless. Insulin is a hormone produced and
secreted into the bloodstream by the pancreas, a glandular organ located
behind the stomach, deep in the abdominal cavity. As it travels through
the circulatory system insulin regulates the level of sugar in the blood—
its most important function—and performs a thousand other tasks. Insulin, by activating or inhibiting various metabolic pathways, can make us
sleepy, hungry, satisfied, dizzy, stuporous, or bloated. It can raise blood
pressure, elevate cholesterol levels (as it did in Jayne Bledsoe's case), cram
fat into fat cells, cause the body to retain excess fluid, damage arteries,
and even change protein and sugar into fat. In the appropriate amount
insulin keeps the metabolic system humming along smoothly with everything in balance; in great excess it becomes a rogue hormone ranging
throughout the body, wreaking metabolic havoc and leaving a trail of
chaos and disease in its wake.

Although medical researchers have known of the beneficial effects of insulin since the 1920s, when it was discovered, they have also generated an enormous amount of data over the past three decades showing that some of the effects are not so beneficial.

Because there are no drugs available that can significantly reduce insulin levels, dietary manipulation is the *only* effective treatment of insulin excess and the diseases it promotes (although exercise helps). That's not to say that high blood pressure, for example, can't be treated by medications; as everyone knows, it can be. But treating high blood pressure treats only the symptom and not the underlying cause.

Hypertension and Heart Disease: A Bad Rap

Twenty years ago in America we were inundated with medical and media hype about the dangers of high blood pressure. The American Medical Association and the American Heart Association combined forces in a campaign to alert the public to the long-term health consequences of undiagnosed and untreated hypertension, namely, heart disease and stroke. People were encouraged to get their blood pressure checked at the earliest opportunity, and booths sprang up in shopping malls and supermarkets to provide this service (much as they do today with cholesterol testing). Various governmental and private funding agencies poured hundreds of millions of dollars into hypertension research, which thousands of eager scientists used to launch projects to discover the cause, cure, and consequences of this disorder.

Epidemiologists had long known that people with high blood pressure die from strokes and heart attacks at a much greater rate than those with normal blood pressure. By treating hypertension on a grand scale, medical scientists reasoned, they could significantly reduce the incidence of death caused by stroke and heart disease. Based on this reasoning and very little hard evidence, since no long-term hypertensive control studies had ever been done, the push was on to get Americans with high blood pressure diagnosed and medicated. At this point the first long-term studies of the benefits of treatment were just being started. Researchers at medical centers across the country were gathering groups of subjects with hypertension so that they could treat and carefully monitor them for the many years necessary for such studies to be valid. Statisticians performed their analytical alchemy and estimated that hypertension controlled with drugs decreased the incidence of deaths from heart disease and stroke—by 40 percent and 25 percent, respectively.

How accurate were the statisticians? Not very, as it turns out. When the results were in, the researchers were astonished. The incidence of deaths due to stroke had fallen by approximately 25 percent—precisely what the statisticians had predicted; the figures for heart disease, however, weren't even close. Rather than the predicted 40 percent decrease, the experts found *no statistically significant decrease* in deaths from heart disease compared to people who were not treated at all. People who ignored their hypertension and went on about their business didn't develop heart disease at any greater rate than those who went to the expense and trouble of taking daily medications and assiduously monitoring their blood pressure. As you might imagine, this discrepancy prompted a lot of head scratching among the scientific establishment— especially in view of the fact that, based on their predictions, 19 million Americans were now spending upward of $4 billion annually on medicines to lower their blood pressure. What happened? How did the calculations go so far afield?

As is typical in medicine, things are not always as simple as they seem. It's tempting to believe the theory: more people with high blood pressure succumb to heart disease than do people with normal blood pressure; therefore, high blood pressure *causes* heart disease. As the researchers examined the data more closely, they found hypertension and heart disease are related through the common denominator of too much insulin—a discovery that spurred a tidal wave of new research. Since the excess insulin caused both the high blood pressure *and* the heart disease (through mechanisms we will explore in coming chapters), it becomes immediately obvious why reducing the blood pressure without reducing insulin levels would have little effect on the progression of heart disease.

A dismal postscript is that many of the medicines—diuretics and beta-blockers—actually *increased* insulin levels as they reduced blood pressure. So, ironically, many hypertensive patients taking medicine in the hope of preventing heart disease were encouraging the real culprit—excess insulin. In a great majority of these cases dietary control of elevated insulin levels could have eliminated *both* the high blood pressure *and* the threat of heart disease.

Elevated insulin is Jayne Bledsoe's problem. Maybe excess insulin is the reason for Dad's relentless progression (even under medical treatment) from high blood pressure to elevated cholesterol to diabetes in our scenario. The diseases that insulin affects directly—high blood pressure, elevated levels of cholesterol and other fats in the blood, diabetes, heart disease, and obesity—are the cause of the vast majority of death and disability in America today. They are the grim reapers of Western civilization. They kill more than twice the number of Americans *each year* than died in World War I, World War II, the Korean War, and Vietnam combined.

How do we know that these disorders are actually caused by diet and not by some other factor or combination of factors? Just as with most aspects of medicine, some degree of uncertainty persists, but we've got a pretty good idea from data from three different research approaches—historical, current epidemiological, and direct experimental. And nothing in this book is theoretical—it's all proven biochemistry found in any standard medical text—it's simply never been put together in this way before.

The scientific evidence will speak eloquently for itself, so let's begin to examine these biochemical connections of diet and disease.

The Bottom Line

Virtually everyone is familiar with insulin as a regulator of blood sugar, and indeed that's its main job in your body. But far beyond that, insulin can be called the *master hormone of human metabolism*, involved in the regulation of blood pressure, the production of cholesterol and triglycerides, and the storage of fat. When insulin levels become too high—a topic we'll devote considerable discussion to throughout this book—metabolic havoc ensues with elevated blood pressure, elevated cholesterol and triglycerides, diabetes, and obesity all trailing along in its wake. These disorders are merely *symptoms* of a single more basic disturbance in metabolism—excess insulin and insulin resistance.

There are no medications that treat excess insulin; a properly structured diet is the *only* means to bring it in line. (The usual low-fat, high-complex-carbohydrate approach won't do it; it has just the opposite effect.) Some medications—especially the beta-blockers and some diuretic medications, the very ones used to treat blood pressure and heart problems—actually make matters worse by causing the body to produce even more insulin, and doctor and patient get caught in the "symptom treatment trap." Using medications to treat these symptoms of metabolic disturbance while leaving the root cause to grow worse is very much like treating a child's fever with aspirin and ignoring the strep infection that's causing it. The fever comes down, but the child invariably gets sicker.

Here's what usually happens: a patient gains weight and subsequently develops high blood pressure, for which the doctor prescribes a mild diuretic and low salt. The patient returns with better blood pressure but now a slight elevation in cholesterol and is put on a low-fat diet. He returns no lighter, with little change in cholesterol, but now his triglycerides or blood sugar have risen, too. The progression occurs because *all* these disorders are related through a single disturbance (excess insulin) that is not only not being alleviated but is actually being aggravated by the treatment.

These disorders occur so commonly in our society that we've become numb to the staggering toll they take: heart disease, high blood pressure, and diabetes kill twice as many people every year as were killed in both world wars, Korea, and Vietnam *combined*.

Grim statistics aside, how do we know that these disorders are actually caused by diet and not by some other factor or combination of factors? Just as with most aspects of medicine, some degree of uncertainty persists, but we've got a pretty good idea from data from three different research approaches—historical, current epidemiological, and direct experimental. And nothing in this book is theoretical—it's all proven biochemistry found in any standard medical text—it's simply never been put together in this way before.

As the story unfolds, the scientific evidence will speak for itself.

Chapter 4

Excess Insulin and the Insulin Resistance Syndrome

The aspects of things that are most important for us are hidden because of their simplicity and familiarity. One is unable to notice something— because it is always before one's eyes. We fail to be struck by what, once seen, is most striking and most powerful.

LUDWIG WITTGENSTEIN
Philosophical Investigations

Consider how different life would be if we didn't have the ability to store excess energy from the food we eat. Like the electric mixer that works only when it's plugged in, we would have to be constantly hooked up to our energy source—food. At first glance, this might not seem like such a bad idea. Many people nibble, snack, and munch their way through the day anyway, so wouldn't it be grand if they could continue without the consequences of obesity, elevated cholesterol, and the other diseases of overconsumption?

One obvious disadvantage would be that we would have to eat more food faster as we increased our intensity of activity. Let's say we're involved in a strenuous activity—swimming, for example. We could stuff ourselves just before we jumped into the water, but that wouldn't help. It would be like keeping the mixer plugged in for two hours before we used it, then unplugging it and turning it on. Nothing would happen because the mixer can't store electricity. So we would have to eat while swimming. It would be cumbersome and inconvenient to have to figure out a way to consume food at all times—even during sleep.

If we ate too much, it might be like plugging a mixer designed for 120 volts of electricity into a 240-volt circuit. What if we got stuck in an elevator and ate our way through all the food we had with us? As soon as the food was gone, we would sputter and choke out our last few moments like a car out of gas. Our survival would depend on always having adequate foodstuffs immediately at hand, and any activity that had the potential to separate us from our food would be fraught with mortal danger.

Our Built-In Battery

How different that existence would be from the one we live, where most people could go for a couple of months without eating a single bite—some even up to a year or longer, depending on their degree of obesity. We can eat ten meals a day or one or none; we can expend prodigious amounts of energy while eating little or no food, or we can eat prodigious amounts of food and expend almost no energy. In short, we have the capacity to use the energy from food we eat to meet our immediate needs and store the rest for later use. We have a built-in battery—the fat we carry on our bodies, which is replenished every time we eat and used for energy when we don't. In fact the amount of fat on the body of an average person weighing 150 pounds contains enough energy to allow that person to walk from Miami to New York City without eating.

Insulin and a few other hormones coordinate the activities of metabolism and ensure that our fat batteries work, making it possible for us to live unfettered by a constant power supply. The metabolic system precisely regulates the storage of excess food energy as fat and the release and breakdown of this body fat for the energy necessary for life. The metabolic system performs these tasks silently and without conscious effort on our part, but it is not foolproof.

The Yin-Yang of Metabolism

Insulin and glucagon are the primary hormones involved in the storage and release of energy within the body. When we eat, insulin drives our metabolism to store the excess food energy for use later. Then, when later comes, glucagon drives the metabolism the other way, letting us burn our stored fat for the energy we need to swim or walk or sleep in the hours long after we've eaten. If we think of insulin as the hormone of feeding and storing and glucagon as the hormone of fasting and burning, it's easy to see how people living in today's America—with its abundance of food and never-stop-eating lifestyle—could be in the insulin-dominant mode most of the time.

Although it performs countless other tasks throughout the body, insulin's chief priority is to keep the blood sugar level from rising too high. Glucagon's main function is to prevent the blood sugar level from falling too low. The importance of this minute-by-minute regulation of the level of sugar in the blood is underscored by the fact that without either one of these hormones we would be dead in a matter of days or perhaps even hours. Without insulin the blood sugar would skyrocket, causing profound metabolic disturbances, dehydration, coma, and death. An absence of glucagon would allow the blood sugar to fall rapidly, bringing on brain dysfunction, somnolence, coma, and then death, because the brain requires blood sugar to operate properly. Because of this critical need to maintain the blood sugar in a narrow physiological band, the body doesn't really much care about the secondary activities of these hormones as long as they keep the blood sugar where it's supposed to be. And that's what gets us in trouble.

When the level of sugar in the blood falls below a critical level, the pancreas is stimulated to produce and release glucagon into the circulatory system. The glucagon travels to the fat cells, where it harvests fat to be burned for energy, and to the liver, where it stimulates the liver cells to produce glucose, or blood sugar. Under the influence of glucagon the liver—which has the capacity to produce about a cup of glucose per day—makes and releases sugar into the blood. As the sugar level in the blood rises back into the normal range, the pancreas slows down its release of glucagon.

Insulin springs into action when the blood sugar starts to climb too high, as it does after a carbohydrate meal. The elevated blood sugar triggers the pancreas to synthesize and release insulin into the bloodstream. This insulin first makes a pass through the liver, where it shuts down any sugar production that may still be going on, then travels on to the rest of the body, where it acts on sensors or receptors scattered across the surfaces of muscle and fat cells. These receptors, when activated by insulin, initiate a series of reactions that pump sugar (along with protein and fat) from the blood into the interior of the cells for use now or storage for later. Insulin stimulates the fat cells to take up fat and sugar from the blood and store it away as body fat, especially in the middle of the body, within the abdomen and around the vital organs. As the sugar goes into the cells and its level in the blood falls, the pancreas reduces its output of insulin. Insulin and glucagon are opposing forces, but both are always present, and both work together. As one increases, the other decreases, and their interplay brings harmony to the metabolic system.

So insulin and glucagon regulate blood sugar. But look at it another way—can blood sugar regulate insulin and glucagon? Obviously it does. If blood sugar goes up, insulin goes up; conversely, if blood sugar falls, so does the insulin level, and the glucagon level rises. It's this mechanism that gives us indirect control over our insulin and glucagon by manipulating our blood sugar level. No matter how hard we try, we can't change our insulin and glucagon directly: we can't use meditation or biofeedback, and we can't take insulin or glucagon pills because these hormones are destroyed in the digestive process. Short of injecting ourselves with these hormones, the only way we can change our insulin and glucagon levels is to change our blood sugar level—which we can do in a hurry.

If you want your insulin level to increase, just drink a sugary soft drink. Your blood sugar will climb, and so will your insulin level—within minutes. It's a little more difficult, however, to increase glucagon levels. You'd somehow have to get your blood sugar level low enough to stimulate the pancreas to release glucagon. The only way to do this quickly is to give yourself an insulin injection. This extra insulin will drive the blood sugar low enough to stimulate the pancreas to release glucagon. Alternatively, you can wait around several hours without eating until your blood sugar falls enough on its own to bring about a surge of glucagon.

In fact, the blood sugar level governs the functioning of the entire metabolic system. It's at the top of the chain of command. When blood sugar rises, it orders the metabolism to proceed along a certain course; when it falls, it gives the opposite orders. If our blood sugar, through the efforts of glucagon and insulin, controls our metabolism, and we can control our blood sugar level by eating or not eating certain foods, doesn't it stand to reason that we can control our metabolism? Indeed we can. In fact this ability to control our metabolism is the foundation of our dietary program.

INSULIN WORKING OVERTIME: THANKS BUT NO THANKS

Insulin—as part of its energy-storing behavior—activates a number of metabolic systems that we would just as soon not have activated, at least not on a perpetual basis. They were designed to operate on an intermittent, as-needed basis, but thanks to the aging process and the typical American diet, they tend to operate overtime. What systems are we talking about? The cholesterol synthesis system, for one. Insulin activates the enzymes that run the cholesterol-making apparatus, resulting in overproduction of cholesterol. Our own cells make cholesterol and lots of it. In fact, 70 to 80 percent of the cholesterol burbling along in your blood vessels was made by your own body. Only 20 to 30 percent came from your diet. Every cell in the body has the capacity to make cholesterol, but most is made in the liver, the intestines, and the skin, with the vast majority coming from the liver cells. Elevated levels of insulin spur these cells to churn out vast amounts of cholesterol, leading to elevated blood levels. You might wonder why nature designed it this way. Storing excess food energy as fat seems reasonable, but why make cholesterol?

Excess food energy increases blood sugar, which increases insulin, which triggers the storage cycle leading to fat accumulation. To store fat and build muscle, the body must make new cells, and insulin acts as a growth hormone for this process. Cholesterol plays a vital role in this building and storing process; cholesterol provides the structural framework for all cells. In fact, if all of the cholesterol in your body were suddenly to vanish, you would dissolve into a puddle just like the Wicked Witch in *The Wizard of Oz* when Dorothy threw the water on her. Unfortunately, *excess* insulin stimulates *excess* cholesterol, and therein lies the problem.

Excess insulin also encourages the proliferation and growth of smooth muscle cells in the linings of our arteries, an activity that causes a couple of problems. The larger muscle cells thicken the arterial walls, making them less elastic and reducing the volume inside the arteries. Less elastic, smaller coronary arteries are more prone to develop plaque and arterial spasm, the underlying causes of heart disease. Because the heart has to develop greater pressure to force the blood through the narrow, thickened arteries throughout the rest of the body, elevated blood pressure results. To compound this problem, insulin also causes the kidneys to retain salt and fluid, which adds to the blood volume, increasing the pressure even more.

Let's not, however, neglect glucagon, its opposite. Because glucagon is the hormone of fat burning and fatty tissue breakdown, it reverses the building and storage processes set in motion by insulin. Under glucagon stimulation, the body gets rid of fat by burning it for energy. Since the body requires no extra cholesterol to help rid itself of cells, glucagon shuts down the production of cholesterol and helps send it on its way out of the circulation. The body doesn't need extra fluid to burn fat, so glucagon prompts the kidneys to get rid of it. Glucagon stimulates the breakdown and disappearance of the smooth muscle overgrowth in the arteries and lessens the incidence of arterial spasm. It's easier to see the whole scenario for these two master hormones in chart form so that you can compare them more easily.

THE ROLES OF INSULIN AND GLUCAGON

INSULIN	GLUCAGON
lowers elevated blood sugar	raises low blood sugar
shifts metabolism into storage mode	shifts metabolism into burning mode
converts glucose and protein to fat	converts protein and fat to glucose
converts dietary fat to storage	converts dietary fats to ketones and sends them to the tissues for energy
removes fat from blood and transports it into fat cells	releases fat from fat cells into the blood for use by tissues as energy
increases the body's production of cholesterol	decreases the body's production of cholesterol
makes the kidneys retain excess fluid	makes the kidneys release excess fluid
stimulates the growth of arterial smooth muscle cells	stimulates the regression of arterial smooth muscle cells
stimulates the use of glucose for energy	stimulates the use of fat for energy

Scanning this chart, it doesn't take a rocket scientist to see that the more time we spend on the glucagon side, the better off we are. Remember, however, that metabolism control is *not* a one-or-the-other phenomenon: all insulin *or* all glucagon. Both hormones are present in the blood all the time. What drives the metabolism to store or to burn is a *dominance* of one or the other.

How Food Affects Insulin and Glucagon

Scientists have fed research subjects all kinds of food in all kinds of combinations, drawn their blood, and measured its insulin and glucagon to discover how foods affect these hormones. The results of these experiments are in the following chart.

INFLUENCE OF FOOD ON INSULIN AND GLUCAGON

TYPE OF FOOD	INSULIN	GLUCAGON
Carbohydrate	+++++	no change
Protein	++	++
Fat	no change	no change
Carbohydrate and Fat	++++	no change
Protein and Fat	++	++
High Protein and Low Carbo	++	+
High Carbo and Low Protein	+++++++++	+

As you can see from the chart, of the three basic constituents of food—fat, protein, and carbohydrate—carbohydrate makes the most profound change in insulin, because it makes the most profound change in blood sugar level. Fat doesn't do anything; as far as insulin is concerned, fat doesn't exist. The combination of carbohydrate and protein, especially large amounts of carbohydrate with small amounts of protein, causes the greatest increase in insulin, a most enlightening fact considering the typical American diet.

What We Eat

What does the typical American eat? How about the old standard: meat and potatoes—carbohydrate and protein. A hamburger and fries—carbohydrate and protein. A pizza, which is basically cheese, meat, and a crust—carbohydrate and protein. Macaroni and cheese—carbohydrate and protein. Think of anything we commonly eat: eggs and hash browns, milk and cereal, pork and beans, chicken and dumplings, peanut butter and jelly, ice cream, chili con carne, lasagne—the list could go on forever; every one of these popular foods is a combination of lots of carbohydrate and some protein. And lots of fat, of course, which we will consider shortly.

Let's forget about the protein for a minute and concentrate on just the carbohydrates that we eat, which do an outstanding job of raising insulin all by themselves. The second National Health and Nutrition Examination Survey (NHANES II) conducted by the National Center for Health Statistics published data in 1983 on the food consumption patterns of Americans.[1] What would you guess as the number-one food consumed by the most Americans? White bread, rolls, and crackers—almost pure carbohydrate. How about number two? Doughnuts, cookies, and cake—more carbohydrate and fat. Number three, alcoholic beverages. All in all, of the top twenty foods Americans eat, eleven are virtually pure carbohydrate, four are a combination of carbohydrate and protein, and only five are pure protein or a combination of protein and fat. These last five represent only 12 percent of the calories we eat.

What *about* the fat and cholesterol we've shrugged off in our discussion so far? Do we not have to worry about them at all? Don't they cause

---

[1] The newest NHANES information (NHANES III) has not yet been completely tabulated, but partial results show a reduction in fat intake, an increase in carbohydrate intake, and an almost 25 percent increase in the incidence of obesity.

some problems? Sure they do, but not nearly the problems that carbohydrates do. And when dietary fat and cholesterol do cause problems, it's usually *because* of the carbohydrate eaten along with them. It is true that fat is the raw material from which the body makes cholesterol, and it is also true that if you add more fat to your diet your cholesterol will increase, *but only if you continue to eat a lot of carbohydrate at the same time that you add the fat.* If you reduce the amount of carbohydrate when you add the fat, not only will you probably not see any increase; you could even see a *reduction* in cholesterol levels.

Although fat is the raw material the body uses to make cholesterol, insulin runs the cellular machinery that actually makes it. If you reduce the level of insulin, the cells can't convert the fat to cholesterol, almost no matter how much fat is available. Eating fat in the absence of carbohydrate and expecting it to be converted to cholesterol is like trying to make your car go faster by putting a larger gas tank in it. In the same way, a high-carbohydrate diet stimulates insulin, which accelerates the cholesterol production of the cells. Therefore, the worst possible diet is a high-carbohydrate, high-fat diet, because not only is a large amount of fat available for cholesterol synthesis, but an abundance of insulin is on hand to run the machinery at full blast. Sadly, the typical American diet is almost all fat and carbohydrate. According to the National Research Council's Committee on Diet and Health in 1985, 46 percent of calories in the average American's diet came from carbohydrate, 43 percent from fat, and a paltry 11 percent from protein: *89 percent of the American diet is fat and carbohydrate.*

Based on these figures and what you now know about insulin, it's no mystery why there's a problem. The average American consumes a high-carbohydrate, low-protein diet that generates maximal insulin levels and, at the same time, loads up on fat, providing all the raw materials necessary for insulin to convert into cholesterol and excess body fat. Unfortunately, when we—or our average American friends—find our cholesterol too high, our blood pressure too high, or our weight too high, what do our doctors tell us to do? Reduce fat and increase carbohydrate. What happens when we follow this advice? Not much. Now you know why.

When you reduce your fat from the national average of 43 percent to 30 percent on the National Cholesterol Awareness Program Step-One Diet, you still have sufficient raw materials for cholesterol synthesis, and if you raise your carbohydrate consumption to 60 percent as that diet recommends, your insulin, which was already high—that's why you had the problem in the first place—goes even higher. While it's true that you are eating less fat, your increased insulin activity more than compensates to keep your cholesterol or high blood pressure pretty much where it was to start with. Once you have an insulin problem, the only way you can successfully treat the effects of it—elevated cholesterol, high blood pressure, etc.—with a high-carbohydrate diet is by going on a low-calorie diet, say 1,000 to 1,200 calories per day, and often it won't work even then. Most people can't, or won't, stay on a diet that calorically restricted for long, because it's unpalatable. Why does the low-calorie, high-carbohydrate diet work at all? Because, ironically, a low-calorie, high-carbohydrate diet actually contains *less* carbohydrate than the typical American diet. Here's why: the average American eats about 2,200 calories a day. Of that total, 46 percent is carbohydrate, which calculates to about 250 grams of carbohydrate per day. The 60-percent-carbohydrate, 1,200-calorie diet provides about 180 grams of carbohydrate per day, 70 grams fewer than the regular diet.

THE SKINNY JUNK-FOOD JUNKIE AND OTHER PARADOXES

Knowing how insulin works can help us analyze and make sense of seemingly contradictory data. The Harris poll completed in 1990 for *Prevention* magazine presents what appears on the surface to be inconsistent data. Americans scored 66.2 out of 100 in this survey on a variety of health-promoting practices, up from 61.5 percent in 1983, the first year the survey was taken. What health-promoting practices? Eating less fat, eating less cholesterol, as we'd expect. The survey reported that although fewer Americans were making an effort to avoid or restrict sugar, sweets, and other refined carbohydrates, all in all our healthful behavior "has improved significantly since 1983, with greater numbers of individuals actively watching key elements of their diet such as their cholesterol level." You would think that with this "significant" improvement in dietary behavior over the past seven years and the reported reduction of fat and cholesterol intake the population would have less high blood pressure and obesity, and fewer cholesterol problems. The survey didn't look into the first two, but it did address obesity. It reported that 64 percent of adult Americans, or about 100 million people, were overweight, up from 58 percent in 1983. If the nutritional establishment is right, and fat and cholesterol are the problems, with more people following such a "healthful" diet you would expect to see a reduction in obesity. The survey found just the opposite.

You may find specific examples that seem to run contrary to the idea that elevated insulin causes the host of problems we've been discussing. We have a friend, for example, who has a son who might as well be connected by hose to a tank of sugar water. This kid always has a can of some kind of soft drink in his hand. He eats candy bars, cookies, cupcakes, and ice cream nonstop. His favorite foods are "spaghetti, pizza, Cap'n Crunch cereal, and toast." He eats at least 500 grams of carbohydrate per day, a figure that converts to over *2 cups* of pure sugar. (*Any* carbohydrate is metabolized exactly like sugar.)

But the kid is rail thin, and his cholesterol is only 135 mg/dl. What's going on? Is he a statistical aberration, like the one relative in every family who smokes and drinks unremittingly, and lives to be ninety-five?

Although he does eat more sugar than many teenagers, this young man is not very different from most youngsters in America today. They all eat way too much sugar and other refined carbohydrates but seem to suffer no ill effects from it. Studies done both in the United States and in England indicate that many children from the ages of about five up to adolescence consume approximately 200 grams, or about 1 cup, of sugar per day. That's 1 cup of pure sugar, not total carbohydrate; total carbohydrate intake is much greater, about twice as much. So the data show that children eat excessive amounts of sugar and other carbohydrate, but anyone who looks can see that the vast majority of children are not fat. And if you checked their cholesterol levels and blood pressure—as we have done— you'd find that almost all would be within the normal range or even low.

Although today's kids are twice as fat as they were a generation ago,[2] you still see relatively few fat kids because most children don't have an insulin problem—yet. But age and their diet and their genes finally catch up with them. After thirty or forty years of growing older on a high-carbohydrate diet, their intricately meshed metabolic gears start to slip, and they begin to develop obesity, high blood pressure, and all the rest. By then they *will* have an insulin problem.

In childhood the insulin–blood sugar regulation mechanism works perfectly. When you're a kid and you eat ice cream or drink a soda loaded with sugar, your blood sugar starts to rise and your pancreas releases a little insulin, which drives your blood sugar back down pronto. The pancreas releases just a small amount of insulin to force the blood sugar back down to normal because in childhood the cells are extremely sensitive to insulin. Small amounts of insulin translate into low insulin levels. And due to this delicate sensitivity, small amounts of insulin easily handle even the outrageous amounts of sugar and other carbohydrates that kids stuff themselves with—but not without a price. That price is a developing loss of sensitivity of the sensors to insulin—a condition known as *insulin resistance*—and chronically elevated insulin levels. And all the disorders that eventually follow.

---

[2] *Archives of Pediatrics and Adolescent Medicine,* 1995.

Insulin Resistance: When Only Too Much Is Enough

When cells become resistant to insulin, the receptors on their surfaces designed to respond to insulin have begun to malfunction. No clear cause for this malfunctioning has yet emerged from ongoing research, but the odds are it will be a combination of inherited tendency and lifestyle abuse. It simply means that the receptors require more insulin to make them work properly in removing sugar from the blood. Whereas before they needed just a touch to lower it, now they need a continuous supply of excess insulin to keep blood sugar within the normal range.

As time goes by, blood sugar rises higher and stays up longer after the carbohydrate meal despite the enormous amount of insulin mustered to lower it. Bear in mind that were your doctor to check blood sugar during this stage of developing insulin resistance, your blood sugar would be perfectly normal. The major silent change taking place is the ever-growing quantity of insulin needed to keep it that way. Only by checking your blood insulin level—a lab test most doctors don't even consider yet—can you determine whether you have an elevated insulin level (the condition called *hyperinsulinemia)* or *insulin resistance. Hyperinsulinemia* means simply having too much insulin in the blood, whereas *insulin resistance* means that the receptors no longer respond properly to insulin. This is the classic story of the chicken and the egg: which came first? Researchers are not yet certain, but the preponderance of evidence points to excess insulin as the culprit.

It's not the little spurts of insulin that we see in children and adolescents after they eat carbohydrates that cause problems; these are perfectly normal. It is the sustained elevated insulin levels—hyperinsulinemia—of the insulin-resistant adult that lead to the high blood pressure, cholesterol elevation, diabetes, and excess weight of midlife. Hyperinsulinemia is the real problem; all the other "problems" are merely the symptoms. If you look back at the chart showing the roles of insulin and glucagon, you can easily see what kinds of mischief hyperinsulinemia causes and how all these symptoms develop. Picture all the processes listed on the left side operating full blast—as they do under full insulin stimulation—and you can imagine the degree of harm being done silently.

Unfortunately, most doctors treat only the symptoms and often in a way that makes the real problem worse. If you go on a low-fat diet, what happens? By decreasing your fat intake you usually decrease your protein intake, because virtually all foods that are protein-rich contain substantial amounts of fat. Meat, eggs, cheese, most dairy products—the best sources of complete dietary protein—are all either taboo or severely restricted on a low-fat diet. With this protein and fat restriction, the only food component left in the diet is carbohydrate, which by default results in your eating a high-carbohydrate, low-protein diet—the very diet that maximizes insulin production. If you had hyperinsulinemia to begin with—and if you have elevated triglycerides and cholesterol and high blood pressure, you can bet that you do—increasing your body's production of insulin isn't going to help. Instead of attacking the root cause of the problem, you'll leave the doctor's office with a prescription for a high blood pressure medicine, a more stringent diet, and perhaps a prescription for a cholesterol-lowering medicine as well.

You are relieved, your doctor is happy, and the drug companies are ecstatic: they have just signed you on as a new customer to the tune of between $50 and $200 per month for life.

If these methods bring about only cosmetic solutions to blood pressure, cholesterol, and other problems, how can we actually treat these disorders and make them go away? All you need to do is treat the hyperinsulinemia, and the other disorders improve or disappear.

The only method available to treat hyperinsulinemia is diet. Fortunately the dietary approach works spectacularly well. You can treat elevated cholesterol with the standard low-fat cholesterol-lowering diet until the cows come home with limited success, but you can reduce your insulin level with our program in a matter of days and see an almost immediate reduction of blood pressure, a significant reduction in your cholesterol or triglyceride levels in a few weeks, and a steady loss of excess stored body fat in the weeks and months ahead.

It's important to remember, however, that even though the regimen works rapidly to return insulin sensitivity to normal in most people, *it works only as long as you follow it*. It doesn't return you to your childhood levels of imperviousness to carbohydrate assault. You must continue to follow the guidelines to maintain the changes; a return to your former eating habits will return you to your former problems. This nutritional structure is successful because it works *with* your metabolic system instead of counter to it; it's been proven again and again around the world.

Better in the Bush: Aborigines and Insulin Resistance

The concept of undertaking nutritional therapy for disease by constructing a diet of reduced carbohydrate is beautifully illustrated in the work of Dr. Kerin O'Dea, an Australian physician, and his colleagues, who have extensively studied the Australian aborigines over the past decade or so. The aborigines are an interesting group in that they develop a high incidence of hyperinsulinemia and type II diabetes when exposed to an urbanized, Western diet. Like a huge number of Americans, they are genetically predisposed to the development of these disorders, but they develop them much more quickly. This situation, although unfortunate for the aborigines, makes them ideal candidates for the study of the relationship between diet and hyperinsulinemia.

Dr. O'Dea began his studies by looking at the baseline insulin and glucose levels of urbanized aborigine subjects who were consuming a Western diet. He found that both the insulin and the glucose levels were significantly elevated, which should come as no surprise when we consider the diet they were eating: "white flour, white sugar, white rice, carbonated drinks, alcoholic beverages (beer, port), powdered milk and cheap fatty meat." This sounds a lot like the diet of the majority of teenagers in America today. When we look at the composition of this diet in terms of the three nutrient types, we find that it is "high in refined carbohydrate (40–50%) and fat (40–50%) and relatively low in protein (< or = 10%)" or almost precisely the same composition as the typical American diet.

Dr. O'Dea then started these people on his experimental diet, which he designed to approximate the original native diet they would consume were they back in the bush: considerable protein, not a lot of fat, and very little carbohydrate. The nutrient composition was "protein 70–75%, fat 20–25%, [and] carbohydrate <5%." He kept the aborigines on this "very low carbohydrate–high protein diet" for two weeks and then rechecked their blood values. He found that his subjects had developed "a small but significant improvement in glucose tolerance which was accompanied by a similar small reduction in insulin response." He concluded that "these findings suggest an improvement in glucose utilization and insulin sensitivity after the high protein–low carbohydrate diet."

This success inspired Dr. O'Dea to undertake what turned out to be a prolonged and exceptionally enlightening study. He gathered a group of middle-aged, hyperinsulinemic, diabetic, mildly overweight aborigine subjects who had been living on a Western diet much like the one just detailed. These subjects agreed to return to "their traditional country in an isolated location" in western Australia for seven weeks, during which they would live the lives of hunter-gatherers.

During the seven weeks that the aborigines lived off the land in the bush Dr. O'Dea and his group kept careful records of the various foods the subjects ate as they wandered from area to area and tabulated them for later analysis. Depending on whether the group was on the coast or traveled inland, the diet varied, with protein ranging from 54 to 80 percent, fat from 13 to 40 percent, and carbohydrate from less than 5 percent to a high of 33 percent. How did these subjects fare on this high-protein, restricted-carbohydrate diet? Their blood glucose levels fell from an average of about 210 mg/dl to 118 mg/dl. Insulin levels dropped almost by half, from 23 mU/ml to 12 mU/ml, near the normal range. Triglycerides, which are storage fat molecules synthesized in the liver under the stimulus of insulin, fell by a factor of three, from 354 mg/dl all the way down to 106 mg/dl. All this improvement came in just seven weeks from a diet that was predominantly (64 percent) animal in origin. (Exercise wasn't a factor in their improvement. Dr. O'Dea determined that the aborigines were surprisingly *less* active in the bush than in the city.)

Dr. O'Dea summed it up succinctly: ". . . all of the metabolic abnormalities of type II diabetes were either greatly improved (glucose tolerance, insulin response to glucose) or completely normalized (plasma lipids) in a group of diabetic aborigines by a relatively short (7 week) reversion to traditional hunter-gatherer lifestyle." Dr. O'Dea discovered by actual experimentation with a group of people afflicted with one of the diseases of civilization the same thing that anthropologists learned by examining the mummy and skeletal data: the carbohydrate-restricted, high-protein diet confers optimal health on its followers.

Where does this leave us? You are probably wondering if you need to start subsisting on snails, turtles, kangaroo, crocodiles, crickets, and other diverse beasts to get your cholesterol down. That would work, but you don't have to go to those lengths. Our regimen provides all the benefits of the hunter-gatherer diet but uses foods that you capture at the grocery store and even in the wilds of the nearest fast-food outlet. All we need do to gain the benefits of the hunter-gatherer diet is to consume a diet that approximates it in nutritional composition, which we can do easily.

The Bottom Line

Insulin and its counterbalancing partner, glucagon, are the master hormones controlling human metabolism. The word *insulin* may immediately call up a mental association with diabetes, and the connection is a valid one. Controlling blood sugar is definitely insulin's most important job in the human body.

Many people—especially those with heart disease, diabetes, high blood pressure, elevated cholesterol, or obesity in their families—have inherited a tendency for the insulin sensors on the cells to malfunction with age, illness, stress, or assault by years of high sugar and starch consumption. As these sensors become sluggish, the condition of *insulin resistance* develops. Because it's crucial to get the sugar out of the blood and into the cells, the pancreas will compensate by making more and more insulin to force the sluggish sensors to respond. Thus begins a vicious cycle of requiring ever more insulin to keep the system going. Finally, some people become so resistant to insulin that the amount necessary to make the sensors respond and clear the sugar from the blood is more than their pancreas can make; that person becomes an adult diabetic.

Excess insulin stimulates a wide variety of other metabolic systems: it encourages the kidneys to retain salt and fluid; it stimulates the production of cholesterol by the liver; it fuels an increase in triglyceride production; it thickens the muscular portion of the artery walls, increasing the risk for high blood pressure; and it sends a strong message to the fat cells to store incoming sugar and fat.

Insulin's actions are countered by the second metabolic hormone, glucagon. Glucagon sends signals to the kidneys to release excess salt and fluid, to the liver to slow down the production of cholesterol and triglycerides, to the artery wall to relax and drop blood pressure, and to the fat cells to release stored fat to be burned for energy. When insulin levels in the blood are high, however, they so overwhelm the system that they suppress glucagon's actions.

Since food is what mainly controls the production of these two hormones, we have been able to create a nutritional structure that maximizes the release of glucagon and minimizes the release of insulin, creating a closer balance between these two hormones. Under these conditions the actions of the glucagon predominate, allowing the metabolism to heal and the malfunctioning sensors to regain their sensitivity. Once this healing occurs, the metabolic disturbances that insulin resistance caused improve or disappear. If elevated, your cholesterol and triglycerides return to normal, your blood pressure returns to normal, blood sugar stabilizes, and you can effectively lose excess stored body fat. All these benefits accrue not by treating the symptoms—the blood pressure, cholesterol problem, overweight, or diabetes—but the root cause, chronically elevated insulin and insulin resistance. There are no medications yet to treat this disorder—the right diet is the only remedy, but it works extremely well.

Chapter 5

The Deadly Diseases of Civilization

Hydra. A monster with many heads slain by Hercules: whence any multiplicity of evils is termed a hydra.

SAMUEL JOHNSON'S DICTIONARY

In Greco-Roman mythology it fell to Heracles (Hercules) as one of his twelve labors to slay the Hydra, an enormous beast with a doglike body and a writhing cluster of snaky heads. Heracles drove the beast from its lair and began to bash at its many heads with his club, but no sooner had he destroyed one head than two or three replacements sprang from its bleeding stump. Heracles doubled his efforts and summoned his nephew Iolus into the fray, and together, with Heracles slashing and bashing the heads and Iolus cauterizing the stumps before new heads could sprout, they reduced the Hydra to its last and supposedly immortal head. Heracles took it off with one mighty swipe, and the deadly Hydra was gone forever.

The myth of the Hydra is a perfect metaphor for the diseases of civilization. Conventional medical wisdom has unfortunately approached the treatment of these interconnected diseases in much the same way that Heracles first attacked the Hydra—one head at a time—usually with the same results: other heads springing up to confound and frustrate doctor and patient. Just as Heracles finally discovered, however, it is only by going for the immortal head—insulin resistance and hyperinsulinemia—that medical science can hope to complete the Herculean task of ridding the patient of the diseases of civilization. Treating one disease at a time will at best merely hold them at bay; at worst it will actually contribute to the formation of other diseases. How? By worsening the underlying insulin problem, which in turn aggravates high blood pressure, diabetes, heart disease, and all the rest. Before we examine this phenomenon in detail, let's look at how several other medical researchers define this common problem.

Norman Kaplan, M.D., head of the Hypertension Division at the University of Texas Southwestern Medical Center at Dallas, published an article in the July 1989 *Archives of Internal Medicine* entitled "The Deadly Quartet" describing his version of the Hydra. Dr. Kaplan first presents the traditional view that glucose intolerance (a precursor of diabetes), hypertension, and high triglycerides (excess fat in the blood) are usually found in conjunction with upper-body obesity.[1] This view holds that as a person develops upper-body obesity the hypertension, glucose intolerance, and excess triglycerides start to become evident, leading to the conclusion that upper-body obesity *causes* these disorders. It makes sense: first you get fat, then you develop all these other problems; therefore the excess fat must be causing them, right?

When Dr. Kaplan examined the data closely, he found that upper-body obesity is not necessarily the cause of the other three *but is simply found in conjunction with them most of the time*. He goes on to demonstrate that hyperinsulinemia, which has been found to coexist with each of these conditions, can be more realistically represented as the root cause of upper-body obesity, glucose intolerance, hypertension, and excess triglycerides—the deadly quartet of his article's title. Excess body fat—the first thing most people notice—doesn't come first; it comes *after* and as a result of the hyperinsulinemia.

The inevitability of this health progression—first hyperinsulinemia, followed by any or all of the related disorders: obesity, hypertension, diabetes, and heart disease—may not be pleasant to contemplate, but you can take comfort in the fact that if all have one root cause and we can effectively deal with that single troublemaker, we can solve them all at once.

Here's another way to look at it. Imagine hyperinsulinemia as a huge iceberg floating along with only its tips exposed. Ralph DeFronzo, M.D., professor of medicine and head of the Diabetes Division of the University of Texas Health Science Center at San Antonio, a pioneering researcher on hyperinsulinemia and insulin resistance, uses this metaphor to explain the disorder. At meetings he draws a picture of a huge iceberg with peaks labeled *hypertension, heart disease, high cholesterol, diabetes,*

---

[1] The distinction between upper-body and lower-body obesity is significant; it's addressed in Chapter 9.

and *obesity* protruding above the water. The great mass of the iceberg extending deep into the water, the part hidden from view, he labels hyperinsulinemia—as doctors and patients chip away at the tips, the great dangerous mass remains hidden from view.

The Hydra, Dr. Kaplan's deadly quartet, Dr. DeFronzo's iceberg—all are simplistic descriptions of the somewhat complex medical problem of hyperinsulinemia, which until recently hasn't even had a name. Gerald Reaven, M.D., professor of medicine at Stanford University and a long-time researcher into the metabolic effects of insulin, finally remedied that shortcoming. In a 1988 article in the journal *Diabetes* on the cluster of metabolic disorders typically found in association with insulin resistance and hyperinsulinemia, he dubbed it *Syndrome X*. Syndrome X includes the following disorders:

- elevated VLDL (a type of blood fat)
- low level of HDL (the so-called "good" cholesterol)
- insulin resistance
- hyperinsulinemia
- hyperglycemia (elevated blood sugar)
- hypertension

Says Dr. Reaven: "The common feature of the proposed syndrome is insulin resistance. All other changes are likely to be secondary to this basic abnormality."

Although the name *Syndrome X* has gained fairly wide usage in the medical literature, we prefer the more descriptive representation of the Hydra's many heads or the iceberg chunking along beneath the surface en route to a metabolic catastrophe. However you choose to think of it, the important thing is to realize that *these diseases of civilization are in reality only different manifestations of one complex disorder.* As we begin our discussion of the individual manifestations, always keep in mind that they are interrelated through hyperinsulinemia and that any one always lurks around the corner from any other. Let's start by considering what is without doubt the most common insulin-driven disorder—obesity.

The O Word: Obesity

For some of us are out of breath, and all of us are fat.

LEWIS CARROLL

How much of a problem is obesity? According to the government, obesity is an enormous problem. The most recent figures, reported in 1995, place the segment of Americans who are "significantly overweight" at 33 percent—nearly a 30 percent *jump* in one decade while the population has *cut* fat consumption. Although the Centers for Disease Control had set goals for a reduction in obesity from the nation's lower-fat efforts, Americans went off in the opposite direction and got even fatter. If you believe your eyes, obesity is virtually epidemic—as anyone who's ever been to a shopping mall knows.

Despite the manifold health problems associated with obesity, people continue to gain weight; despite the many disadvantages obesity inflicts on its victims on the job, the cultural stigma against them, the plethora of weight-loss centers, books, and products available, more people than ever are overweight. Why?

HOW WE GET FAT

Obesity is defined simply as the accumulation of excess fat on the body; obesity has nothing to do with excess weight. Based on the standard height-weight tables, Arnold Schwarzenegger would be considered over-weight, but he obviously isn't overfat or obese.

Although it's almost always attributed to excess calories, obesity is more related to the multifaceted actions of insulin and glucagon on the storage of fat. As any juvenile-onset diabetic can readily attest, in the ab-sence of insulin one can eat and eat and eat while continuing to lose weight; it's not just a matter of how much is consumed but the result of a complicated interplay among insulin, glucagon, and what and how much is consumed. These two hormones exert a profound influence on all the metabolic pathways, but especially on those involved in the burn-ing and storing of fat and the development of obesity.

When you eat food, your body either breaks it down and burns it for energy or stores it away as body fat in the fat cells (or as glycogen, the storage form of glucose, in the muscles) for later use. Both functions oc-cur simultaneously, and although both the storing and burning pathways are active to some degree all the time, one pathway usually predominates. What is important is the net direction of fat flow over time—i.e., are you mainly storing fat or mainly burning it for energy? Which pathway pre-dominates most of the time? If you mainly store it, you develop obesity; if you mainly burn it, you lose weight.

The flow of fat is composed of the fat you eat, the fat released from storage in your fat cells, and the fat you make from excess protein and carbohydrate. Yes, the body can make fat from carbohydrate and plenty of it. That's why you can't eat fat-free cookies and ice cream and potato chips and expect to lose fat! Remember our friend the pig—pigs are omnivorous and have basically the same metabolic biochemistry we do. And nothing fattens a pig like corn.

Obviously if the direction of fat flow is from our mouths to our fat cells for storage, we are going to gain fat; if this pathway predominates, in time we will become obese. Conversely, if the fat flows in the opposite direction, from the fat tissue to the muscle cells and other tissues to be burned for energy, we won't; in fact we will lose weight. If our goal is to remain—or become—slender and fit, obviously this second pathway is preferable. But if the flow of fat just keeps on rolling along into the fat cells, can we get it to change course? The exciting answer is yes, and here's how.

IT WENT THATAWAY: DIRECTING THE FLOW OF FAT

Insulin and glucagon, the hormone twins, are the primary regulators of these metabolic pathways and actually direct the flow of fat down one pathway or the other. By altering the ratio of insulin to glucagon—*which we can do through our selection of foods*—we can determine which pathway predominates. Instead of allowing our biochemistry to control us, we can control it.

Taking as our starting point the fat in the blood, let's walk through the fat metabolism pathways and follow the flow of the fat molecules. Fat travels through the blood in a form called *triglyceride,* a molecule composed of three fatty acids. At the surface of the cells enzymes break down the triglyceride molecule, and the fatty acids can enter the cells.

Once inside the cells, fat reaches its first hormonal regulation point—the mitochondria. These tiny sausage-shaped power plants within the cells burn the fat—but only if the fatty acids can actually get into the power plant. To do that they need carnitine, which operates a little shuttle system to bring the fat in for oxidation. Insulin inhibits this fat-carnitine shuttle system, saying, in effect, "Hey, we're full; we don't need any more energy. Send that extra fat to the fat cells." Which is precisely what happens when there's too much insulin: the fatty acids turn back into triglycerides and move back into the blood. Glucagon in contrary fashion *accelerates* the shuttle, rapidly moving fat into the mitochondria. Glucagon's signal: "We need energy; let's start breaking that fat down and getting it in here to the furnace."

Muscle, liver, kidney, lung, heart, and other cells break down fat and burn it for energy, but it's a different story with the fat cells. Fat cells merely store the fat molecules. Residing on the surface of the fat cells are two enzymes—both regulated by insulin and glucagon—responsible for herding fat into or out of the fat cells. The first, *lipoprotein lipase,* transports fatty acids into the fat cell and keeps them there. (Lipoprotein lipase, as we shall see shortly, also plays a major role in the rapid regaining of lost weight that plagues so many dieters.) The other, *hormone-sensitive lipase*, does just the opposite—it *releases* the fat from fat cells into the blood. As you might imagine, insulin stimulates the activity of lipoprotein lipase, the fat-storage enzyme, and glucagon inhibits it; glucagon stimulates the fat-releasing enzyme, and insulin inhibits it.

Figure 5.1 illustrates the favored pathways in the insulin-dominant state that occurs immediately after eating and for several hours thereafter—*or exists the majority of time in people with hyperinsulinemia.* As you can see, fat flows toward the fat cells, where it is warmly welcomed, taken in, and held tightly until insulin levels fall, bringing about its release. *In the insulin-dominant mode, fat storage prevails.*

In the glucagon-dominant mode, Figure 5.2, fat flows away from the fat cells. Fat released from the fat cells enters the other cells and gets shuttled into the mitochondria, where it is completely burned for cellular energy. Along with this fat from the fat cells any dietary fat—whether consumed as fat or converted from carbohydrate or protein—also flows into the mitochondria for oxidation instead of into the fat cells to be stored.

Just a glance at these diagrams makes clear why hyperinsulinemia creates and sustains the obese condition—and why so many Americans are overweight. As long as the stimulation of insulin persists, the fat can't really get out. If the situation changes, however, and insulin levels decrease, under the stimulation of glucagon the flow of fat reverses and the fat mass diminishes.

THE BUILT-IN NO-WIN SITUATION

We know that 95 percent of people who manage to lose weight will not be able to keep it off. Amazingly, obesity remains much less treatable than the vast majority of cancers, a grim statistic in and of itself. Are 95 percent of the overweight doomed to live out their lives swaddled in layers of fat?

In a brilliant and controversial essay on intelligence published in the winter 1969 issue of *Harvard Educational Review,* Arthur R. Jensen, a professor of psychology at the University of California at Berkeley, wrote: "In other fields, when bridges do not stand, when aircraft do not fly, when machines do not work, when treatments do not cure, despite all conscientious efforts on the part of many persons to make them do so, one begins to question the basic assumptions, principles, theories, and hypotheses that guide one's efforts." Most physicians, dietitians, and nu-

FIGURE 5.1

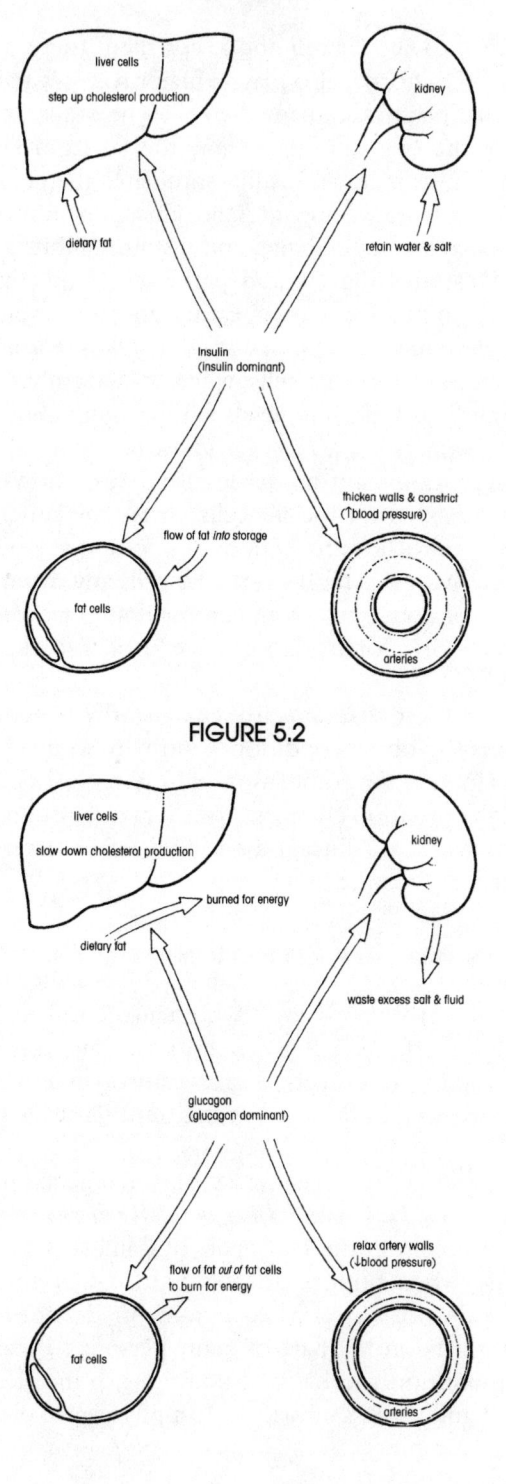

liver cells

step up cholesterol production

dietary fat

kidney

retain water & salt

Insulin
(insulin dominant)

flow of fat *into* storage

fat cells

thicken walls & constrict
(↑blood pressure)

arteries

FIGURE 5.2

liver cells

slow down cholesterol production

burned for energy

dietary fat

kidney

waste excess salt & fluid

glucagon
(glucagon dominant)

flow of fat *out of* fat cells
to burn for energy

fat cells

relax artery walls
(↓blood pressure)

arteries

tritionists have been locked in the notorious clean and well-lit prison of a single idea for decades. These experts have been treating obesity with low-calorie, low-fat, high-complex-carbohydrate diets, then standing around wringing their hands, watching 95 percent of their patients regain their weight. Perhaps inevitably they blame the patient for the failure.

The evidence seems clear that the low-fat, high-carbohydrate diet—the standard obesity therapeutic agent—is flawed in principle, out of sync with biochemical reality. So why not try something different?

Several recent studies point the way. Scientists studying the rapid-regain phenomenon have fingered lipoprotein lipase, the fat-storage enzyme mentioned earlier, as one of the primary villains. It turns out that the biological activity of this enzyme increases prodigiously immediately *after* weight loss. That's right, *the very act of losing weight strengthens and makes more potent the enzyme that is in great measure responsible for the overweight state to begin with.* Although it no doubt has an evolutionary purpose, this is a sorry state of biological affairs: while working hard to lose weight, you reinforce the biochemical underpinnings of your obesity. Add to this the fact that insulin by itself *further* activates the already hyperactive lipoprotein lipase and you begin to understand why 95 percent regain.

What standard treatment is brought to bear against this combined force? The only weapon in the arsenal, *the low-fat, high-complex-carbohydrate* diet, a diet that *stimulates* the release of insulin. Expecting a formerly obese person with a history of hyperinsulinemia not to gain fat on a carbohydrate-rich diet is like throwing gasoline on a fire, then wondering why it flares. In fact, it's amazing that even 5 percent of successful dieters manage to keep it off. But that may correlate with the percentage of overweight people who *don't* have hyperinsulinemia and insulin resistance.

What about our goal, to divert the flow of fat away from the fat cells? Although we can't control lipoprotein lipase directly, we can control it *indirectly* by controlling the metabolic hormones—insulin and glucagon—that modulate it. By keeping insulin levels low, we can remove any stimulation this hormone provides; by keeping glucagon *elevated,* we can continue to inhibit lipoprotein lipase and thus counteract the stimulatory effect brought on by the weight loss. The nutritional plan in this book lowers insulin and raises glucagon levels, the ideal combination both to achieve and to *maintain* a lower fat mass. We've seen it happen in thousands of our patients, and in our experience it's the *only* approach that works.

Diabetes

Diabetes. A morbid copiousness of urine; a fatal colliquation by the urinary passages.

SAMUEL JOHNSON'S DICTIONARY

Almost 2,000 years ago physicians first wrote of diabetes, describing it as a disease causing its sufferers to urinate frequently and in great quantity and to have a great thirst. These early physicians watched helplessly as their patients consumed enormous volumes of fluids that seemed to pour through them unstopped, became progressively more ill and emaciated, and finally died. The disease causing this wretched condition they named *diabetes,* which means "to run through like a siphon." It took 1,600 years before physicians realized that along with vast quantities of body fluids their diabetic patients were losing sugar in their urine. Thomas Willis, a professor at Oxford University in the seventeenth century, wrote of his experience with diabetic patients that their urine was "wonderfully sweet, as if imbued with honey or sugar." He added to the name the Latin term *mellitus,* meaning "sweetened with honey."[2]

Although *diabetes mellitus* is accurate in targeting a couple of the primary symptoms, it's a useless description of the underlying disease mechanisms. By naming diseases by their signs and symptoms, early physicians often created confusion, leading to misspent effort by those who followed. Diabetes is a case in point. Today we subdivide diabetes mellitus into two separate and distinct diseases—type I and type II diabetes—with two different pathological causes but essentially the same symptoms. Sixty or seventy years ago, however, physicians believed that all diabetes was the same—there was just a difference in severity. Some people got it in childhood or early adulthood, suffered a progressively rapid course, were unresponsive to treatment, and died within a few years. Others developed it much later, had much less severe cases, and could be "cured" or at least treated fairly successfully by diet. Both groups of patients produced large amounts of sweet urine and so were diagnosed as having diabetes mellitus.

Physicians now recognize that although both disorders are called *dia-*

---

[2] You may be wondering how Professor Willis knew his patients' urine was "wonderfully sweet" without actually tasting it. He did taste it. In fact, up until the middle of the 1800s physicians routinely tasted their patients' urine to check for diabetes mellitus.

betes the circumstances and pathology leading to their development are entirely different. Type I diabetes, the more rapidly serious of the two, usually develops in childhood or adolescence when a virus or other toxic substance destroys the insulin-producing cells in the pancreas and requires aggressive treatment with insulin in shot form. It is a disease of insulin lack. In contrast, type II diabetes develops later in life, can usually be treated with diet and/or oral medicines, and is a disease of insulin *excess*. It seems strange that the same disease can be caused by both an excess *and* an insufficiency of insulin, but that is precisely the case.

Although our dietary plan is in most cases the ideal nutritional regimen for optimal health in those with type I diabetes, it is not the total treatment. Since their damaged pancreases can produce no, or at best very little, insulin, these patients require injections of insulin daily to meet their metabolic needs. Should they not receive their insulin, they face serious illness and even death in fairly short order. The treatment of this complex disease is beyond the scope of this book, but a brief discussion of the pathology involved illustrates well the indispensable role insulin plays as the overseer and regulator of metabolism. Our attention has so far focused so exclusively on the disorders of insulin excess that you may believe that insulin has no redeeming qualities or that glucagon is a metabolic panacea. A quick look at type I diabetes will dispel this notion in a hurry. Type I diabetes is a disorder of insufficient insulin and unrestrained glucagon excess, and as such it serves to clarify the importance of a regulated *balance* between insulin and glucagon.

TYPE I DIABETES: GLUCAGON RUN AMOK

The best way to understand type I diabetes is to look at Figures 5.1 and 5.2 in the last section. Recognize that in healthy nondiabetics both these forces are at work at once and in balance. But in type I diabetics, with no insulin to hold it back and only glucagon to stimulate its release, fat pours out of the fat cells into the blood as in 5.2. For the same reason any incoming dietary fat can't get into the fat cells and so joins with the fat rushing from the fat cells and heads toward the tissues for disposal. As this blood, laden with fat, courses through the liver, the fatty acids enter the liver cells and then, without insulin to stop them, easily enter the mitochondria for breakdown. In contrast to other cells, liver mitochondria process fatty acids differently in that they don't burn the fatty acids for energy but instead partially break them down into molecules called *ketone bodies* and release them into the circulation. Normally the ketone bodies produced in the liver cells travel through the blood to the muscle and other tissues that burn them for energy. In type I diabetics, however, the enormous quantities of ketone bodies generated by the massive fat flux far exceed the needs of the tissues and outstrip the body's capacity to jettison them via the urine, the stool, and the breath. As the ketone bodies, which are acids, accumulate in the blood, the blood becomes more and more acidic until the victim is in the throes of a metabolic nightmare called *diabetic ketoacidosis,* which leads to coma, then death if not treated quickly.

This reverse flow of fat makes it impossible for a person without insulin to gain weight. Indeed the first symptom a person with undiagnosed type I diabetes usually experiences is an unexplained weight loss in the face of constant hunger and greater-than-normal food intake; *it's not unusual for such a person to lose 30 or 40 pounds in a month or two.*

TYPE II DIABETES: THE SLOW ROAD

Type II diabetes represents approximately 90 percent of all cases of diabetes, and although less immediately sinister than its type I counterpart, it is every bit as deadly over the long run. Like heart disease, high blood pressure, and obesity, type II diabetes doesn't develop overnight but requires years of underlying metabolic disturbance before the symptoms become apparent. As a result, since most cases of type II diabetes surface during middle age, the disorder is often referred to as *adult-onset diabetes.* The development and diagnosis of the type II variety usually follows a weight *gain,* a fact easily explained by the difference in insulin dynamics between the two disorders.

In both cases blood sugar is elevated but for different reasons. The blood sugar level rises in type I because there is no insulin present to hold it down by moving it into the cells; blood sugar goes up in type II because the cells have become so resistant to the effects of insulin that even large amounts can't adequately move the sugar out of the blood and into the cells. In type II diabetes there may exist the paradoxical situation in which both insulin and blood sugar are elevated— at least for a while. In the early stages insulin is always elevated, but as the disease progresses insulin levels often decrease as the pancreatic beta cells (the cells that produce the insulin) fatigue or "wear out" from constantly producing insulin at prodigious rates under the stimulation of the increasing blood sugar. During the early stages, which can last for years, the constantly elevated insulin levels give rise to high blood pressure, heart disease, elevated cholesterol, and obesity—all disorders that afflict type II diabetics with great frequency. During the later stages of the disease the elevated blood sugar damages the kidneys, eyes, blood vessels, and nerves in the same way it does in type I diabetes.

Type II diabetes is without doubt of genetic origin; if your parents have or had it, then the odds are high that you will inherit the predisposition to the disease. If you follow the proper diet, you can ward off the onset of type II diabetes or even reverse its damaging effects. Conversely, in the susceptible person, dietary imprudence can certainly hasten the development and worsen the severity. Our diet is the optimal nutritional regimen for patients with type II diabetes because by correcting the underlying insulin resistance it lowers the abnormally elevated blood sugar levels, begins to repair any pancreatic damage, and can restore the tissues to normal.

From Insulin Resistance to Type II Diabetes

This vicious cycle begins slowly and develops over many years. Beginning with a genetically susceptible person, years of insulin bombardment brought on by teenage dietary and lifestyle abuse finally take their toll on the insulin sensors in the tissues and they begin to become resistant. To make the system work, the pancreas cranks out more insulin and thus begins the upward creep of chronically elevated insulin. Ultimately enormous levels of insulin may be required to keep the blood sugar within the normal range in the face of severe insulin resistance. In the majority of cases this is as far as the progression goes: insulin remains elevated, doing its damage through enhanced cholesterol synthesis, arterial thickening, increased fat storage, and all the rest but still managing to keep the blood sugar controlled. In genetically predisposed people, however, the condition progresses further, leading first to glucose intolerance, then ultimately to type II diabetes.

Consider a person with severe insulin resistance, who to keep blood sugar normal must produce huge amounts of insulin every day. At some time his overworked pancreas will reach the point at which it can no longer accommodate a bigger need—it's already making as much insulin as it possibly can. If the sensors continue to develop even more resistance to insulin, what will happen? His blood sugar level will begin to rise, because he can no longer step up insulin production to overcome the increased resistance necessary to force his blood sugar back into line. At the limit of pancreatic insulin output type II diabetes is just around the corner. If the person in our example were to undergo a glucose tolerance test now, it would be abnormal.

You might think that under these circumstances the blood sugar would continue to rise gradually as the insulin resistance gradually worsened. And that would be the case except for another of the nasty little feedback systems that often arise when the metabolism starts to get out of kilter. *Glucose at high blood concentrations is toxic to many tissues, including the pancreatic beta cells.* Under constant overstimulation by the excess glucose the beta cells may finally give up and cease producing insulin altogether—a condition called *beta cell fatigue* or *beta cell burnout.* As the blood glucose rises and exceeds a certain threshold—typically 140 mg/dl—for a period of time it actually destroys the ability of the beta cells to produce insulin. Falling insulin levels exert less control over the rising blood glucose, which then climbs higher and faster, further damaging the beta cells, which in turn produce even less insulin, reducing control over blood glucose even further—you can easily color in the rest of the picture. High blood sugar or hyperglycemia then becomes not only a manifestation of diabetes but a self-perpetuating cause of the disorder as well, leading to the paradox in which the victim is *both* diabetic *and* hyperinsulinemic.

Once the patient's blood sugar reaches diabetic levels, it begins to cause many but not all of the problems of type I diabetes: sugar spills into the urine, causing frequent urination and increased thirst, and the increased blood glucose causes degenerative complications of the eyes, nerves, kidneys, and blood vessels. As long as the patient's beta cells are producing some insulin, the patient avoids the dangerous ketoacidosis of type I diabetes because the insulin prevents the stored body fat from rushing out and converting to ketone bodies under the influence of unopposed glucagon. If, however, enough beta cells fatigue and insulin production falls sufficiently, glucagon can predominate and all the problems of type I diabetes ensue. Usually the beta cells continue to make more than enough insulin to prevent ketoacidosis, indeed enough insulin to cause all the symptoms of insulin excess, including hypertension, excess cholesterol production, obesity, and heart disease, the disorders with which most type II diabetes victims are afflicted. Typically most physicians focus on these disorders—the tips of the iceberg—instead of the cause of the problem, aberrant insulin metabolism.

Once again by aiming efforts at the underlying hyperinsulinemia people can reverse and often rid themselves of another of the major diseases of civilization. Even those with type I diabetes can markedly lower their insulin doses and attain much better control over their blood sugars with our plan—but *only under the supervision of a physician.*

Dr. Richard K. Bernstein, a diabetologist in Mamaroneck, New York, is the author of *Diabetes: Type II* (originally published by Prentice-Hall), an excellent primer on the merits of carbohydrate restriction as applied specifically to diabetes types I and II.[3] He believes that strict adherence to a low-carbohydrate diet is the cornerstone of all diabetic therapy and is of primary importance in the maintenance of the tight blood sugar control necessary to provide a normal productive life span to victims of both types of diabetes.

Hypertension

To be sure, hypertension is a silent killer, and the first major symptom may be death.

KENNETH COOPER, M.D.

Our patient Tom Edwards came in weighing about 315 pounds and was taking three different medications to control his high blood pressure, which at 160/105 still wasn't particularly well controlled. We had just started treating weight-loss patients with the protein-sparing modified fast described in Mike's earlier book *Thin So Fast,* and we hadn't yet used it on anyone with a serious blood pressure problem. Back in our do-it-like-everyone-else days we treated many overweight patients with blood pressure problems by putting them on low-calorie diets. As their weight came down slowly (which it usually did *if* they stayed on the diet; getting them to stay on it was the hard part), so did their blood pressure. On successive visits a month or so apart we'd gradually reduce their blood pressure medications, sometimes getting them completely medication free if they lost enough weight. There was no reason to assume Tom would be any different.

We didn't yet know about the dramatic insulin-lowering properties of this new nutritional approach, in fact at that point we didn't know that

---

[3] Dr. Bernstein, a long-suffering type I diabetic, has a fascinating history. He developed his methods of treatment by experimenting on himself during his predoctor days, when he was an engineer. He realized the benefits of the carbohydrate-restricted diet and tight control of blood sugars but was unable to penetrate the medical establishment despite his astounding success because his methods were not consistent with accepted medical wisdom. Rather than tilt at windmills, the 45-year-old Mr. Bernstein enrolled in medical school to give himself credibility. He wrote his first book while in medical school and since obtaining his M.D. degree he continues to write and has a private practice specializing in the treatment of diabetes. If you or someone you care about has either type of diabetes, get Dr. Bernstein's book. It contains a wealth of information on all aspects of diabetes care and is written by someone who truly knows his subject. We can't recommend this book highly enough. The new edition will be published by Little, Brown in 1997.

insulin was involved in anything other than blood sugar control. We didn't take him off any of his medications but told him we would be able to as soon as he lost some of his weight. Tom called three days into the program.

"Doc, I'm dizzy," he said. "When I get up out of a chair I almost pass out. When I stand on my feet for a while at work I get so spacey-headed I feel like I'm going to faint."

We told him to come to the office right away. When he arrived, the nurse found his blood pressure to be 100/60—an unduly low figure compared to the pressures he had been running—and his weight had dropped to 309 pounds. Six pounds is a lot of weight to lose in only three days for most people, but not for someone weighing in at 315. Most of his early weight loss was fluid loss, but we couldn't square it with the dramatic fall in blood pressure. Even using potent diuretic drugs, we hadn't gotten that kind of response. Mike told him to quit taking one of his medications, and his symptoms improved as his blood pressure went up a little. He was back in a few days with the same symptoms. Within the first two weeks of his diet his blood pressure had fallen to the point that we took him off all but one of his medicines and that one at reduced dosage. By this time he had lost only 13 pounds or so, less than 5 percent of his body weight, and we couldn't figure out what was going on.

Shortly after this experience we attended a scientific meeting at which a researcher from Switzerland gave a paper on the effects of insulin on fluid retention. His data showed that a rapid reduction in serum insulin levels would bring about a rapid and substantial diuresis. And of course that would mean a rapid and substantial decrease in blood pressure as well—exactly what happened with Tom Edwards. This revelation explained some other strange phenomena we had experienced with patients on the modified fast, changes that took place way too soon after starting to be in any way related to the minuscule weight losses. It also launched us on our study of the wide-ranging actions of insulin, insulin resistance, and hyperinsulinemia.

HOW INSULIN DRIVES UP BLOOD PRESSURE

Excess insulin causes high blood pressure in basically three ways: it causes fluid retention, alters the mechanics of the blood vessels, and increases nervous stimulation of the arterial system. Let's examine these processes in order, starting with insulin's propensity to raise blood pressure by driving the body to retain excess fluid.

Along with transporting nutrients to the tissues and hauling waste products away, the blood bathes the cells with electrolytes in the proper mix and concentration. These electrolytes—sodium, potassium, chloride, bicarbonate, and others—are critical for normal cell function and are, like blood sugar, maintained within a narrow range. The kidneys filter the blood that runs through them, removing waste products and regulating the concentration of the electrolytes. Here's another of the body's great balancing acts. If the blood contains too much sodium, the kidneys pull it out, deposit it in the urine, and send it to the bladder to be removed; if there is too little, the kidneys assiduously conserve what there is and remove just enough fluid to ensure the proper concentration of sodium in the blood.

Diuretics work by forcing the kidneys to get rid of more sodium than they normally would. As the kidneys eliminate this sodium they jettison fluid along with it to maintain the blood concentration of sodium within the proper range.

Insulin has exactly the opposite effect: it forces the kidneys to retain sodium—even when there's too much and the kidneys would rather get rid of it. To maintain the sodium concentration in the blood at the proper level, the kidneys must then retain excess fluid to dilute the excess sodium. More insulin means more sodium retention and therefore more fluid retention. As the body retains more fluid and the blood volume increases, the blood pressure begins to rise and can in due course reach dangerous levels, requiring treatment. The typical first-line therapy is the administration of diuretics to override the effects of insulin, forcing the kidneys to release excess sodium and fluid, returning the blood pressure to normal. Or the patient can use nutrition to reduce the elevated insulin levels and achieve the same results in a less costly fashion.

Insulin also increases blood pressure by altering the mechanics of the vascular walls, namely, by making the arteries less elastic. Recall from the last chapter that insulin acts as a growth hormone on the smooth muscle cells in the walls of the arteries and that as the insulin level increases the excess stimulation of these smooth muscle cells causes them to enlarge. As these smooth muscle cells grow, they increase the thickness of the arterial walls, making them stiffer and less supple while at the same time decreasing the volume within the arteries. The heart then has to exert more force to push the blood through these narrowed, more rigid arteries, resulting in elevated blood pressure.

The third way insulin causes elevated blood pressure is by stimulation of the nervous system, leading to the increased release of norepinephrine, an adrenalinelike substance, into the blood. Adrenaline is a neurotransmitter whose effects we've all experienced during times of stress, excitement, or after a bad scare. If you narrowly avoid an automobile accident, you typically feel flushed, notice your heart beating faster, and have a shaky, uncomfortable feeling—all brought on by the sudden outpouring of adrenaline. Not only does this rush of adrenaline cause these uneasy feelings; it drives up the blood pressure at the same time. Elevated insulin levels acting through unknown mechanisms engender an increase in blood norepinephrine that, although not of the magnitude of the rush occasioned by the near disaster, nevertheless raises blood pressure and causes an increased heart rate, placing the heart under continuous stimulation and keeping the blood vessels constricted.

The three ways insulin induces and sustains high blood pressure all complement one another. Insulin-spawned adrenaline acts to constrict insulin-thickened, less supple arterial walls, while at the same time the entire vascular system tries to cope with all the excess fluid retained by the insulin-stimulated kidneys. It's difficult to imagine how the blood pressure *wouldn't* rise under these conditions.

Heart Disease

More commonly the arterio-sclerosis results from the bad use of good vessels.

SIR WILLIAM OSLER, M.D.

Heart disease, the last head of the Hydra, is responsible for more death and disability than the rest of the heads combined. Hyperinsulinemia exerts its sinister influence on the heart in a number of ways: by increasing the blood cholesterol in ways we'll examine in Chapter 7 and by acting directly on the coronary arteries, making them more prone to occlusion, spasm, and clot formation. Before delving into the precise ways in which insulin acts, let's take a moment to review what medical science knows about the progression of coronary artery disease and heart attack first from a clinical and then from a cellular perspective.

WHAT IS A HEART ATTACK?

A heart attack occurs when, for whatever reason, the blood flow to an area of the heart is cut off or severely diminished. The heart is nothing but a large muscle that contracts rhythmically, pumping blood throughout the body. How hard does this muscle work? Imagine that you are holding a 5-pound weight in your hand and you begin to flex your arm at the elbow, bringing the weight to your shoulder. Your biceps, the muscle on the front of your upper arm, is doing most of the work during this exercise. The various arteries servicing your biceps carry oxygen- and nutrient-enriched blood to the working muscle as the veins bear away the waste products and deoxygenated blood. If you flex your arm repetitively faster and faster, you will ultimately reach the point at which the oxygen needs of the hardworking biceps exceed the capacity of the arteries to supply it. When your muscle begins to get inadequate amounts of oxygenated blood, it begins to hurt, more than likely prompting you to discontinue the exercise and allow your muscle to recover. Now, if your arm were hooked up to some kind of device that beeped electrical impulses into your biceps to make it contract involuntarily regardless of the pain involved, you can imagine the consequences. The pain would rapidly become excruciating. If the stimulation continued, some of the muscle fibers would begin to die, and ultimately the entire muscle would be damaged irreparably and fail. Your arm would dangle uselessly at your side, unable to contract despite the relentless beeping of the electrical stimulator.

Only in the nightmarish fiction of a Stephen King novel might this torture be inflicted on a human arm; in real life it is inflicted on human hearts daily. The heart has a built-in, mindless stimulator, the *sinoatrial node*, that beeps out an electric current across the body of the cardiac muscle about 72 times per minute. (Just try contracting your biceps a little faster than once per second and you will realize what an amazing muscle the heart is. It contracts at this rate—or even much faster if, for example, the body needs more oxygen due to exercise or fever—day in and day out, awake or asleep, never resting until the day you die.)

Due to the enormous demands for energy required to continuously contract 72 times per minute throughout life, nature has endowed the heart with an extensive circulatory system, the coronary arteries that wrap around the heart carrying large quantities of oxygen-rich blood to all segments of the muscle. If one of these coronary arteries—as a result of blood clot, spasm, or plaque growth, for instance—fails to supply a portion of the heart with enough blood to meet its demands, the heart is in trouble. But the sinoatrial node continues to stimulate the heart muscle, including the segment that is now receiving inadequate oxygenated blood. And as with our biceps, the heart muscle that can't quit beating to rest becomes racked with agonizing pain—the pain of a heart attack. If the blockage is severe enough and continues long enough, the segment of heart served by the involved coronary artery becomes irreversibly damaged and dies.

Along with the severe pain, the aftermath of coronary arterial blockage typically includes shortness of breath, weakness, nausea, drenching sweat, and the feeling of impending death. Medical science has defined and attached names to all the different degrees and manifestations of this phenomenon: angina pectoris, the pain associated with the lack of heart muscle oxygenation; myocardial ischemia, the situation in which the heart muscle receives inadequate oxygen, but before it is permanently damaged; and myocardial infarction, death of a segment of heart muscle. For our purposes we can lump all these together under the rubric of heart disease.

As long as the coronary arteries provide adequate supplies of oxygen-rich blood to the heart, it will pump on forever. The problem arises when the flow of blood to an area of the heart is cut off or reduced significantly. How does this happen? Usually by occlusion of a coronary artery created by the buildup of plaque—cholesterol-filled fibrous growths—on the inner linings of the arteries involved. Plaque forms over a long period of time, progressing in a stepwise fashion, starting with the infiltration of cholesterol into the lining of the artery and proceeding to the development of the mature lesion. And amazingly, insulin, once again, exerts its influence at several points along the way. Just how it does this will become clear when we examine this sequence from the beginning.

THE SCAVENGER'S FEAST: HOW PLAQUE IS FORMED

Five basic processes, each building on the one before, are responsible for the formation of plaque:

1. the infiltration of cholesterol into the arterial wall
2. the alteration of the entrapped cholesterol
3. formation of foam cells
4. formation of fatty streaks
5. conversion of fatty streaks to plaque

The process begins when LDL cholesterol (LDL) makes its way through the endothelium, the layer of cells lining the interior surface of the arterial wall. (See Chapter 7 for a complete discussion of LDL cholesterol, the so-called "bad cholesterol.") The development of plaque occurs beneath the inner lining in an area called the *subendothelial space.* The more LDL that circulates in the blood, the more LDL particles get through to the critical space beneath. If the lining has been damaged in some way—a common one is from cigarette smoking—the process proceeds even faster.[4] Insulin increases the formation of plaque at this earli-

---

[4] This is the mechanism by which cigarette smoking is thought to increase the formation of plaque. Toxic agents make their way from the smoke through the lungs and into the bloodstream, where they proceed to damage the endothelial linings and allow large amounts of LDL to get through unhindered.

est stage by helping increase the concentration of LDL in the blood, as we'll discuss in Chapter 7.

Once the LDL particles penetrate the barrier, certain specialized white blood cells, called *macrophages* or *scavenger cells,* can migrate into the area to ingest them. Bloated from their LDL dinner, these cells take on a grayish, foamy appearance—at which point they're called *foam cells.* In the presence of abundant LDL beneath the lining layer, many macrophages move in and eat themselves into the foam cell state; the many foam cells then coalesce to form the *fatty streak,* the first visible sign of plaque formation.

But there's a crucial point here: the macrophages won't ingest the LDL *as long as it is normal.* So even though more LDL in the blood means more beneath the endothelial layer, nothing happens unless the LDL particles are in some way chemically altered or otherwise damaged. Were this not so, medical science would have its smoking gun in the high-blood-cholesterol-leads-to-increased-heart-disease debate. For years scientists have grown human macrophages in a culture medium and observed their activity in the presence of various substances. If the macrophages encounter normal LDL, they ignore it regardless of the amount presented to them. If, however, the LDL is chemically altered before being added to the culture, the macrophages hit it like a trout hitting a fly. Somehow the altered LDL turns on the feasting response of the macrophage, leading to foam cell conversion and vascular damage.

We don't know exactly how this alteration occurs, but two theories seem the most reasonable. Macrophages grown in culture ingest LDL that has been either oxidized (typically by free radicals, sharklike molecules that indiscriminately attack and damage other molecules) or glycolated (irrevocably bound to sugar). Both these processes—oxidation and glycolation—occur naturally in the body, increase with aging, and are themselves risk factors for coronary artery disease, so it is more than likely that one or the other—or both—is the driving force behind the alteration of LDL, making it so appetizing to macrophages.

Although the fatty streaks make the endothelium bulge slightly into the interior of the artery, they don't cause enough narrowing to significantly restrict blood flow. But once the fatty streak is in place, plaque formation proceeds in earnest. Smooth muscle cells from a layer deeper in the artery migrate into the fatty streak. Some begin growing there, producing a connective tissue containing collagen and other fibrous molecules, while others actually differentiate into macrophages and become foam cells themselves. The engorged foam cells die, releasing their cholesterol into the center of the developing mass.

The end result of this process is the lesion called *atheromatous plaque* (*atheroma* means a "porridgelike" mass, which is how the lesions actually appear). This plaque encroaches into the artery, restricting blood flow and sometimes completely obstructing the artery. Easily visible to the naked eye, an atheromatous plaque is a soft yellowish nodule on the inside lining of an artery. When sliced open, these lesions reveal a soft, greasy, granular core. As the plaque develops further, bleeding can occur within it, producing a sudden ballooning of the lesion that can obstruct blood flow through the artery and cause a heart attack. The lesion may become calcified, causing the artery to become rigid and brittle. It may start to crack, ulcerate, and discharge debris into the bloodstream or, more ominously, to form clots on the ulcerated surface. These clots form the blockage that is typically the ultimate cause of most heart attacks.

Where Does Insulin Come In?

Insulin exerts its influence at several points along the plaque development progression, starting with elevated levels of LDL cholesterol in the blood. Although arterial damage and heart disease can occur in the face of normal—or even low—blood cholesterol, elevated LDL levels usually hasten its onset. And insulin, by its action on the cholesterol synthesis pathway located within the cells, helps to create and sustain excess amounts of LDL in the blood.

Insulin also increases the proliferation of smooth muscle cells in the artery and their migration into the area of plaque formation. This not only accelerates the development of plaque but increases the thickness and rigidity of the arteries as well. Once these smooth muscle cells migrate into the developing fatty streak and plaque growth continues, insulin stimulates the increased synthesis of collagen and other connective tissue that make up a large part of the forming mass. At the same time insulin enhances cholesterol synthesis within the plaque lesion, the source of its greasy appearance.

As you can see, the only stage in this pathway that insulin *doesn't* affect (or at least hasn't yet been shown to affect) is that of LDL modification. Although insulin itself apparently doesn't play a direct role in the alteration of the LDL molecule, making it a target for the macrophages, the metabolic changes that go along with insulin resistance and hyperinsulinemia do. As blood sugar rises, increased amounts of glucose are irreversibly attached to LDL molecules, altering their structure and making them attractive to the macrophages; free radicals form and attack other LDL molecules—a process enhanced by an insulin-resistant environment—rendering them susceptible to the same fate.

Insulin and Plaque—A Direct Correlation

In the early 1960s a research team led by Dr. Anatolio Cruz in a now-classic experiment demonstrated the changes wrought by chronically elevated levels of insulin. His team injected insulin into the large arteries in the legs of dogs: each day each dog was injected with insulin in the artery of one leg and the same-size dose of sterile saline in the other. This procedure was followed daily for almost eight months. Upon examination the arteries injected with the insulin were found to have a pronounced accumulation of cholesterol and fatty acids along with a thickening of the inner arterial lining; the opposite arteries, injected with saline, remained normal. Dr. Cruz induced these profound changes with a relatively small dose of insulin given only once a day for a little over seven months. Picture the changes he might have found had he been able to keep the insulin level consistently elevated for several years! With this in mind it's not difficult to imagine the changes in our own coronary arteries after many years of chronic hyperinsulinemia.

Can You Undo This Damage?

Are we doomed to live with the current state of our coronary arteries barnacled with plaque, or can we reclaim them? We can reclaim them, but not overnight. The development of plaque takes time, and so does its regression; it's a process that takes years, not months. It can also be done only in the face of a *lowered insulin level.*

In the words of one researcher, a consistent finding in animal studies is that insulin "inhibits regression of diet-induced experimental atherosclerosis, and insulin deficiency inhibits development of arterial lesions." In other words, if you want to clean up your coronary arteries, you can't do it in the presence of hyperinsulinemia. Unfortunately, when plaque has reached the point of calcium deposition, hemorrhage, and excess fibrous tissue formation, it is irreversible despite insulin lowering; even at that point, however, dietary intervention can forestall further formation. And if plaque hasn't reached the final stage, our program, by removing the harmful stimulation of insulin in excess, allows the arteries to recover, slowly become more supple, and ultimately rid themselves of the dangerous cholesterol deposits beneath their inner linings. Another head of the Hydra severed by aiming for the immortal one.

When the Deadly Quartet Isn't a Foursome

If hyperinsulinemia indeed causes all these disorders we've been discussing, why doesn't everyone with hyperinsulinemia have high blood pressure, heart disease, diabetes, and obesity? How, for example, can a person have hyperinsulinemia, elevated cholesterol, and high blood pressure and not be overweight? We know that insulin causes the storage of fat, so a person with greatly elevated insulin levels is bound to be overweight, right? Not necessarily. Take the case of Linda Mot. Ms. Mot is a slender (5'8" tall, 110 pounds) 44-year-old woman with high cholesterol. She'd been to another physician who had recommended that she start medications to remedy the problem, but she wanted a second opinion. We began by asking her about her diet.

"What do you usually eat? What are your favorite foods?"

"Well, I don't eat a lot of fats," she assured us. "I try to eat a balanced diet with lots of different foods."

"What's your favorite food?"

"Anything with chocolate in it," she answered without hesitation.

"So, you eat a lot of sweets along with your balanced diet?"

"Oh, yes, I love sweets, especially chocolate," she answered, "and I've always considered myself fortunate in that I could eat them without worrying. All my friends have to watch their weight and either don't eat junk food or do and feel guilty about it. I can eat all the cake, pie, doughnuts, and especially chocolate candy and ice cream that I want and never gain a pound. I guess I'm really lucky."

"Do you have any other health problems besides the cholesterol?"

"I've had some problems with high blood pressure, but that's all okay now because my doctor gave me some pills for my fluid retention that keep the blood pressure down."

"Fluid retention?"

"Yeah, I don't ever gain any weight—you know what I mean; I don't get fat—but I do have a problem with holding on to fluids. My ankles swell a little, sometimes I can't get my rings on, my eyes get puffy, that sort of thing. But the water pills get rid of it and keep my blood pressure down to boot."

"Does your father have heart problems?"

"Yes . . . how did you know?"

Ms. Mot's blood pressure was moderately elevated, and her blood tests revealed a total cholesterol of over 300 and an insulin level that was 56 mU/ml, *almost twice the highest limit of normal by the lab's standards and over five times the limit of what we consider normal.* We set about revising Ms. Mot's diet, not an easy task since she was confronted with a major diet overhaul and had all her life eaten everything she wanted. People who have never had a problem with excess weight have the most difficult time sticking with any kind of diet because dieting has never been a part of their mind-set. Ms. Mot was no exception to this rule, but she has persevered—with an occasional chocolate debauch—and her insulin level has come down along with her blood pressure and cholesterol. Although her blood values haven't quite reached normal yet, she has completely eliminated her problem of fluid retention and hasn't had to take a "water" pill since she started our dietary plan.

Getting back to our original question, why does the slender Ms. Mot—who falls into a category we call *normal weight, metabolically obese*—have most of the problems associated with hyperinsulinemia yet no excess weight, while others who are overweight may not have high blood pressure or elevated cholesterol? Why do some have diabetes or high blood pressure only, while others have the whole full-blown syndrome of hyperinsulinemia?

The answers to these questions lie in the genetic basis of these diseases of civilization. It is well known that these diseases run in families, and when all the studies are in it will be apparent that hyperinsulinemia does too. Depending on our own unique genetic makeup, we each have different propensities to develop these disorders once our insulin levels begin to climb.

WHEN YOUR GENES CATCH UP WITH YOU

Some fortunate people are genetically programmed so that even in the face of a lifetime of reckless eating they don't develop much insulin resistance. Most of us, however, are not so lucky and do gradually develop some degree of insulin resistance and hyperinsulinemia. Our genetics then determine what happens after our insulin levels go up: some of us inherit genes that program us to develop high blood pressure; others will develop diabetes; most will gain weight; and an unfortunate group will develop the whole full-blown cluster of disorders. If your parents developed high blood pressure and diabetes as they began to age, chances are they had underlying hyperinsulinemia and your odds are greater of developing the same problems. Although you can't do anything to change your genes, you can at least be aware of the source of the problem and take steps to avoid or remedy it.

By attacking the individual diseases, we physicians and patients are at best playing a delaying game; only by focusing our energies and treatments on insulin resistance and hyperinsulinemia can we hope to kill the Hydra instead of merely replacing one of its heads with another. Unfortunately, we can't just take a pill and lower our insulin levels; the only way is by changing the foods we eat, by changing our diet to one that is closer to what nature designed us to eat in the first place. The good news is that once we do undertake the proper dietary treatment the proof that we're on the right track is usually dramatic and not long in coming. Thanks to the profound biochemical activity of the correct foods, hyperinsulinemia usually disappears in a hurry, taking with it most of its untoward side effects. Your body will simply heal itself if you give it the right fuel.

The Bottom Line

The major diseases of Western civilization—obesity, high blood pressure, heart disease, elevated blood fats, and diabetes—have a common bond. In truth these diseases that afflict, disable, and kill so many people in America today aren't diseases at all; they're symptoms of a more basic single disorder: hyperinsulinemia (excess insulin) and insulin resistance. Here's how the problems develop:

When you eat, your body breaks down the food into its basic components—protein, carbohydrate, and fat—and absorbs them into the bloodstream, causing a rise in blood sugar. This rise signals your pancreas to make and release insulin that attaches to sensors in the tissues, enabling the sugar to come out of the blood and move into the cells, where it can be either burned for energy or stored away for later use (as fat in the fat cells or as glycogen in the muscles). Years of dietary and lifestyle abuse in susceptible people can lead to malfunctioning of the insulin sensors and the progressive development of chronically elevated insulin levels. This sluggish system favors the storage signals for fat and sugar, leading to the development of excess body fat. Continued dietary abuse (with excess carbohydrate) can finally result in such severe resistance to insulin (insulin sensors so sluggish) that no matter how much insulin your pancreas can make, it's no longer enough to make the system work. The combined forces of the high insulin and the rising blood sugar damage the pancreas and limit its ability to produce insulin, which then sends the blood sugar level skyrocketing, and adult-onset diabetes (type II diabetes) results.

The excess insulin works in several ways to cause elevation of blood pressure: it prompts the kidneys to hold on to salt and fluid; it promotes growth in the muscular layer of the artery walls, making them thicker and less pliable; it increases the levels of norepinephrine, an adrenalinelike substance that raises the heart rate and constricts the blood vessels. Many cases of hypertension in this country can be laid at the door of hyperinsulinemia and insulin resistance.

In heart disease insulin also plays several key roles in causing the formation of hard plaque that blocks the arteries, obstructs blood flow through them, and leads to heart attack. Insulin increases the liver's production of LDL cholesterol, increases the thickness and rigidity of the artery walls, and favors the laying down of the cholesterol beneath the artery lining, where it can harden and create blockage.

The bad news is that all these disorders are related—if you suffer from one, another might be in your future. The good news is that by simply restructuring your diet to reduce excess insulin and restore the insulin sensors to their normal sensitivity, you can undo much of the damage. Blood pressure, blood cholesterol and triglycerides, and blood sugar respond very quickly to dietary correction. Thickening of the arteries and early plaque formation takes years of insulin control to correct; in the late stage, even with the best nutritional control, it's doubtful that you can dissolve a rock-hard obstructive plaque. Still, you'd be preventing further damage by using this program. But the beauty of this concept is in the awesome power of food to correct these disorders. If you simply give your body the proper nutritional tools, it will take them and heal itself.

Chapter 6

The Microhormone Messengers: Meet the Eicosanoids

You can view eicosanoids as the biological glue that holds together the human body. In that regard they are the most powerful agents known to man, yet they are totally controlled by the diet.

BARRY SEARS, PH.D., author of *The Zone*

You may never have heard of eicosanoids before, but understanding how they work in your body is as important to your health as understanding hyperinsulinemia.

Early in Goethe's *Faust* the devil appears to Dr. Faust, who inquires of him, "Who are you?" Mephistopheles replies, "Part of that force which would do evil evermore, and yet creates the good." This exchange could be applied to eicosanoids, a gang of at least 100 powerful hormonelike substances that control virtually all physiological actions in your body. The most important thing about eicosanoids is to keep them in balance. If you have too little of one, too much of another, eicosanoids can send your body hurtling down the slippery slope of biochemical evil toward arthritis, blood clots, and dozens of other dangerous conditions. In fact, they play a major role in *most* diseases, including heart disease and cancer. When they're balanced, the system hums along smoothly in perfect health. In fact, Dr. Barry Sears, a prominent researcher in the area of eicosanoids and diet, describes the maintenance of the dynamic balance between the various eicosanoids as the *definition* of optimal health. The most exciting thing about eicosanoids is that you can control these powerful agents simply by making the right food choices.

The bad news is that many things we *can't* exert much control over—aging, viral illnesses, and stress to name a few—drive our body's production of eicosanoids in the wrong direction, leading to arthritic aches and pains, blood clots, arterial constriction, heart disease, dry skin, and a host of other problems: in short, all the signs and symptoms of aging and stress. The good news is that our nutritional regimen reverses many of these changes, leading to dramatic health improvements difficult to correlate with a simple change in diet. As you progress on our program you should begin to notice many of these changes caused by the shift to more "good" eicosanoids: increased luster and body in your hair, increased skin moisture and suppleness, increased endurance, sounder sleep, to mention just a few. We began to notice these changes in our patients years ago and, in fact, were puzzled by them—before we fully understood the role diet plays in eicosanoid modulation.

Patients would start on the program and return for their follow-up visits reporting that rashes they'd had for ages had cleared up.

"Why did my rash go away?" they would ask.

"We don't really know, but we're glad it did," we would reply.

"How come my allergies are better?"

"Why don't my knees hurt as much anymore?"

"Why did my headaches go away?"

"Why did my nails stop splitting?"

"How come my asthma got better?"

"We don't know, we don't know, we don't know."

But after seeing these changes occur time and time again as patients reduced their insulin levels, we became confident enough to change the dialogue a little and make it more proactive.

"Well, Mrs. Smith, this little rash on your arms will more than likely disappear once you get going on your program and get your insulin down."

"Really? How come?"

"We don't really know; it's just a good side effect of the program."

Now that we understand eicosanoids and their effects, not only can we predict with a fair degree of confidence exactly what kinds of changes and improvements our patients are likely to experience; we can also tell them why. We draw them a simple diagram, point out the critical points along the eicosanoid synthesis pathway, tell them what specific foods to avoid, and explain why it's so important to get their insulin levels under control. As you progress through this chapter, you will learn about the power of diet to control eicosanoids, and you'll understand the good changes you'll begin to experience in your own body.

What Are Eicosanoids?

You're probably thinking, *If these eicosanoids are so potent, why have I never even heard of them?* Even your doctor may not be familiar with the term: this is cutting-edge research. But you've probably heard of at least one type, prostaglandins, first discovered in secretions of the prostate gland about sixty years ago. Prostaglandins, along with their cousins prostacyclins, thromboxanes, and leukotrienes, are known collectively as *eicosanoids* because they are all compounds composed of twenty carbon atoms (Greek *eikosi,* twenty). If you've ever taken an aspirin—or any other of a large number of drugs—you've done so specifically to interfere with the formation of prostaglandins and other eicosanoids. If you've ever had a headache, menstrual cramps, abdominal discomfort from ulcers, swelling or inflammation, or a rash, you have likely been the victim of too many of the wrong eicosanoids.

Although prostaglandins and the other eicosanoids act in many ways like hormones, there is one critical difference that explains why we've understood so little about them until recently. Hormones, which are produced in specific glands and travel through the blood, can readily be measured by blood tests. Eicosanoids, on the other hand, are produced inside the cells, act inside the cells, and vanish in fractions of seconds, much too quickly to be detected easily. Development of exceptionally sophisticated instrumentation has allowed scientists to identify more than 100 different eicosanoids—in fact, the 1982 Nobel Prize was awarded for research in eicosanoids.

What Do Eicosanoids Do?

Eicosanoids exert powerful physiological effects at extremely low concentrations. How powerful? Comparing the physiological effects of fiber (which has been touted widely for its many health benefits) to those of eicosanoids would be, to use a baseball analogy, about like comparing the home run power of, say, Woody Allen to that of Babe Ruth. Fiber isn't even in the same ballpark with eicosanoids. Fiber exerts a slight chemical and bulking effect in the colon, whereas eicosanoids control and direct the regulation of such diverse functions as blood pressure, blood clotting, the inflammatory response, the immune system, uterine contractions during birth, sexual potency in men, the pain and fever response, the sleep/wake cycle, the release of gastric acid (the potent new antiulcer drugs now under investigation are eicosanoid modulators), the constriction and dilation of airways in the lungs and blood vessels in the tissues, and many others. In short, eicosanoids exert major effects on just about everything that goes on in the body. As a result, numerous drugs work by increasing or decreasing the body's synthesis or response to eicosanoids. We mentioned aspirin earlier, so let's consider that as an illustration.

Doctors have recommended aspirin forever to relieve pain and reduce fever. More recently, however, they've begun prescribing it to reduce the risk of heart attack and, most recently, to reduce the risk of colon cancer. How can one inexpensive, simple drug do all this? Because aspirin is a potent inhibitor of eicosanoid synthesis. Certain eicosanoids are responsible for pain, fever, increased blood clotting and constriction of arteries, as well as increased cell growth and intestinal secretions, and by blocking the synthesis of these eicosanoids aspirin eliminates or reduces the problems they cause. The downside of aspirin, however, is that it doesn't block the production of *only* the offending eicosanoids; it blocks the production of many others as well. This generalized blockade results in the development of the unpleasant side effects we associate with aspirin: stomach pain, severe ulcer problems, and allergic reactions. Aspirin itself doesn't do any of these things; it simply causes the change in the eicosanoid balance that does the actual work—or damage.

Your Diet and the Eicosanoid Factory

Drugs are not the only modulators of eicosanoid production: food plays an even greater role. In fact of all the things you can do to alter your eicosanoid balance, regulating your insulin and glucagon levels with diet is the most potent. And with what you've already learned about insulin, it should come as no surprise that it is a major stimulant of the production of the wrong kinds of eicosanoids. Since the structure of the diet—particularly the carbohydrate content—determines the level of insulin, following our program allows you to regulate eicosanoid synthesis without using drugs. The fat content of the diet also plays a significant role in the production of eicosanoids. The essential fatty acids that are the building blocks of eicosanoids come from the diet—i.e., no essential fatty acids, no eicosanoids. An *essential fat* is one required to sustain life that can't be made by the body's own biochemistry and consequently must be obtained from the diet. Linoleic acid is the only truly essential fat; all the others can be made from other substances or made from linoleic acid.

Fortunately linoleic acid is commonly found in many foods, so unless you starve or go on a *totally* fat-free diet you are likely to get all the linoleic acid you need.

A plentiful dietary source of fatty acids in combination with the appropriate ratio of insulin and glucagon provides the optimal circumstances for the production of beneficial eicosanoids. Basically, with a few modifications that we'll deal with later in the chapter, you can think of this system as a factory where linoleic acid is the raw material, insulin and glucagon the processors, and eicosanoids the finished products. Each of our billions of cells houses these little factories turning out the various eicosanoids that regulate the function of these cells and, consequently, the tissues and organs these cells compose.

Heroes and Rogues: Two Kinds of Eicosanoids

Eicosanoid end products fall into two basic groups that have opposing functions:

"THE GOOD"	"THE BAD"
Series one eicosanoids:	Series two eicosanoids:
act as vasodilators	act as vasoconstrictors
act as immune enhancers	act as immune suppressors
decrease inflammation	increase inflammation
decrease pain	increase pain
increase oxygen flow	decrease oxygen flow
increase endurance	decrease endurance
prevent platelet aggregation	cause platelet aggregation
dilate airways	constrict airways
decrease cellular proliferation	increase cellular proliferation

It should be pretty obvious that we want more of the series one eicosanoids. It should also be apparent that eicosanoids play a major role in most diseases—either a disease-enhancing role or a disease-suppressing role. Take heart disease, for example: when you combine the blood vessel narrowing (vasoconstriction), the decreased oxygen flow, and the increased platelet aggregation (clot formation), caused by the series two eicosanoids, you have the setup for a heart attack. Most cardiac drugs work to offset these effects of the series two eicosanoids. Cancer offers another example: cancer occurs when cells lose their ability to regulate their own division and replication, and the cells begin to proliferate madly in an uncontrolled fashion. Series one eicosanoids suppress this rogue cell growth and are being investigated extensively for use as cancer chemotherapeutic agents; series two eicosanoids *promote* tumor growth. Victims of asthma and bronchitis who suffer tightness of the small airways in their lungs need more series one eicosanoids to reverse this airway constriction; series two eicosanoids make it worse.

Strange as it may seem, you wouldn't want to have all good and no bad; you do, however, want to have more good than bad. The bad serve a useful purpose—blood clotting when we get cut, for instance—you just don't want to be overwhelmed with them. Your goal is to do whatever you have to do to make more good than bad eicosanoids so that the balance is shifted toward the good side most of the time. Of all the means available to accomplish this goal, we can say without hesitation that following our nutritional program is the most potent. It provides the necessary essential-fat building blocks to make plenty of eicosanoids while at the same time keeping insulin and glucagon—the most powerful forces in eicosanoid synthesis—in the appropriate range to maximize the output of good eicosanoids.

Controlling the Eicosanoid Production Line

Now for some serious science: you don't have to internalize this technical information to make eicosanoids work for you, but if you're curious, here's how it all works. If it's more science than you're looking for right now, jump ahead to the next section, where there's vital information about fatty acids.

There are three points along the eicosanoid synthesis pathway where we can exert dietary influence over the eicosanoid end products. The first control point is at the start of the process, where linoleic acid, the raw material for eicosanoid synthesis, enters the system. The second is by altering the synthesis process itself in a way that results in the production of predominantly good eicosanoids. The third is by restricting the dietary intake of arachidonic acid, a precursor of many of the bad eicosanoids. Figure 6.1, a schematic representation of the eicosanoid synthesis pathway, shows how our program affects these control points.

The first step in eicosanoid synthesis is getting the raw material—linoleic acid—into the production line. Linoleic acid is a ubiquitous fat found in practically all foods, so you should have plenty available unless you've been on a slash-and-burn, extreme-low-fat diet for a long time. The problem then is not the amount of available linoleic acid but getting it into the system. The key to getting sufficient linoleic acid into the pathway is the critical gatekeeper enzyme—*delta 6 desaturase.* If this enzyme is active and working properly, linoleic acid flows continuously into the system, providing the material for all the eicosanoids your body needs to make. Inhibiting the action of this enzyme denies entry to adequate amounts of linoleic acid, and deficient eicosanoid production results. The first step in modulating your eicosanoid balance is to ensure that you have plenty to work with, which you can do by keeping this gatekeeper enzyme happy and working efficiently. You can do this by catering to its wants while avoiding, as much as possible, those things that slow it down. The following chart lists the major factors affecting this enzyme.

FACTORS THAT INFLUENCE GATEKEEPER ENZYME ACTIVITY

SPEEDS UP GATEKEEPER	SLOWS DOWN GATEKEEPER
Dietary protein	Aging
	Stress
	Disease
	Trans fatty acids
	Alpha Linolenic Acid
	High-carbohydrate diet

A quick glance should alert you that the deck is not exactly stacked in your favor in terms of getting sufficient linoleic acid into the pathway. On the positive side the nutritional regimen we recommend will provide you with plenty of protein, so by following it you're doing all you can to activate the enzyme pumping linoleic acid into the system. The next step is to eliminate those things that slow down the gatekeeper enzyme's activity.

It's pretty obvious that you can't really do anything about aging. You can try to control your stress levels by meditating and using other relaxation techniques, removing yourself from stressful situations, and just kicking back and relaxing, but as a practical matter stress is something most of us must endure as part of the fast-paced American way of life. You can do everything possible to stay disease free, but you're still going to be laid low by the occasional cold or flu and sometimes by even more serious afflictions. Since these three factors—aging, stress, and disease—are pretty much beyond your control, you're left with the remaining three factors, all dietary and over which you do have control, to effect the synthesis of eicosanoids.

FIGURE 6.1

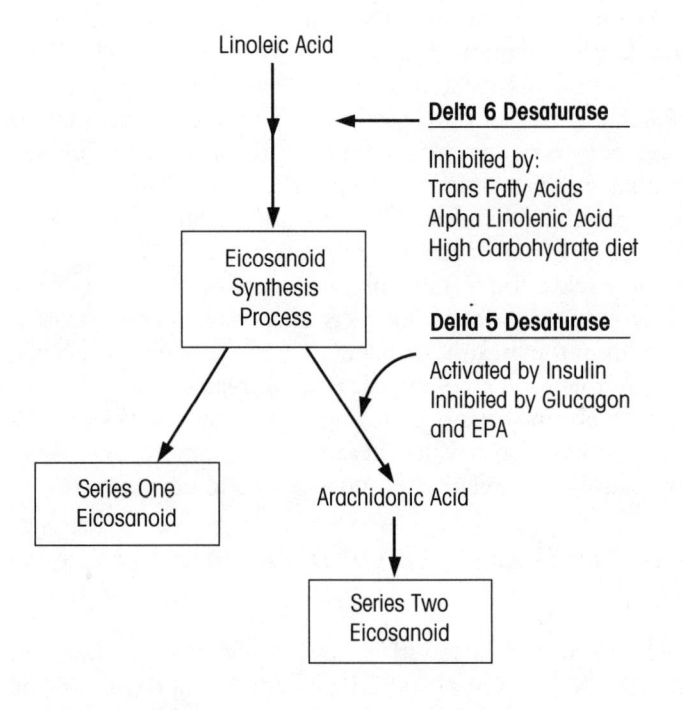

ACCENTUATE THE POSITIVE; ELIMINATE THE NEGATIVE

Trans fatty acids: Butter vs. Margarine

Trans fatty acids are made when polyunsaturated fats are partially hydrogenated. Polyunsaturated fats have multiple double-carbon bonds in their structure. The instability of these bonds makes polyunsaturated fats more liquid, whereas fats that contain single carbon bonds "saturated" with hydrogen atoms are more solid. The fat that you find around the edge of a steak, for instance, is solid at room temperature and is predominantly a saturated fat; butter, also a saturated fat, is solid at room temperature. Corn oil, a polyunsaturated fat of vegetable origin, is liquid at room temperature. To make corn oil solid so that with the addition of artificial flavoring it can be used as margarine, it must be partially hydrogenated, an operation that forces hydrogen into the oil molecules under high temperature and pressure and in effect artificially saturates it. That's why it remains solid on the dinner table. If that's all that happened, there wouldn't be much of a problem, but unfortunately artificially hydrogenating the fat permanently alters the structure of the double-carbon bonds to an unnatural configuration (called the *trans configuration* in chemical parlance). In the process, what was once a good-quality polyunsaturated oil is converted to a hybrid called a *trans fatty acid*. The virtue of trans fatty acids from a food manufacturing and processing perspective is their stability and longer shelf life along with the fact that the fat molecules thus changed pack together better to make a more solid substance. (*Partially hydrogenated* is the villain here; fats labeled *hydrogenated* are not a problem.)

Trans fatty acids, found not only in margarine but in any of the thousands of commercial food products that have been partially hydrogenated, cause the health damage they do because they inhibit the formation of the good eicosanoids. For this reason margarine—that very substance Americans have been eating to save themselves from heart disease—can *increase* the risk for heart disease, cancer, and all the other problems caused by a relative abundance of bad eicosanoids.

Alpha Linolenic Acid (ALA): All Oils Are Not Created Equal

This omega-3 fatty acid found in the oils of various plants also slows down the gatekeeper. Canola oil (10 percent ALA), flaxseed or linseed oil (57 percent ALA), black currant oil (14 percent ALA), and soybean oil (7 percent ALA) are its primary sources. To avoid undermining your body's production of good eicosanoids, you need to minimize your consumption of the oils containing ALA, and that means limiting your intake of canola oil and soybean oil. Over the past few years there has been a boom in canola oil consumption because of reports that monounsaturated fats decrease the risk of heart disease. Indeed canola oil contains 60 percent monounsaturated fat, which is good, but it also contains 10 percent ALA, which is not so good. We have switched to olive oil; it has more flavor, contains more (82 percent) monounsaturated fat, and has no ALA. If you don't like the flavor of olive oil, try light olive oil. For recipes that won't work with the distinctive olive flavor, use sesame oil (the light one, not the dark toasted Asian sesame oil); it contains 46 percent monounsaturated fat, no ALA, and has a much more delicate taste. If you just can't bring yourself to abandon canola oil, you can offset the negative effects of the ALA by scrupulously avoiding trans fatty acids and carbohydrate excess and by keeping your protein intake up. In fact, of all the things you can do to enhance the production of good eicosanoids, eliminating canola oil is probably the least important.

Not so, however, with flaxseed oil, another oil many people consume for its supposed health benefits. Promoters of flaxseed oil—a reputed panacea for a variety of disorders—tout as one of its virtues its ability to help relieve the pain and inflammation of arthritis. You will recall that a bit earlier we discussed how aspirin, the archetypal drug for arthritis relief, works through an indiscriminate blocking of eicosanoid production, both good and bad, and that the shift away from so many bad ones eases the pain, but at the expense of potentially unpleasant side effects. By virtue of its high ALA content, flaxseed oil is a sort of biological version of aspirin: it blocks the synthesis of all eicosanoids, giving some relief to arthritis victims in the short run. You may be thinking at this point, *So what? If it gives relief, isn't flaxseed oil okay, at least for arthritis sufferers?* It would be if it were the only means available to afford relief, but it's like using a nine-pound hammer to kill a fly: it kills the fly, but it does a lot of other damage, too. With the techniques you learn in this chapter you'll be able to fine-tune your eicosanoid pathway to reduce inflammation, enhance immune function, and all the rest without having to resort to the blunt-instrument approach of flaxseed oil and other health food store remedies we've yet to deal with.

Another oil containing some ALA—soybean oil—is hard to avoid entirely since it's incorporated into most processed foods. Fortunately, it has a low percentage of ALA, so a little of it won't slow down your eicosanoid factory much. Just make sure that it isn't partially hydrogenated soybean oil, or you'll have trans fatty acids compounding the problem.

The following chart lists most commonly used oils and their composition. In general, select oils for cooking that contain a high percentage of monounsaturated fatty acids and little or no ALA.

FATTY ACID PERCENTAGES OF COMMONLY USED OILS

OIL	SATURATED	MONOUNSATURATED	LA	ALA
Almond	9	65	26	0
Canola	6	60	24	10
Corn	13	27	57	2
Flaxseed	9	16	18	57
Hazelnut	7	76	16	0
Olive	10	82	8	0
Peanut	18	49	29	0
Safflower	8	13	79	0
Sesame (light, not Asian)	13	46	41	0
Sunflower	12	19	69	0
Walnut	16	28	51	7

High-Carbohydrate, Low-Protein Diets: Trouble at the Gate

According to several studies, high-carbohydrate, low-protein diets inhibit the activity of the gatekeeper enzyme, leading to deficient eicosanoid production. High-carbohydrate diets compound the problem because they also stimulate the release of excess insulin, an even more serious problem for good eicosanoid synthesis, which we'll discuss in due course.

To ensure that you get the linoleic acid into the production pathway needed to synthesize all the eicosanoids necessary for optimal health, you must consume a diet of at least 30 percent protein, while avoiding trans fatty acids, ALA, and high-carbohydrate intake. But that's not the whole equation; it's only the first part. If you follow these steps, you will have all the raw material in the system that you need to make plenty of eicosanoids; the next step is to make certain these raw materials are converted to the *right* eicosanoids.

CONTROLLING INSULIN AND GLUCAGON

The most critical step in the entire eicosanoid synthesis process is the next one, the one over which we have the most nutritional control—directing the flow in either the good or bad direction. The direction of the flow is under the control of a second critical enzyme called, confusingly enough, *delta 5 desaturase*. This enzyme, when activated, shifts the synthesis process away from the good and toward the production of primarily bad eicosanoids; conversely, inhibiting this enzyme increases the production of good eicosanoids. As with all enzymes, this one has its own particular set of activators and inhibitors. And guess what? Insulin is a major activator. That's right, elevated levels of insulin send the production of bad eicosanoids soaring. What inhibits this enzyme? Glucagon, of course, which always works in opposition to insulin. In fact, short of drug therapy, of all the things that can modulate your eicosanoid balance insulin and glucagon are the most potent. Control them and you control your eicosanoids.

If we look at this from a dietary perspective, we can begin to make even more sense out of the current state of ill health gripping our society. The low-protein, high-carbohydrate diets most people try to follow first compromise the entry of adequate linoleic acid into their eicosanoid factories and then by increasing insulin and decreasing glucagon actually drive whatever gets in toward the production of the bad eicosanoids, causing aches, pains, vasoconstriction, platelet aggregation, and all the rest. The nutritional plan described in this book, however, does just the opposite. The increased protein content stimulates the entry of adequate raw material into the pathway, while the lowered insulin levels and the increased glucagon levels drive the production in the good direction, reversing the problems caused by an overabundance of bad eicosanoids. Knowing what you know so far, it's easy to understand the unexpected benefits our patients experienced when they began our program.

The Fish Oil Rescue

Eicosapentaenoic acid (EPA) is another substance that works like glucagon to divert the production of eicosanoids in the good direction; it just doesn't work nearly as well. EPA, an omega-3 fatty acid found in the oil of such cold-water fish as mackerel, herring, and salmon, adds another measure of dietary control over the eicosanoid balance. It also provides another example of how eicosanoids—and science—work in real life.

You have no doubt read that fish oil helps prevent heart disease. Somewhere along the way researchers stumbled onto this phenomenon—which we now know is eicosanoid related—and decided to study it. They gave subjects varying amounts of fish oil for varying lengths of time and checked them for platelet aggregation, vasoconstriction, all the other components of heart disease, and the development of heart disease itself. The results were frustratingly inconclusive: sometimes, in some subjects, fish oil worked like a charm; in others it showed no benefit. For anything to be scientifically valid it must be reproducible in the majority of cases; the case of fish oil was a hit-or-miss proposition at best. What happened?

Now that we know the role the EPA found in fish oil plays in eicosanoid modulation, we can see the problem these researchers were up against. Heart disease is a complicated, multifactorial problem, but for purposes of illustration let's confine our discussion to just a couple of the underlying actions contributing to the disorder. Platelets aggregate around a tiny injury on the lining of the coronary artery and form a clot. The artery may then constrict, further reducing the blood flow to the heart tissue beyond. As we have seen, both these actions are a consequence of bad eicosanoids, so if we can deliver an overwhelming force of good eicosanoids to the area, we should be able to reverse these changes, or so thought the researchers using fish oil rich in EPA for the purpose. But let's say that one group of subjects was following the standard low-fat, high-carbohydrate diet (which you now know means low protein as well). These people would be running their eicosanoid factories in the wrong direction because of their elevated insulin and lowered glucagon levels. Since EPA isn't nearly as potent as glucagon in driving the eicosanoid flow in the good direction, just about all the fish oil in the world would have trouble overcoming the forces driving eicosanoid production in the wrong direction. You would not expect these subjects to have a positive result. People who ate more protein or who had no insulin problems would likely show different results. These subjects would have a smaller insulin response to the diet and consequently would be making both good and bad eicosanoids in a fairly balanced fashion. The addition of fish oil to the diets of these subjects would then be enough to drive their eicosanoid production predominantly in the good direction, manifested in decreased platelet aggregation, diminished vasoconstriction, and all the rest—in short, positive results showing the benefit of fish oil as a therapeutic agent.

So, you have two groups of patients showing different results with the same amount of EPA. The reason: the metabolic hormonal effects of the difference in their underlying diets. This factor confounds many studies that are otherwise vigorously controlled. You can't get meaningful results unless you make sure to control for the extremely powerful druglike effects of food on insulin and glucagon—a step most researchers forget or don't understand.

Because of the relative weakness of fish oil as an agent to drive eicosanoid synthesis, we like to use it mainly as a fine-tuner. If our patients aren't getting the full benefit of the positive eicosanoids driven by the dietary reduction of insulin, we sometimes add fish oil to the regimen. We also use fish oil to counter the effects of dietary arachidonic acid, the third and final variable in the eicosanoid equation.

ARACHIDONIC ACID: NATURE THROWS US A CURVE

Arachidonic acid is one of those curves nature loves to throw at us just to keep us from being able to wrap everything up nicely and simply. Arachidonic acid (AA) is a fatty acid essential to life but also incredibly destructive in excessive amounts. Lab animals injected with large amounts of all other fatty acids go on about their business with no apparent ill effects—those injected with arachidonic acid are dead within moments. AA is made in the eicosanoid synthesis pathway and is the immediate precursor of the bad eicosanoids. If you keep your insulin down and your glucagon up, you should make very little arachidonic acid, but—and here's the curve—arachidonic acid doesn't come from just the eicosanoid pathway; it also comes in directly via the diet. Unfortunately, the dietary variety can also transform into bad eicosanoids. So, you may be asking, *I can do everything right, watch my carbohydrate intake, keep my insulin down, and still be sabotaged by dietary AA?* Yes,

Are You Sensitive to Arachidonic Acid?

The main symptoms associated with too much AA (or sensitivity to it) are:

- chronic fatigue
- poor or restless sleep
- difficulty awakening or grogginess upon awakening
- brittle hair
- thin, brittle nails
- constipation
- dry, flaking skin
- minor rashes

but *only* if you're particularly sensitive to arachidonic acid and eat a large amount of it.

AA is found in all meats, especially red meats and organ meats, and in egg yolks. It probably hasn't escaped your notice that these foods are the same ones that most people identify as being loaded with fat and cholesterol. Despite popular opinion, though, it's not the saturated fat and cholesterol that cause most of the problems associated with these foods: it's their arachidonic acid content—for those who are sensitive to it.

The AA in meat is located both in the muscle tissue and in the fat. The quantities are higher in red meat because red meat has more fat, which, at least in today's domestic feedlot animals, contains high levels of AA. Animals have the same eicosanoid synthesis cascade that we do, and when they are grain-fed and fattened, the high-carbohydrate grain stimulates their insulin just as it does ours. Fats are stored in fatty tissue in the same ratio that they occur in the blood, so cattle—and people—having large quantities of circulating AA will store large quantities as well. The good news is that range-fed cattle and wild game have much less fat to begin with, and what fat they have contains little AA. You can add wild game to your diet by following in the footsteps of your ancestors and bagging it in the field or by purchasing it from one of the purveyors listed in the appendix. But the easiest first step in avoiding dietary AA is to avoid as much visible fat as possible on your meat, especially red meat.

Does this mean you should avoid beef entirely if you're sensitive to arachidonic acid? (See page 85 to find out if you are.) Not at all. Here are a couple of techniques that will decrease the amount of AA you get in the beef you eat. First, after you trim as much of the visible fat as you can, *grill* your steaks. This method of cooking reduces the amount of AA in beef by about 35 percent. You can also follow our favorite way to marinate a steak that is not only healthful but actually makes the beef taste better—we've provided that method in the box below. Most alterations you make in foods for health reasons really take a toll on taste, but not this technique for steak. The only drawback is that it takes a little advance preparation, so it doesn't work for spur-of-the-moment meals.

A Trick for Reducing Arachidonic Acid in Steaks and Roasts

Trim all the visible fat from the steak, then place it in a large resealable plastic bag along with a mixture of 1 cup of red wine and 1 cup of olive oil or light sesame oil (or any other oil you like as long as it contains no ALA). Allow the meat to marinate in this mixture in the refrigerator for a full 24 hours, flipping the bag and contents over a couple of times. Take the steak out, drain it for an hour or so, discard the marinade, rub the beef with some pepper or other spices to your taste, then grill it. You won't believe the taste. The wine acts as a solvent to leach out a fair amount of the saturated fat in the steak, which is replaced in part by the monounsaturated fat in the olive oil or other oil you use. These oils permeate the steak, giving it a juicy, succulent taste that you have to experience to believe—and make it more healthful to boot. You can use this technique with roasts as well. You won't get quite the same arachidonic acid decrease you will with the steak because you will be roasting the meat instead of grilling. Roasts taste even better if you make cuts all over the meat and insert slivers of garlic.

No advance work is necessary to decrease your arachidonic acid consumption from egg yolks. Make omelets using one or two whole eggs and the remainder egg whites. Or use one egg and add ricotta or tofu to scramble it. Try to remove yolks from egg recipes as much as you can because the yolks are very high in arachidonic acid. If you must eat a lot of eggs and you're AA sensitive, add some fish oil to your diet.

What about sautéing and frying? You now know how the trans fatty acids in margarine prevent the building blocks from getting into the eicosanoid production pipeline, so we want you to avoid margarine. Many polyunsaturated fats undergo a trans alteration during the high temperatures required for panfrying, so your health will also be best served by avoiding those. We need heat-stable fat that also imparts great taste, and the substance that fits the bill is butter.

I Can't Believe You Said Butter

That's right, the much-maligned butter is much better for you than almost anything else under these circumstances, because it is a naturally saturated fat—no trans fats to gum up your eicosanoid factory. But it can

Clarified Butter

Clarified butter, a mainstay in the culinary repertoire of great chefs everywhere, is also called *ghee* in some recipes. You can purchase ghee already prepared in Indian markets. To make your own:

1. Place a pound of unsalted butter, cut into large pieces, in a saucepan over medium heat.

2. As the butter melts and begins to bubble, reduce the heat to a level at which small bubbles continue to surface. These bubbles bring the yellow-white milk solids to the top, where you can skim them off and discard them.

3. After 10 to 15 minutes of bubbling and skimming, you will have taken most of the milk solids off the top or they will have congealed on the bottom.

4. At this point, strain the hot melted butter through cheesecloth. *Voilà!* You have clarified butter.

5. Pour the clarified butter into an airtight container and store it in the refrigerator for up to 6 weeks.

6. Whenever you need to panfry or sauté, put a few teaspoons of it into your skillet. You can also mix clarified butter with a little olive oil, light sesame oil, or other fairly heat-stable oil and have an unmatched taste sensation.

be made even more useful by clarifying it (so it won't burn) using the method described on page 87.

Remember that all of these precautions are necessary only if you have a problem with arachidonic acid. If you follow an insulin-lowering diet—the most important change you can make as far as modulating your eicosanoids is concerned—and you solve all your health problems to your satisfaction, eat all the red meat and eggs you want. If you do everything else right, keep your insulin levels low, and still have a problem (with hypertension, for instance), maybe you're exceptionally sensitive to dietary arachidonic acid. You might want to try reducing your intake and see what happens (see page 86).

The Case of Mr. G

Mr. Gorden is forty-seven years old and extremely sensitive to dietary arachidonic acid. He came to see us initially for weight loss—he weighed over 350 pounds. On examination we found him to have high blood pressure, 180/115, and high cholesterol, over 300 mg/dl. We started him on an insulin-lowering weight-loss diet. When he returned in a week for follow-up, he had lost nine pounds, but his blood pressure was down only slightly. A few weeks later he had lost more than fifty pounds, and his cholesterol was much improved, but his blood pressure, though somewhat improved, was still elevated. His diet diaries showed that he ate several eggs and at least one serving of red meat every day. We instructed him to substitute fish and chicken for his steak, gave him the recipe for beef preparation described in the box on page 86, and recommended that he make his scrambled eggs using only one yolk. He did, and within two weeks his blood pressure was normal. He had been making enormous quantities of vasoconstricting eicosanoids from dietary AA, causing his elevated blood pressure.

Fine-Tuning Your Eicosanoids

You can fine-tune by paying attention to how you feel and what kind of symptoms you are experiencing. Do any of the symptoms listed in the box on arachidonic acid apply to you?

If you've been on the plan for a while and you are still experiencing any of these symptoms, you probably need to reduce your AA consumption and/or increase your intake of EPA. Remember, EPA works in the same way as glucagon to drive eicosanoid production in the good direction, so if you're following your insulin-lowering, glucagon-enhancing diet and not getting quite the results you expect, you can boost glucagon's efforts with EPA. To increase your consumption of EPA you can eat mackerel, salmon, herring, or other cold-water ocean fish several times a week, or you can take fish oil capsules.[1] The standard dose of EPA in the typical fish oil capsule is 180 milligrams—not a lot. To get enough EPA to achieve results, you will need to take at least four to six capsules a day, more if you've strayed from your diet and don't have glucagon working for you at full capacity. Fish oil capsules may be purchased from most drugstores and all health food stores.

One easy way to monitor how you're doing is to notice your bowel movement frequency and composition. Good eicosanoids tend to increase the flow of water into the colon, whereas bad eicosanoids made from AA tend to reduce water flow into the colon. The more water in the colon, the looser the stools. If you're constipated, you probably need a little more EPA; if you develop diarrhea, you need less EPA. Another bowel sign that reveals your eicosanoid balance is whether your stools float or sink. Increased water flowing into the colon produces stools that are less dense and tend to float.

As you begin to get your eicosanoids in balance by controlling your insulin and by increasing your intake of essential fats, you should notice increased luster and body in your hair, your skin should become more moist and supple, your endurance should improve, and you will probably sleep much better. We've noticed many of these changes in our patients as they have begun following our program, even before taking any extra essential fats at all.

---

[1] When you purchase fish oil capsules, make sure they are labeled *cholesterol free*. Fish tend to concentrate many pollutants, including heavy metals and PCBs, in their fat, and this fat is where fish oil comes from. The refining process that removes all these pollutants also removes the cholesterol, so if the label says *cholesterol free*, you can be sure that the oil you are buying is pollutant free.

The Bottom Line

Your body works as a balance of opposing forces. At the most basic level control of these forces—whether your blood vessels dilate or constrict, you have pain and inflammation in a joint or none, you breathe freely or wheeze, you sleep well or poorly, you suffer allergies or don't react, to name a few—occurs through cell-to-cell messenger microhormones called *eicosanoids*. Your body manufactures two families of these messengers—those beneficial to your health and those detrimental to it—by making alterations to one essential dietary fat. Whether the fat becomes a "good" messenger or a "bad" one depends primarily on your diet.

Your first task is to eat a diet that provides you with plenty of linoleic acid—the essential fat from which all the eicosanoid messengers are made. The best dietary sources for ensuring you always get plenty of this raw material to build eicosanoids are naturally pressed oils. We recommend olive oil, but other good oils are almond, hazelnut, safflower, light sesame, sunflower, and walnut. Oils that have been altered by the manufacturer to make them more stable for sale (cheap cooking oils are heated to keep the polyunsaturated fats in them from spoiling, and this damages the oil irrevocably) or to change them from their natural form to something else (liquid vegetable oil is artificially saturated by manufacturers to make it become margarine or shortening, again damaging the oil) contain trans fats that interfere with normal eicosanoid production.

The next step in production is getting that raw material onto the assembly line, and a number of factors beyond your control influence this step: aging, stress, and disease (but also trans fats and a high-carbohydrate diet) all slow down entry of the linoleic acid into the eicosanoid production pathway. Dietary protein enhances entry of linoleic acid to the pathway. Following the guidelines of our program, you will be eating the proper balance of protein, carbohydrate, and fat to ensure that the raw material gets into the system.

Once it does, whether it becomes primarily a "good" messenger or a "bad" one depends again on diet. Excess insulin from a high-carbohydrate diet favors the formation of "bad" eicosanoids; so does the dietary fatty acid arachidonic acid (AA), found in red meat and egg yolk, which the body turns directly into the "bad" eico-sanoids. Although you don't have to avoid these AA-containing foods unless you seem to be especially sensitive to AA (see page 85 for more information), you can reduce your consumption of this fatty acid by using a few tricks of food preparation we describe for you on pages 86 and 87.

Fish oil (omega-3 fatty acid) helps to offset the detrimental effects of AA by slowing down the production of bad eicosanoids coming off the assembly line. You can use fish oil capsules to supplement your intake of dietary fish oil found in cold-water ocean fish: mackerel, herring, salmon, tuna.

Eating a diet like the one we recommend maximizes your production of "good" messengers and favors a balance of eicosanoids to optimize your health.

The important points to remember are:

1. The most potent means to restore your eicosanoid balance and keep it there is to follow an insulin-lowering diet such as ours.

2. Next in importance is to avoid as much as you can partially hydrogenated fats and ALA to ensure adequate supplies of eicosanoid building blocks getting into the production line. Use olive oil instead.

3. Keep an eye on your dietary arachidonic acid, especially if some of your health problems such as hypertension don't completely disappear with steps 1 and 2.

4. Fine-tune your essential fat status by adding EPA (fish oil) as described.

Although the control points in the eicosanoid synthesis pathway are the critical ones that we can modulate with diet, the whole system requires certain vitamins and trace elements for optimal performance. Essential fats are absolute magnets for free radical attack. Unless you've been lost at sea for the past year or so, you know that free radicals cause all kinds of damage and that antioxidants fight them off. Vitamins, minerals, and trace elements are vital to this process. Once you understand how they work and put them into play as part of your overall insulin-lowering, good-eicosanoid-enhancing program, you will truly have the ultimate dietary strategy for perfect health.

Chapter 7

Cholesterol Madness

Thus we should beware of clinging to vulgar opinions, and judge things by reason's way, not by popular say.

MONTAIGNE (1533–1592)

If the sixteenth-century French essayist Montaigne were alive today, he might write about the various groups who are whipping the world into an anticholesterol frenzy in much the same way he did about certain philosophers of his time: "[they] have created in their feeble imaginations this absurd, gloomy, querulous, grim, threatening, and scowling image, and placed it on a rock apart, among brambles, as a bogey to terrify people." Cholesterol is indeed a bogey and one that terrifies people beyond reason. We are obsessed with it. Obsessed to the point that, like the Eskimos who have in their language twenty-seven different words for *snow,* we have come up with almost as many to describe cholesterol. We have HDL cholesterol (which can be further subdivided into HDL_2 and HDL_3 cholesterol), LDL cholesterol, VLDL cholesterol, IDL cholesterol, and a whole slew of others if you start differentiating by apoprotein type (apoproteins are protein structures found on the surface of the various cholesterol complexes).

Although the average American is not likely to be conversant with this arcane language of cholesterol research, he's certainly alert to the specter of high cholesterol and all its sinister ramifications. In fact most people recall the results of their last cholesterol test faster and with greater accuracy than their hat size. Cholesterol levels have become the ultimate measure of health and fitness—to be bragged about if low and confessed to if elevated.

And, of course, cholesterol has become big business. Whenever mass paranoia starts to brew, a legion rises up ready to exploit it. The food processing industry and its advertisers now emblazon the containers of edibles as diverse as soft drinks and cornflakes with the superfluous statement "contains no cholesterol." Cholesterol angst is not lost on the various governmental and private research funding bodies responsible for underwriting all kinds of medical research. These groups disburse hundreds of millions of dollars to eager research labs throughout the world, allowing them to pursue the secrets of cholesterol in ever-more-intricate studies. As a measure of this scientific interest, more than a dozen Nobel Prizes have been awarded for cholesterol's study.

Why all this fuss? What exactly is cholesterol? Should you be concerned about it? Where does it come from? How do you get rid of it, or how, at the very least, do you control it? You're about to learn everything you need to know to make an accurate assessment of your own health as it relates to cholesterol, and you'll learn how you can dramatically lower your cholesterol level—if it's elevated—without using drugs and without going on a bare-subsistence, low-fat diet. In fact, if you are a careful reader, by the time you finish this chapter you will know more about cholesterol than 95 percent of the physicians in practice today. You won't learn all the esoteric terms for all the minute components of the various cholesterol complexes, but you will gain an understanding of the actual workings of the cholesterol regulation system that will put you way ahead of most doctors.

It is absolutely essential that you understand this information, and we urge you to read this chapter carefully, but we understand that the material is complex and somewhat detailed. Jump ahead to The Bottom Line at the end of the chapter to get the gist of things first, then come back and digest this crucial information at a more leisurely pace. It is in some ways the most important chapter in the book, not because we believe cholesterol is such an important problem but because everyone else does. Virtually all the criticism you will hear from people about this nutritional plan will arise from their mistaken perceptions about cholesterol. In order to be able to properly respond to that criticism, you need to have a firm grasp of cholesterol metabolism and understand why the plan works. (Here comes the nitty-gritty science, so now's the time to skip ahead if you're so inclined.) Let's begin by taking a look at the cholesterol molecule and the little glitch in the body's cholesterol regulatory system that causes all the problems.

Cholesterol: Essential for Life

Despite the mounting fervor against it, the average American doesn't know exactly what cholesterol is but is quite certain that it's dangerous.

The consensus on cholesterol seems to be *the lower, the better,* but as we shall see, this is not always the case. Far from being a health destroyer, cholesterol is absolutely essential for life.

Although most people think of it as being a "fat in the blood," only 7 percent of the body's cholesterol is found there. In fact, cholesterol isn't really a fat at all; it's a pearly-colored, waxy, solid alcohol that is soapy to the touch. The bulk of the cholesterol in your body, the other 93 percent, is located in every cell of the body, where its unique waxy, soapy consistency provides the cell membranes with their structural integrity and regulates the flow of nutrients into and waste products out of the cells. In addition, among its other diverse and essential functions are these:

Cholesterol is the building block from which your body makes several important hormones: the adrenal hormones (aldosterone, which helps regulate blood pressure, and hydrocortisone, the body's natural steroid) and the sex hormones (estrogen and testosterone). If you don't have enough cholesterol, you won't make enough sex hormones.

Cholesterol is the main component of bile acids, which aid in the digestion of foods, particularly fatty foods. Without cholesterol we couldn't absorb the essential fat-soluble vitamins A, D, E, and K from the food we eat.

Cholesterol is necessary for normal growth and development of the brain and the nervous system. Cholesterol coats the nerves and makes the transmission of nerve impulses possible.

Cholesterol gives skin its ability to shed water.

Cholesterol is a precursor of vitamin D in the skin. When exposed to sunlight, this precursor molecule is converted to its active form for use in the body.

Cholesterol is important for normal growth and repair of tissues since every cell membrane and the organelles (the tiny structures inside the cells that carry out specific functions) within the cells are rich in cholesterol. For this reason newborn animals feed on milk or other cholesterol-rich foods, such as the yolks of eggs, which are there to provide food for the developing bird or chick embryos.

Cholesterol plays a major role in the transportation of triglycerides— blood fats—throughout the circulatory system.

A quick review of this list should give you a better idea of what cholesterol does and dispel any notion that it's a destroyer of health to be feared and avoided at all costs. Far from being a serial killer, cholesterol is absolutely essential for good health; without it you'd die. Without cholesterol we would lose the strength and stability of our cells, rendering them much less resistant to invasion by infection and malignancy. In fact, a grave sign of serious illness, such as cancer development or crippling arthritis, is a *falling* cholesterol level.

Where does cholesterol come from? Although some cholesterol indeed does come from food, the vast majority (80 percent) is produced by the body itself. In fact, every cell in the body is capable of making its own cholesterol. Most don't, however, and rely instead on that made in the liver, intestines, and skin, with the liver responsible for the lion's share of the production. Due to the body's need for large amounts of cholesterol, a feedback loop exists so that whenever dietary intake decreases the liver's synthesis increases. And, in opposite fashion, when the diet is rich in cholesterol, the liver synthesizes less. This self-regulation helps explain the baffling research finding that blood cholesterol levels vary only minimally in the face of enormous variations in dietary intake. As a matter of fact most people, contrary to what you read and hear daily, can consume almost unlimited amounts of cholesterol without significantly increasing their blood cholesterol levels. That being the case, people having excessive blood cholesterol levels—and many do—must have a problem with the ability of their bodies to regulate cholesterol levels internally. That is precisely the case. *The key to lowering elevated cholesterol levels is not in the restriction of dietary cholesterol or fat but in the dietary manipulation of the internal cholesterol regulatory system.* Unfortunately, there's a glitch in the works that causes all the problems.

The Fly in the Ointment

Nature endowed—or inflicted—us with a minor design flaw that creates most of the problems we have with excessive cholesterol: *cholesterol levels are regulated only inside the cell.* Why is this a design flaw? Because problems arise due to excess cholesterol in the blood, yet the cholesterol level in the blood isn't regulated—there is no feedback loop to signal the need for the body to lower cholesterol levels in the blood when they get too high.

The cells of the body require a steady supply of cholesterol to build and repair cell membranes and to carry out all the other tasks required of them to make life possible. Where does the cholesterol for all this construction come from? Basically two sources: the cell either extracts cholesterol from the blood or makes its own or both. The important thing is that the interior of the cell needs plenty of cholesterol, so the interior is where the cholesterol sensors are located. Falling cholesterol levels within the cell trigger these sensors to fire off messages to the production machinery within the cell to increase the supply—make it or get more from the blood. By these means the level of cholesterol inside the cell is maintained tightly within a narrow optimal range. The point to remember is that the sensors that dictate cellular need for cholesterol are *inside* the cells (primarily of the liver), not out in the bloodstream.

When cholesterol causes its artery-clogging mischief, where does that occur? In the walls of the arteries supplying the heart and the major arteries supplying the body and brain, *not* in the cells with cholesterol sensors. This system glitch is analogous to having a big powerful air conditioner in a house and putting the thermostat that controls it into a small, hot, airtight closet. The cooling machinery could be cranking out enough cold air to form icicles on the woodwork throughout the house, but the thermostat in the closet would never know. As far as it knows, the air is hot and needs cooling, so it calls for more cold air, and in spite of the icicles forming on it, the air conditioner keeps huffing and struggling along to pump cold air out.

The cholesterol plaques choking the interiors of the arteries are like the icicles in the house. Deposits of cholesterol fill the arteries, but the sensors inside the cholesterol-producing cells never know it because they, like the thermostat in the closet, are concerned only with cholesterol levels within the cell, not what's going on outside in the arteries. What are these feedback controls, these cholesterol sensors that often work against us? And what can we do to escape or confound this apparent design glitch? There is a way.

HOW CHOLESTEROL GETS AROUND: INTRODUCING THE LIPOPROTEINS

A few years ago patients came into our office wanting to know their cholesterol levels; now that's not enough. Now most patients want to know their *total* cholesterol levels along with their LDL and HDL levels and the various ratios of all the above. At this stage of the cholesterol awareness game, most people know that LDL is the "bad" cholesterol and HDL is the "good" cholesterol but don't have an inkling of what HDL and LDL actually are. Although it's possible to live a long and prosperous life without ever knowing what LDL and HDL are, it's important to be familiar enough with them to see how they, along with cholesterol in general, fit into the insulin, glucagon, and insulin control equation—especially if elevated cholesterol or heart disease runs in your family or is a problem for you.

You can think of the various lipoproteins as envelopes that enclose cholesterol and triglycerides, making them soluble in blood so that they can be transported to the tissues. Since neither cholesterol (a waxy, fatty solid) nor triglycerides (the storage form of fat) are soluble in blood, the only way they can get around is to be wrapped up in and carried by a substance that is soluble in the blood. The lipoproteins fit the bill.

LDL is the abbreviation for *low-density lipoprotein,* while *HDL* stands for *high-density lipoprotein.* The names of these complex molecular compounds tell us nothing about what they do but are instead reflective of their densities: how light or heavy they are. The lightest of all the blood fats are the triglycerides. In a slurry of blood fats they would float to the top, like cream. Next lightest are the very-low-density lipoprotein (VLDL) molecules. These are carriers of some triglyceride and a little cholesterol. Next heavier is low-density lipoprotein (LDL) molecules that carry mainly cholesterol. And finally are the densest, heaviest molecules of all, the high-density lipoprotein or HDL.

A Day in the Life of a Lipoprotein

Your liver cells make and release VLDL (very-low-density lipoprotein) into the bloodstream as a molecule composed mainly of triglyceride but with a little cholesterol. As this young particle circulates through the blood, it matures by acquiring more cholesterol. The mature VLDL particle ferries triglycerides to the body tissues to be burned for energy or stored. The cholesterol-rich remnants left after most of the triglyceride has been released becomes a low-density lipoprotein (LDL) molecule that is practically all cholesterol. This cholesterol-rich LDL, the so-called "bad" cholesterol, circulates through the bloodstream and is the primary means the body has for transporting cholesterol to the outlying tissues. Three fates can befall these LDL particles: they can be removed from the circulation by the liver—as we shall see, a critical operation in the maintenance of normal cholesterol levels; they can be requisitioned by other tissues needing cholesterol; or, unfortunately, they can be deposited in the arteries. Figure 7.1 summarizes the sequence of events in the life of a lipoprotein.

LDL: The Heart Disease Heavy

Since LDL is the main culprit in the development of coronary artery disease, the secret of cholesterol control is in knowing how your body deals with LDL and how you can influence the cells to remove as much LDL from the blood as possible. How do the cells remove LDL from the circulation? With LDL receptors.

Remember, cholesterol is regulated from *within* the cell, and when the level inside the cell falls, the cell either makes more or procures more from the blood outside the cell. The cell gets the cholesterol from the

FIGURE 7.1

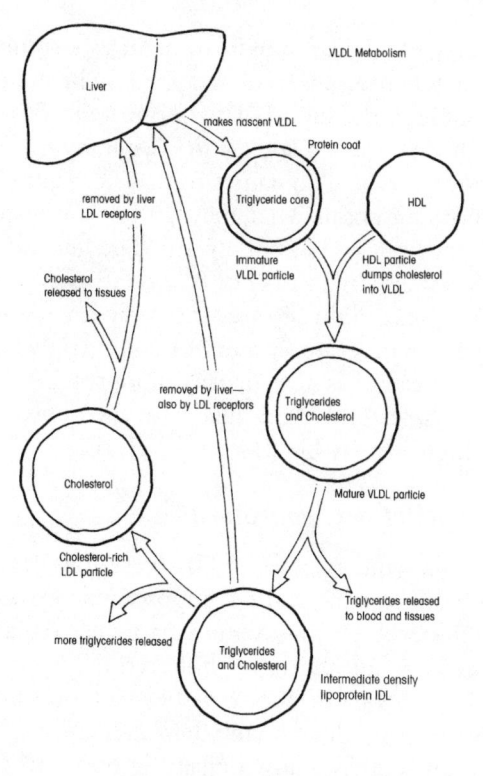

blood by sending structures called *LDL receptors* to the surface of the cell to grab the cholesterol-filled LDL particles and pull them into the interior of the cell, where the cholesterol is removed and used for cellular functions. Remember those obscene winged monkeys in the movie *The Wizard of Oz*, the ones the Wicked Witch sent to get Dorothy and Toto? They swooped down, grabbed Dorothy and her dog, and carried them back to the castle to be used for the witch's evil purposes. LDL receptors work in much the same way. When the cell sends out the call for cholesterol, forces within the cell manufacture these receptors and send them to the surface of the cell, where they lie in wait for the next LDL particle circulating through the blood, which they grab and pull into the interior of the cell. Once inside the cell, the LDL receptor releases the LDL particle and heads back toward the surface to grab another one. The enzymatic machinery within the cell then removes the lipoprotein envelope from the LDL particle and harvests the cholesterol core for synthesis of cellular products. Clearly the more LDL receptors we have scavenging cholesterol from the blood and hauling it into the cells, the better off we are.

Please Don't Take My LDL Receptors Away

Some of the first and most important work done on the relationship between heart disease and cholesterol focused on the LDL receptors. Researchers found that some people who developed heart disease at an extremely early age—often in the teens or early twenties—had a disorder in the genes responsible for telling their cells how to make LDL receptors, and consequently they could not remove LDL from their blood. Their blood LDL levels rose exceedingly high, causing them to develop blockages in their coronary arteries decades before people without this rare genetic disorder.

Their misfortune pointed up the importance for people not so afflicted to do whatever they can to ensure that their cells are teeming with the hardworking LDL receptors that keep their blood LDL within the normal range and reduce their risk of heart disease.

Of Mice and Men

In fact, it seems reasonable to suppose that if we could somehow rev up the production of our LDL receptors our cells could clear the cholesterol from our blood even in the face of a diet high in saturated fat and cholesterol. Recently a team of scientists including Drs. Michael Brown and Joseph Goldstein—recipients of the Nobel Prize for their discovery of the LDL receptor—working at the University of Texas Southwestern Medical Center at Dallas tested this idea in the laboratory.[1]

These researchers developed a strain of mice that produced *human* LDL receptors in their livers at a rate about five times that of the mouse LDL receptors in the livers of the normal mice used as experimental controls. On the normal laboratory diet the mice with the increased number of LDL receptors—the experimental strain of mice—maintained blood cholesterol levels that were 50 percent less than those in the normal controls, a finding that would be expected considering the increased number of LDL receptors. The surprise came when the scientists fed both groups of animals a diet high in saturated fat and cholesterol. As anticipated, the levels of LDL in the blood of the normal mice zoomed upward, while there was *no increase* in the level of LDL in the blood of the experimental mice. In the words of the authors of the study, ". . . increasing LDL receptor expression above its normal level in the mouse *can prevent hy-*

---

[1] Yokode, M., et al., "Diet-Induced Hypercholesterolemia in Mice: Prevention by Overexpression of LDL Receptors," *Science* 250 (November 30, 1990): 1273-75.

percholesterolemia [elevated blood cholesterol] *even in the face of a diet that contains large amounts of cholesterol, saturated fats, and bile acids."* (Emphasis added.)

That's easy, you say, in mice, but can *we* increase the production of LDL receptors in *our* cells? Yes, we can. To understand how, we need to look at the other half of the within-the-cell cholesterol regulation equation. Remember, the cell obtains cholesterol from two sources: it either makes it, or it sends the LDL receptor to fetch it from the blood. We've seen how the LDL receptor works; now let's consider how the cell makes cholesterol.

The Cholesterol Factory

When the signal goes out that the cholesterol level inside the cell is getting low, the cell, along with making more LDL receptors, starts to crank up the production machinery within itself to make more cholesterol. This assembly-line process chugs along, churning out cholesterol and adding it to that brought in by the LDL receptors, until the cell has a sufficient quantity to perform its tasks, then the process slows until the cell runs low again and calls for more. Since the cell's cholesterol comes from these two sources, which are both regulated by the cell, it makes sense that if, for whatever reason, one of the two processes slows down, the other will pick up the slack. This is precisely what does happen. Following this line of reasoning, if we could somehow slow down the rate at which our cells make cholesterol internally, they would have to increase the number of LDL receptors they send to the surface to pull more LDL from the blood. Again, this is exactly what happens; in fact the most potent cholesterol-lowering drug available today—lovastatin (Mevacor)—works on this principle.

The cholesterol synthesis pathway inside the cells is like a production line in a factory. The raw materials are brought in and in a series of steps shaped and fashioned into the final product. There is one step in the line—called the *rate-limiting step*—that determines how fast the production runs and controls how much gets produced. It is at this crucial step—an enzyme with the unwieldy name *3-hydroxy-3-methylglutaryl-coenzyme A (HMG-CoA) reductase*—that the cholesterol drug lovastatin intervenes. It slows down this step and decreases the amount of cholesterol produced. Less cholesterol within the cell indirectly increases the production of LDL receptors that rush to the surface to pluck the LDL cholesterol out of the bloodstream, bringing about a swift and significant lowering of LDL cholesterol in the blood. Unfortunately, it doesn't work its magic without side effects or without expense. Lovastatin has caused liver problems, muscular disorders, gallbladder disorders, rashes, and psychiatric disturbances to name a few and at the maximal recommended dose costs in the neighborhood of $200 per month for life. Despite this formidable list of side effects, because it works so quickly and dramatically, it keeps the cash registers ching-ching-chinging in pharmacies all across the country. Wouldn't it be great if there were a way to get the same cholesterol-lowering results without having to resort to drug therapy? There is.

Controlling Cholesterol with Insulin and Glucagon

If you pick up any medical biochemistry textbook and turn to the section on cholesterol synthesis, you will learn that a couple of hormones affect the activity of the rate-limiting enzyme HMG-CoA reductase. What hormones? Our old friends insulin and glucagon. Insulin stimulates HMG-CoA reductase, while glucagon inhibits it. Knowing this, it starts to make sense that people with insulin resistance and elevated insulin often also have elevated cholesterol levels. The high levels of insulin continuously stimulate production of cholesterol, leading to an abundance within the cells. With plenty in the cells, there's no reason to send LDL receptors to the surface to get more, so the amount of LDL in the blood rises and remains elevated.

Glucagon, as is its custom, does exactly the opposite. It inhibits the activity of HMG-CoA in much the same way that lovastatin does and brings about similar results. As glucagon slows down the production of cholesterol within the cell and the supply inside begins to run low, the cell sends its trusty LDL receptors to the surface to harvest LDL cholesterol from the bloodstream, resulting in less LDL cholesterol in the blood. Once again we see how by regulating insulin and glucagon levels we can correct or improve problems that are seemingly unrelated to insulin and blood sugar—in this case blood cholesterol. Our nutritional plan relies on food to balance insulin and glucagon and reduces blood cholesterol levels in exactly the same way that lovastatin does, but without the unpleasant side effects and hefty expense. And that's not the end of the story. This regimen acts in a number of other ways to improve the blood lipid picture, which we'll examine shortly. Before we do, you need to become familiar with one more actor in the cholesterol drama—HDL.

Heroic HDL

If LDL is the villain in the cholesterol drama, then high-density lipoprotein (HDL) is surely the hero. HDL scavenges cholesterol from the tissues, including the linings of the coronary arteries, carries it through the blood, and hands it off to the VLDL particles circulating in the bloodstream, ultimately converting it to LDL. So the transportation of cholesterol is not along a one-way street: LDL carries it toward the tissues for deposition, while HDL gathers it from these tissues and carts it back the other way to the cells of the liver, where it is disposed of. Since both processes occur simultaneously, the amount of cholesterol in the tissues depends on the relative amounts of LDL and HDL in the blood. It's like a freeway leading to and from a major city. At 7:30 A.M. on Monday morning the half heading into town will be congested, but there will still be some traffic on the side heading away from the city. The increased population of the city during the workday, which changes moment by moment, is the sum of the people entering the city minus the ones leaving. If you have a lot of LDL and not much HDL, then the preponderance of the cholesterol traffic is going to be toward the tissues; if, on the other hand, you have a greater amount of HDL, the flow goes in the opposite direction. With these facts, medical researchers have been able to quantify risk for heart disease based on the ratios of these lipoproteins.

My "Bad" Looks Good, But My "Good" Looks Bad

If you have your cholesterol checked in your doctor's office or, more likely in these days of cholesterol madness, at a shopping mall, you will find your results listed under the heading "Total Cholesterol." The number you see there is the sum of all the different lipoprotein envelopes that are carrying the cholesterol—the measurement of all the cholesterol carried in the blood as LDL, VLDL, and HDL.[2] Just as a screening test, total cholesterol isn't too inaccurate because the lion's share (about 70 percent) of it is carried by LDL. If the total cholesterol reading is high, then the odds are that the LDL is high also; conversely, if the total fig-

---

[2] Actually it is a combination of five lipoproteins, but we will concern ourselves only with VLDL, HDL, and LDL.

ure is low, the LDL is too. But, there can be exceptions, and that's why most physicians use the fractionated HDL and LDL figures to diagnose and treat our patients.

Medical researchers have investigated and compared the rates of heart disease development to the levels of the individual lipoproteins. You shouldn't be surprised to learn that the higher the level of LDL, the greater the risk of heart disease, and the higher the HDL, the lower the risk. What if both are high or both low? Just such situations do occur, so we prefer to look more at the ratio of the two rather than at either one individually. Two benchmark standards have been established:

1. Total cholesterol divided by HDL should be below 4.
2. LDL divided by HDL should be below 3.

Let's look at a couple of examples to see how this works.

If your total cholesterol is 240 mg/dl (a figure that would have been in the low normal range just a few years ago but today makes people think they can almost feel their coronary arteries clogging with cholesterol) and your HDL is 60 mg/dl, your ratio is 240/60, or 4, which is okay. If you can raise your HDL to 70 mg/dl even though your total cholesterol stays the same, you are in good shape with a ratio less than 4. Conversely, if you find yourself with a total cholesterol of 180 mg/dl, before you start patting yourself on the back, check your HDL. If it's 30 mg/dl, your ratio of 6 is too high; you need to raise your HDL. Looking at the other ratio, if your LDL is only 120 mg/dl (the upper limit of normal is considered to be 129 mg/dl) but again your HDL is only 30 mg/dl, your ratio is 4, above the benchmark of 3 for LDL/HDL. This is a case where the "bad" (LDL) looks good, but the "good" (HDL) looks bad.

DIET AND CHOLESTEROL QUIZ

Let's consider a scenario involving cholesterol and diet. Using your knowledge of the ratios we've been calculating, decide what you would do. You go to your doctor's office for a physical exam, and he finds that your total cholesterol is 240 mg/dl. He tells you that he has a diet guaranteed to reduce your cholesterol to 200 mg/dl if you will follow it. You do follow the diet and come back to see him in two months. Your total cholesterol is now 200 mg/dl. Are you happy? What if your HDL was 60 mg/dl on your first visit? That makes your total cholesterol–to–HDL ratio 4 (240/60), a good number. What if when you come back in two months your HDL has fallen to 45? Now your ratio is 4.4 (200/45).

Your ratio has worsened even though your total cholesterol figure has fallen, because your HDL fell at a greater rate. Your risk for heart disease—the reason you went on the diet in the first place—has now *increased* because your ratio has worsened. Would you be pleased with your new diet?

An interesting hypothetical case, you might say, but what doctor would actually start a patient on a diet that would cause such changes, a diet that would lower HDL more than it would total cholesterol? Well, tens of thousands of doctors put hundreds of thousands of patients on just such a diet each and every day. The diet in the example is the standard high-carbohydrate, low-fat diet that doctors everywhere prescribe for their patients with elevated cholesterol.

The "Controversial" High-Complex-Carbohydrate Diet

As the data on diet and cholesterol continue to accumulate, the evidence indicates that the high-complex-carbohydrate, low-fat diet doesn't live up to its billing as a cholesterol solution. Most studies show that although these diets lower total and LDL cholesterol somewhat, they lower HDL cholesterol by a greater percentage, leading to a worsening of the ratios that are more important than the individual measurements by themselves. A study published in the February 1991 issue of the *Journal of Clinical Endocrinology & Metabolism* illustrates this concept nicely.

The research group led by Dr. Mark Borkman of Sydney, Australia, studied young (average age thirty-seven), normal-weight, nondiabetic subjects of both sexes to determine the effects of diet on various blood parameters. The subjects followed one of two diets—either a high-carbohydrate diet or a high-fat diet—for a three-week period, then followed the other diet for the next three-week period. After each dietary period the researchers examined the subjects and analyzed their blood.

The high-carbohydrate diet was designed to follow the current standard nutritional recommendations and was over 50 percent carbohydrate and under 30 percent fat. It was "based on foods rich in starch and indigestible carbohydrate (whole-meal bread, pasta, rice, and potatoes), fruit and vegetables, nonfat dairy products, and lean meat." (Sound familiar?) The high-fat diet was mainly "full cream dairy products, eggs, butter, and fatty meats, with restriction of starch foods, vegetables, and fruit." Despite this "restriction," the subjects on the high-fat diet managed to consume 31 percent of their calories as carbohydrate, or roughly 175 grams of carbohydrate per day, so this hardly qualifies as a rigorous carbohydrate-restricted diet—an important point because had the carbohydrate been a little more restricted, the results would have been even more impressive.

When the researchers tabulated the results of the study, they found that the total cholesterol dropped from an average of 191 mg/dl on the high-fat diet to about 159 mg/dl on the high-carbohydrate, low-fat diet, a 17 percent decrease; the LDL cholesterol dropped from 139 mg/dl to 111 mg/dl, a 20 percent decrease; and the HDL cholesterol from 42 mg/dl to 32 mg/dl, a 24 percent decrease. The ratios are shown in the following chart.

CHOLESTEROL COMPARISONS STUDY

	HIGH-CARBOHYDRATE DIET	HIGH-FAT DIET
Total cholesterol	159 mg/dl	191 mg/dl
LDL cholesterol	111 mg/dl	139 mg/dl
HDL cholesterol	32 mg/dl	42 mg/dl
Total cholesterol/HDL	4.97	4.55
LDL/HDL	3.47	3.31

If you consider the results of this study and others like it solely from the perspective of what the high-carbohydrate, low-fat diet does to the total and LDL cholesterol, you will conclude that the high-carbohydrate diet lowers cholesterol significantly. But when you throw in the HDL figures, the picture changes considerably. The total cholesterol/HDL and LDL/HDL ratios can be thought of as rough indicators of the flow of cholesterol into and out of the tissues: the higher the number, the greater the flux of cholesterol *into* the tissues—the situation we want to avoid if we are concerned about heart disease. You can see from this table that although the total and LDL cholesterol are lower in the blood of the subjects on the high-carbohydrate diet, the actual flow of cholesterol into their tissues is higher. The authors address this issue in their summary: "These results suggest that practically achievable high carbohydrate diets . . . have net effects on lipoprotein metabolism that may be unfavorable."

These results and others like them have gotten the attention of the medical research community; now the high-carbohydrate, low-fat diet is beginning to be referred to as the *controversial* high-carbohydrate, low-fat diet. Unfortunately most medical researchers have marinated for so long in their antifat, procarbohydrate bias that they can't change their perspective. At meetings and in their writings they continue to promote the standard fare while admitting that it's controversial, but it's the best we have right now. But *is* it the best we have right now? Is there anything better? Absolutely, but before we turn our attention to the way this better diet controls cholesterol, let's fill in one last piece of the cholesterol puzzle.

Most people assume that the lower they can keep their cholesterol, the better; they much prefer a cholesterol of 100 mg/dl to one of 220 mg/dl. As you probably realize, they would be in error. There is an ideal cholesterol range that you should shoot for, one that is as dangerous to go below as to go above, but many health-conscious people continue on in pursuit of ever-lower levels in the misguided notion that they are extending their life spans by conquering cholesterol. These people are making a serious error because they have seen only half of the data.

The Other Half of the Cholesterol Story

The higher your cholesterol, the more likely you are to die with heart disease or stroke. That's the gist of information promulgated by medical research and the cholesterol-lowering drug manufacturers. They demonstrate their data with graphs like those in Figure 7.2.

In truth, mortality from heart disease probably does increase as cholesterol increases and decrease as the level of cholesterol continues to fall—to a point. But this graph is only half the story. Heart disease is not the only cause of death in this country—people do die from other causes. What the multihundreds of millions of dollars in research studies designed to demonstrate a reduction in deaths from heart disease as cholesterol levels decrease *fail to prove* is that reduction of cholesterol to very low levels leads to a decreased rate of death overall. The actual complete graph showing death from all causes (not just heart disease or stroke) as related to blood cholesterol levels looks more like Figure 7.3.

As your cholesterol level falls below a certain point, you jump out of the frying pan of heart disease risk and into the fire of death by all sorts of other diseases. What kind of diseases? Cerebral hemorrhage, gallbladder disease, and many types of cancer, for which falling cholesterol is a marker.

As you can see, the ideal cholesterol level is in the area where the U-shaped curve bottoms out, in the 180 mg/dl-to-200 mg/dl range. Avoid trying to get it lower; don't trade one serious health problem for another.

FIGURE 7.2

HEART DISEASE DEATHS VS. BLOOD CHOLESTEROL LEVELS

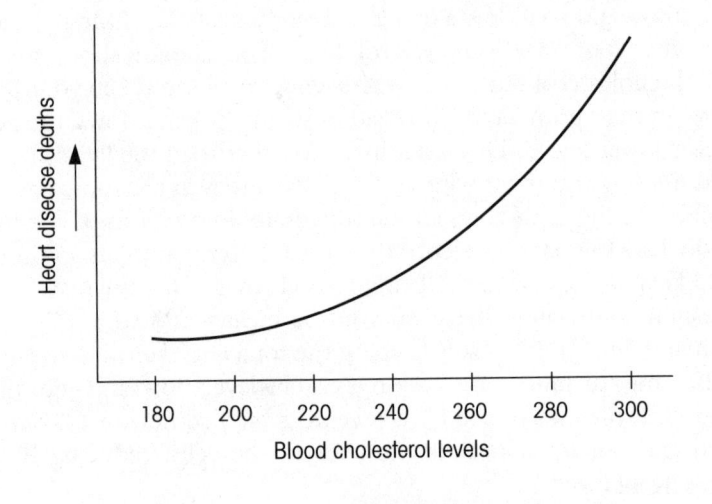

FIGURE 7.3

DEATHS FROM ALL CAUSES VS. CHOLESTEROL LEVELS

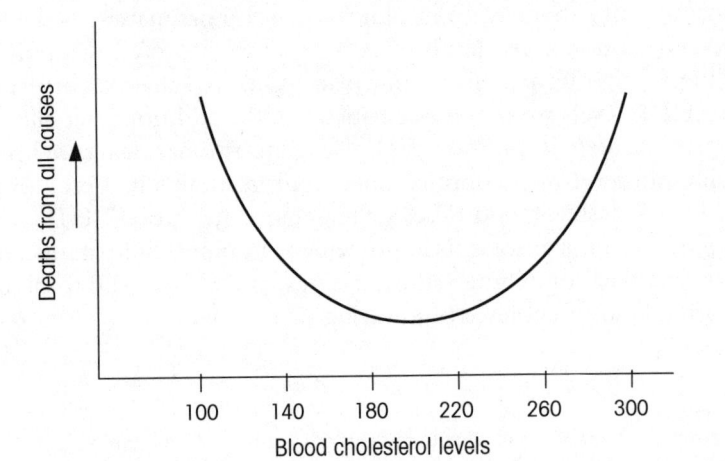

Putting It All Together

Given what you now know about the various lipoprotein groups, it's clear that you ought to follow a diet that keeps your LDL cholesterol low while keeping your HDL cholesterol high. You should shoot for an LDL/HDL cholesterol ratio of 3 or less, endeavoring to keep your total cholesterol in the optimal range instead of blindly tearing down the path toward ever-lower levels. This is all fine, and other than the last sentence we would find no argument with any of this from even the most vociferous members of the high-complex-carbohydrate, low-fat camp. But how do you do it? How can you corral your cholesterol into its optimum range and keep it there while still eating foods that you enjoy?

Our insulin-controlling diet gives you the means. It lowers LDL and raises or maintains HDL, usually keeping the total cholesterol in the ideal 180-to-200 mg/dl range. By keeping insulin levels low and glucagon levels high, our plan keeps the LDL receptors busy retrieving LDL from the blood and pulling it into the interior of the cells, reducing blood LDL cholesterol levels.

Recall that when Dr. Reaven of Stanford published his findings on insulin resistance and hyperinsulinemia (Syndrome X) one of the features he described was a low HDL. Medical science has yet to provide us with the underlying biochemical reason for this lowered HDL, but it's present in the majority of patients with insulin resistance. Fortunately, as the levels of insulin go down, the levels of HDL rise: we've noted this positive change in patient after patient on our plan.[3] One explanation for the increase of HDL levels we see in our patients is the additional fat allowed on our plan: *dietary fat increases HDL.*[4] Our nutritional structure brings the cholesterol level to its optimal range and maintains it there, lowers "bad" LDL cholesterol, and raises or maintains the "good" HDL cholesterol—the result is an overall improvement in blood lipid status. And it does it on a diet containing red meat, eggs, and cheese—all forbidden on any other kind of cholesterol-lowering diet.

---

[3] Occasionally the HDL will fall a little, but this fall is always accompanied by a much greater fall in the LDL and total cholesterol, so the ratio of total cholesterol divided by HDL improves.

[4] This is also the reason HDL goes down during a low-fat diet. But because HDL decreases in greater proportion than does the LDL, such low-fat diets can actually worsen those all-important ratios.

Seeing Is Believing

Reluctant is a mild word to describe the feeling most physicians would have about prescribing a diet high in red meat and eggs for patients with a cholesterol problem. We'll admit that it caused us some worry the first time we did it, even though we knew from the research that it *should* work. But the proof of any nutritional regimen's worth is in the laboratory results down the line. And the biochemically correct nutritional plan we developed for our patients with elevated cholesterol succeeded beyond our expectations. We've described this insulin-controlling plan to other physicians who tried a few patients on it very reluctantly at first. As their experiences mirrored ours, and their patients' blood cholesterol levels plummeted just as ours had, these physicians became enthusiastic supporters of the program. Along with the experiences of these colleagues, we often read in medical journals of other physicians who stumble onto a diet that controls insulin and its consequences without really understanding what's happening. They are so amazed at the cholesterol-controlling abilities in the face of what seems to be a diet that would increase cholesterol that they publish their findings.

Much was made of an article that appeared in the March 28, 1991, issue of the *New England Journal of Medicine,* about an elderly gentleman who ate twenty-five eggs per day yet had a normal blood cholesterol level. You may have read this story in your newspaper, because all the wire services picked it up, and several nutrition writers offered their views on the freakishness of it. The consensus seemed to be that this was a special case, like the relative everyone seems to have who smoked four packs a day and lived to be ninety-five. Here are the details:

An eighty-eight-year-old man living in a nursing home ate twenty-five or so eggs per day and had done so for the past thirty years of his life. His physician had documented this fact and reported that despite his eating habits the gentleman's cholesterol had always been in the normal range. The apparent inconsistency of this situation—as far as most physicians are concerned this would be akin to smoking a carton of cigarettes per day for thirty years and having a normal chest X-ray—attracted the attention of a medical researcher at the University of Colorado medical school, who examined this patient and reported his findings. Upon questioning, this slender (6'2", 185-pound) elderly man stated that he followed a standard diet with a wide variety of foods, which he supplemented (for reasons unknown to himself) with a couple of dozen eggs per day. His blood levels of cholesterol were: total cholesterol, 200 mg/dl; LDL, 142 mg/dl, and HDL, 45 mg/dl; his LDL/HDL ratio was 3.16. The body of the article went on to discuss the reasons this man's cholesterol levels were normal despite his intake of 5,000 mg of cholesterol per day (about seventeen times the normally recommended amount). The author concluded that the patient made less cholesterol, absorbed less cholesterol, and got rid of more cholesterol biochemically than the average person, and was thus spared the consequences of his two-dozen-eggs-per-day habit.

We were troubled by this article when we first read it because we couldn't reconcile his normal cholesterol with the diet this gentleman ate. If he were consuming a "normal" diet as the article reported (particularly nursing-home fare), then he was no doubt getting plenty of carbohydrates. His insulin should have been up and consequently his cholesterol as well. After pondering this for a while, it occurred to us that if this man were eating twenty-five eggs a day he couldn't possibly be eating much else. After all, twenty-five eggs represents about 2,000 calories per day, a more-than-adequate amount for a sedentary man of eighty-eight. We corresponded with the author of the article, and indeed, the nursing home confirmed our prediction that "the quantity of these [other] foods is limited."[5] Since the eggs contain no carbohydrate whatsoever and the other foods are limited, it's our guess that this gentleman consumed about 50 or 60 grams of carbohydrate per day along with his eggs, an amount that correlates precisely with Phase II of our plan. Knowing this along with all the mechanisms we have discussed, it's no surprise that this patient's cholesterol stayed within the normal range—he simply went on his own bizarre version of an insulin-controlling diet.

We found another such serendipitous consumption of a diet similar to our plan, this time by multiple patients, reported in the *Southern Medical Journal* in January 1988. In this case a New York physician, H. L. Newbold, M.D., treated a group of patients who had food allergies by placing them on a specific diet to eliminate certain foods thought to cause their allergic problems. In Dr. Newbold's words:

> At the time of the initial visit, each patient was eating an ordinary, varied American diet. All patients had an elevated serum cholesterol. [The average total cholesterol of the study group was 263 mg/dl, with a range of 224–327 mg/dl. The average HDL was 57.1 mg/dl.]
>
> I discovered that each patient could best tolerate beef rib steaks. For varying periods, these patients ate mostly unaged beef rib steaks. Some patients could occasionally tolerate lamb, pork, or chicken in place of the rib steak, but they

---

[5] Personal correspondence with Fred Kern, M.D., the author of the article.

ate them no more often than once every three or four days. Rarely, they ate cuts of beef other than rib steaks.

Patients were instructed to have their butchers leave a percentage of fat on the steaks. They were told to eat as much of the fat as they could comfortably tolerate.

These patients were told to supplement their basically meat diet with a small amount of raw fresh vegetables and raw fruits—a restricted version of our program. Before you read this chapter, what would you think of a diet like this one? You would guess it would send the cholesterol levels of these poor patients screaming upward. Almost anyone in today's low-fat world would think that. What happened? Dr. Newbold explains: "After eating a diet high in beef fat for three to eighteen months, the average serum cholesterol fell to 189 mg/dl." The cholesterol levels of these patients declined from 263 to 189 mg/dl while the HDL levels increased from 57.1 to 62.7 mg/dl. Once again we see people going on the "wrong" diet and lowering their cholesterol levels by 28 percent while increasing their HDLs by almost 10 percent—a drop in total cholesterol–to–HDL ratios from 4.6 to 3. Not too bad!

Clearly, as these studies show, you can reduce and control your cholesterol levels without having to resort to the old hidebound, low-fat, low-cholesterol diet. You can partake of a wide variety of fruits and vegetables on our program while at the same time eating the red meat, eggs, and cheese that you may have been avoiding in an effort to lower your cholesterol. Don't be misled by the misguided efforts of your friends and relatives who don't understand the workings of cholesterol metabolism as you do. Continue with your plan and let your lab results speak for themselves.

The Truth About Fiber

Fiber has been touted as a means of reducing weight and the risk of developing colon disorders and cancer, as a remedy for constipation, as a preventer of hemorrhoids, and, thanks to *The 8-Week Cholesterol Cure*, as part of a cure for elevated cholesterol and heart disease risk. After an extensive survey of current medical research literature on the role of fiber in human health, we came to one certainty: no one really knows exactly what fiber is, what it really does, or how it works. But there is consensus on the notion that fiber does improve bowel function by adding bulk to the stool and speeding it more quickly along. These properties prevent or lessen constipation and discourage the formation of hemorrhoids.

The story on cholesterol reduction is less clear, with some studies showing a reduction from fiber intake while others do not. There probably is some benefit here in that fiber may bind with cholesterol in the intestine and prevent its reabsorption.

Fiber does help to stabilize blood sugar by slowing down the absorption of dietary carbohydrates. Slower absorption may blunt the blood sugar rise and the insulin response to it, resulting in a lower, more constant blood sugar level.

Although great hoopla surrounded the news that fiber exerts some protective effect in preventing colon cancer, based on the huge Harvard Nurses Study, in truth, the difference in colon cancer between those women who ate the most fiber and those who ate the least was three cases, an insignificant number.

Our nutritional regimen gives you a wide variety of choices of fruits and vegetables that will provide you with far more fiber— without the metabolically active carbohydrate—than all the bran muffins you could eat. For instance, a bowl of raspberries contains more fiber than ten of the basic-recipe bran muffins described in *The 8-Week Cholesterol Cure* and almost no usable carbohydrate.

Because the fiber content of foods is not metabolically active, you can subtract the grams of dietary fiber from the total carbohydrate content of foods you eat. We call what's left, the Effective Carbohydrate Content of Food (ECC). We've compiled charts of effective carbohydrate grams for a wide range of foods (see Chapter 10).

Peruse those charts and notice that the vegetables giving the best carbohydrate value are the green leafy ones and the cruciferous ones (because they're rich in fiber). The worst are potatoes, corn, and dried beans. Among the fruits, berries of almost all kinds are the best carbohydrate/fiber bargain; bananas and raisins are among the worst.

In fact, using our ECC chart, we find that you could have 1 cup broccoli, 1 cup cabbage, 3 celery ribs, 1 cup green beans, 1 cup lettuce, $1/2$ cup mushrooms, 1 cup zucchini, 1 cup spinach, and 1 cup raspberries spread throughout the day, giving you only 27 grams of metabolically active carbohydrate and 16.3 grams of fiber, most of it of the soluble variety. You could add a couple of slices of light bread and still have eaten only 40 grams of usable carbohydrate and a total of 21.3 grams of fiber—almost 100 percent more than the average American diet. This is hardly stringent in terms of amount of food, vitamin content, mineral content, volume, fiber, or any other parameter.

The ECC charts in Chapter 10 will guide you naturally toward foods that contain more fiber and less starch, because that's where you'll get the most food for the lowest carbohydrate intake. And if you simply can't or won't eat any of the high-fiber fruits and vegetables, and you become constipated, you can always add fiber by using the commercial vegetable fiber powders, such as Konsyl or Nutriflax.

How much fiber do you need? For good health people usually need *at least* 25 grams a day. In the past, restricted-carbohydrate diets have been criticized for not providing enough fiber. Is this a valid concern? Yes, but not with our plan, which provides ample fiber.

The Bottom Line

In America people have become accustomed to thinking of cholesterol as an evil destroyer of health. The average American is not even sure what cholesterol is exactly; only that it's "fat in your blood" and "it's dangerous." In fact, nothing could be further from the truth: cholesterol is absolutely essential for life, and falling levels of cholesterol are a grave sign, often a marker for cancer.

Cholesterol isn't even really a fat; it's a pearly white waxy alcohol with a soapy feel. Every cell in your body requires cholesterol to maintain the structural integrity of its cell membrane, to control the flow of water and nutrients into the cell and waste products out. Your nerves and your brain require cholesterol for normal electrical signal transmission.

Your body uses the cholesterol molecule as a building block for many important hormones: the sex hormones (estrogen and testosterone) and your body's natural steroid, hydrocortisol.

Cholesterol in the bile your liver makes aids in the digestion of fatty foods and helps you absorb fat-soluble vitamins A, D, E, and K from food. Cholesterol gives your skin the ability to shed water.

Every cell in your body can make it. In fact, only about 20 percent of the cholesterol in your blood comes from your diet. Your body (primarily your liver) makes the vast majority (80 percent). To ensure your cells always have plenty, if there's not enough coming in, the cells pick up the slack and make more. That's why simply cutting back on dietary cholesterol often doesn't cause much of an improvement in blood cholesterol levels.

The standard low-fat-diet approach to treating cholesterol actually causes the cells of your body to have to make *more* cholesterol for vital functions. Control over how much the cells make lies *within the cells* themselves. When the supply in the cell runs low, the cell can either make more cholesterol or send messengers to the surface of the cell to collect some from the bloodstream.

Insulin plays a key role here: it revs up the cells' cholesterol-manufacturing machinery, building up a surplus within the cell, making it unnecessary for the cell to retrieve any from the bloodstream, and thereby allowing excess cholesterol to build up in the blood.

By eating a diet that reduces insulin levels, as our program does, you reduce the signal telling the cells to make cholesterol; they *must* harvest it from the blood to have enough, and your blood cholesterol levels—especially the "bad" LDL—fall rapidly. Even while eating a diet that contains red meat, egg yolk, cheese, butter, and cream, as long as you control your insulin output, your cholesterol will remain in the healthy 180-to-200 mg/dl range with the LDL/HDL ratio under 3. And the extra dietary fat will actually raise the HDL—"good" cholesterol—level in your blood.

Chapter 8

Vitamins, Minerals, and Potassium

Nicotinic acid cures pellagra, but a beefsteak prevents it.

HENRY E. SIGERIST, medical historian

For your body to function optimally, your diet must include sufficient amounts of micronutrients—vitamins, minerals, and potassium. In this chapter you will learn what they are and how much of which ones you need for good health.

More than 4,000 years ago the Chinese recognized that people became ill with a disease called *beriberi* when they relied on a diet of polished rice. Some substance, they didn't know what, in the rice husks prevented this illness. We now understand that polishing the husks away removes all the thiamine (vitamin B_1) from the rice, and thiamine deficiency causes *beriberi*. From this early discovery of vitamin deficiency's role in causing disease to the recent studies showing the power of antioxidants and phytochemicals to protect us against cancer and heart disease, health practitioners of every stripe, from mainstream physicians to snake oil salesmen, patent medicine peddlers, nutritional gurus, and scientific researchers, have searched for that "magic bullet" cure-all micronutrient that will alleviate human suffering and disease. As this vitamin debate rages, it has often left the health-conscious public confused. Should you supplement your diet with vitamin and mineral tablets or rely on the micronutrients in the foods you eat? If you do supplement, what should you take and how much? Is the RDA (Recommended Dietary Allowance) enough to promote optimal health, or should you take more? Which vitamins and minerals, in particular, might be beneficial in the metabolic disorders related to insulin resistance?

First, the RDA for vitamins and minerals: we speak from the camp of those researchers, clinicians, and scientists who feel that although a diet that provides the RDA of all essential vitamins and minerals will certainly keep most people from developing serious deficiency diseases, these levels are woefully inadequate to ensure optimal health and peak performance. For example, the RDA of vitamin E is about 10 milligrams per day, but several recent studies have shown this antioxidant to be protective against heart disease (and a number of other diseases of aging) only if taken at doses six, ten, even *forty* times the RDA.

Rest assured that our program—even in its strictest phases—provides you ample opportunity to consume every essential vitamin, mineral, and nutrient in quantities that meet or exceed the RDA, but whether you do so will depend on your own taste preferences. Like George Bush and his aversion to broccoli, we all tend to consume the foods we like in quantity and avoid those we aren't quite so fond of even though they might be rich in beneficial micronutrients. Because our purpose here is to help you regain your health and overcome the problems that "civilized" eating has inflicted on you, we ask that you ensure the micronutrient adequacy of your diet by supplementing it with a complete general multiple vitamin and mineral tablet and potassium.

For good general health you need adequate amounts of all the vitamins and minerals. Certain vitamins and minerals, however, have a special bearing on insulin resistance and the disorders caused by it.[1]

The Vitamins

In general vitamins function in your body as facilitators in certain chemical reactions. For example, your body must have vitamin C (ascorbic acid) to build strong collagen, the main structural protein in the body that makes the framework for bone, muscle fiber, tendon, ligament, skin, hair, and scar tissue to heal wounds. Without adequate vitamin C the collagen that's made is weak and of poor structural quality. It tears easily. When people become deficient in vitamin C, they bruise easily, their teeth loosen and fall out, they lose their hair, their gums bleed, their wounds don't heal well, their joints weaken, and finally they usually hem-

---

[1] To answer your questions about using vitamin and mineral supplementation to prevent or treat conditions other than insulin-related ones, look for *The Doctor's Complete Guide to Vitamins and Minerals* by Mary Dan Eades, M.D. (New York: Dell, 1994).

orrhage (from weak blood vessel walls) and die. The disease this vitamin deficiency causes is called *scurvy*, and it nearly destroyed the navies of many countries until the British recognized that they could prevent it by making sure their sailors ate plenty of limes and lemons while at sea.

This preventive measure created a popular misconception that citrus fruits are the only good dietary source of vitamin C, but Arctic explorer Vilhjalmur Stefansson conclusively proved that wrong in the late 1920s. Fresh, lightly cooked meat and fish, he found, contain enough of a vitamin C–like substance (as well as all other critical micronutrients) to prevent scurvy and other deficiency diseases. The *Journal of the American Medical Association* documented that Stefansson, who spent one full year on a drastic diet of nothing but fresh meat and water not only did not die as predicted but emerged fitter, leaner, with lower cholesterol counts (about the only laboratory marker for heart disease available in the late 1920s), and healthier in every regard.

However, unless you can obtain a steady supply of very fresh meat and you like to eat it cooked rare, you will need to get your vitamin C from other sources. According to the RDA, your daily intake of vitamin C should be a modest 60 milligrams per day, about the amount contained in a medium orange. For most people that will be enough to prevent the development of scurvy. But that's just one side of the equation. What amount of vitamin C would it take to optimize health? That's the question that occupied Nobel Prize laureate Dr. Linus Pauling for the last four decades of his illustrious career. Reasoning that since humans are one of only four species (along with other primates, guinea pigs, and the fruit-eating bat) that have lost the ability to make vitamin C, we ought to obtain from our diets at least as much as other species make on their own—and he concluded that the RDA is pitifully inadequate. We need not 60 milligrams but more on the order of 6,000 to 20,000 milligrams. Based on body size, Dr. Pauling calculated his own daily dose at 20,000 milligrams (20 grams), which he took religiously. And during the last decades of his life—he died recently at age ninety-three—he devoted his resources and time to an intense study of this vitamin's role in prevention and treatment of diseases ranging from the common cold to atherosclerosis to cancer. We recommend that you supplement your diet with a daily intake of at least 1 gram (1,000 mg) of vitamin C and along with it vitamin E and beta-carotene, forming the group called the *antioxidants*. Vitamin C stays in the body for only twelve hours, so if you want to go beyond the 1-gram recommendation, split your dose and take it morning and night.

THE ANTIOXIDANTS

All day, every day, this modern world assaults us with harmful substances—air pollution in the form of smog and industrial toxins, secondhand cigarette smoke, additives and other chemicals in our food and water, pharmaceuticals, radiation—but the commonest and potentially most damaging of all is a substance we must have for life: oxygen. While you may not be accustomed to thinking of oxygen as harmful—and rightly so since it's generally beneficial—you should also remember that exposure to oxygen can turn a pickup truck into a rusty heap of iron, a succulent apple slice into an ugly piece of brown mush, and a tiny spark into a raging inferno. There is a duality in this substance; it can both create and destroy. Oxygen fuels the metabolic fire that burns within us and gives us life, but it can also cause widespread damage—by a process called, naturally enough, *oxidation* (the same process that rusts out the truck) and through the formation of reactive substances called *free radicals*. What does all this have to do with the metabolic mayhem of insulin resistance?

It's oxidation of cholesterol molecules that renders them more reactive and more likely to lay down in the artery walls, forming plaque and causing heart attacks. Oxidation of essential fats alters their structure and disrupts their entry into and flow along the eicosanoid pathway, leading to the overproduction of "bad" eicosanoid messengers, leading to blood clotting for heart attack and stroke or to inflammatory messengers causing painful joints or to allergy messengers that promote asthma or hives. It's oxidation of other body tissues that ages them, leading to the development of arthritic damage, wrinkled skin, and cataracts, and it's oxidation that damages the cells, promoting the development of cancers.

How does oxidation do these things? The human body is made up of billions of cells, and those cells are made up of billions of atoms, and those atoms are composed of charged particles called *protons* and *electrons*. The positively charged protons exist in the middles (or nuclei) of the atoms, with the negatively charged electrons whirling in pairs in orbit around the middle. Normally all the positive and negative charges balance, all the electrons are happily paired, and the atom exists in a state of electrical neutrality. But to function, to create energy for life, we must upset this balance by shuffling these electrons from atom to atom in a controlled way. When an atom loses one of its electrons, it becomes electrically unbalanced, with more positives than negatives. When it takes on this charge, we call it a *free radical*—one of its electrons is alone, or free, in its orbit. This free radical becomes very reactive, on the prowl for an electron to replace the one it lost, potentially setting off a chain reaction of electron robbing. As long as the process remains controlled, all is well. But the uncontrolled development of too many of these free radicals—from toxins, cigarette smoke, pollution, and the like—can lead to cell damage, promoting the development of disease and accelerating the aging process.

Antioxidants, as their name implies, help to prevent the damaging effects of oxygen and other free-radical-forming substances on your body's tissues, and thus they reduce your risk of disorders ranging from heart disease to cancer. For example, recent medical research has shown that deficiencies of the antioxidants vitamin C and beta-carotene (the vitamin A forerunner) may contribute to the development of high blood pressure and that vitamins C and E help to reduce the risk of heart disease caused by atherosclerosis in the blood vessels supplying the heart (and elsewhere).

You will find vitamin C in foods such as sweet peppers, broccoli, citrus fruits, melons, strawberries, tomatoes, raw cabbage, leafy greens (spinach, mustard, and turnip greens), and fresh meat and liver. Good sources of beta-carotene are carrots, cantaloupe, spinach, broccoli, winter squash, and apricots. Seeds, nuts, and the oils derived from them, especially sunflower seeds and almonds, are the richest food sources of vitamin E. Following our dietary guidelines, you will gravitate naturally toward these kinds of foods since they are also the vegetable and fruit sources with the lowest carbohydrate content and the most fiber. If you like these foods and eat them often, wonderful. You should always get plenty of the antioxidants, other vitamins, and minerals you need from food. Don't worry about getting too much vitamin C; the more the better because you can't store it and it won't hurt you. If—like a few of our patients over the years—you prefer such "vegetables" as ketchup, potatoes, corn, dried beans, rice, and pasta, don't let a day pass without supplementing your intake of all the antioxidants—beta-carotene and vitamins C and E. These foods may be vegetables, but in the main they are starches, just like bread and cereal—and you know by now that they're to be severely restricted. Remember the Egyptians?

THE ESSENTIAL B VITAMINS

In addition to the critical antioxidants, your diet must include all the other vitamins, but especially those in the B group. To make optimal use of the protein, carbohydrate, and fat in the foods you eat, to turn these raw materials into muscle, blood, enzymes, and energy, your body must have a steady supply of all the vitamins that make up the B vitamin complex. This group—niacin, thiamine, riboflavin, and vitamins B_5, B_6, and B_{12}—works interdependently, so when you supplement one of them, you should supplement *all* of them; take B complex, not just vitamin B_{12} or B_6. For the B vitamin group to function efficiently, you must also have plenty of folic acid. Like vitamin C, the B vitamins and folic acid are water-soluble, so you must replace them daily, either in the foods you eat or in supplement form.

You will find the richest food sources for B vitamins in meats: in organ meats, such as liver and kidney; in muscle meats, such as beef, pork, veal, and chicken; in seafood, especially oysters and clams, but also in ocean fish, such as tuna and salmon; in egg yolk; and in cheese and milk, especially dry milk. Other good sources of B vitamins include walnuts, peanuts, sunflower seeds, sesame seeds, and avocados.

FOLIC ACID FOR STRONG BODIES

Folic acid, which occurs primarily in liver, green leafy vegetables, and brewer's yeast, helps your body build protein and blood, the cornerstone of a healthy, strong, lean body mass. Your body also needs plenty of this vitamin to be able to absorb B vitamins. Taking birth control pills depletes the folic acid stores, so especially for young women who use this form of contraception taking extra folic acid is important to healthy fat loss and nutritional rehabilitation.

The Minerals

IRON: THE CASE FOR EATING RED MEAT

If you've been avoiding eating red meat, not for philosophical or religious reasons but because you've been told it's not good for you, rejoice! Not only does red meat provide you with lots of high-quality protein and an abundance of every member of the B vitamin complex, but it's also a rich source—perhaps the best source—of iron. The iron in red meat, called *heme iron,* is bound to protein, a form the human gastrointestinal tract can absorb more easily and completely. For this reason vegetarians and others who do not eat red meat tend to develop iron deficiencies and anemia even though their diets may contain plenty of iron from grain and vegetable sources. While spinach and other dark green leafy vegetables contain a lot of iron, it's bound to compounds (called *phytates*) that the human intestine can't absorb. Iron deficiency and protein malnutrition, caused by a meatless diet and a reliance on grain, account for widespread mental retardation in third-world countries and developing nations around the world.

If you avoid red meat for cholesterol reasons, see Chapter 7.

Just as the intestine will absorb protein-bound heme iron better than other forms, so will it absorb other necessary minerals when they are combined with protein. The reason for this better absorption lies in how minerals enter the intestine.

MAKE OURS CHELATES, PLEASE

Most minerals—particularly those in many inexpensively manufactured vitamin and mineral tablets—occur as salts. In a salt the mineral combines with other elements; for example, iron as ferrous sulfate combines with sulfur and oxygen. When these mineral salts enter the stomach, the salts break apart into individual elements called *ions*.[2] The mucous coating of the stomach lining is slightly charged, and it attracts these positively and negatively charged ions in much the same way that opposite poles of magnets attract. Beneath the mucous coating each of the cells of the lining of the stomach has a tiny channel—called the *ion channel*—that will admit a single ion at a time. Because the ions compete with each other for entry into the channel, the amount of any mineral that gets through depends on how much of it is in the stomach at the time and whether anything else is in the stomach.

Technology has offered us a way to bypass the bottleneck of the single ion channel. The process, called *chelation*, wraps each mineral ion in a jacket of amino acids, the building blocks of protein. The disguise works; the stomach lining absorbs these amino acid–chelated minerals as if they were protein. They don't have to stand in line to be admitted through the single ion channel. By using mineral chelates, you can completely and efficiently absorb all the minerals necessary for optimal health in much the same way your intestine will better absorb the heme form of iron. For this reason we ask that when you choose a vitamin and mineral supplement, you look carefully to be certain that it contains minerals as amino acid chelates. That way you'll know you will get—and get the benefit of—what you've paid for. You'll find several vitamin and chelated mineral supplements recommended at the end of this chapter.

---

[2] Don't be confused by our recommendation of taking potassium as a salt. The electrolytes—potassium, sodium, and chloride—function as ions.

THE OTHER MINERALS

Iron is only one of many minerals your diet should include. While all the trace minerals—particularly boron, iodine, molybdenum, and zinc—are important to your general health, of special importance to the metabolic disorders related to insulin resistance are the following minerals.

Chromium

The insulin receptor, the structure on the surfaces of your cells that actually becomes resistant to insulin, requires chromium to function properly. Deficiency of chromium is rampant—it affects 90 percent of the American population—because a diet high in starch and sugar puts a heavy demand on the insulin system to handle the incoming carbohydrate load, and that high demand depletes chromium. Restoring your chromium levels to normal will almost certainly require you to take a supplement since it will take a daily dietary intake of 200 micrograms to do the job and even the richest source, brewer's yeast, contains a meager 2 micrograms to the gram (liver and black pepper provide even less). Strenuous exercise also causes a chromium drain, so your need to replace this mineral will be especially high if you've been carbo-loading pasta, potatoes, and fat-free bagels before you run, bike, or swim.

Chromium's crucial role in maintaining proper insulin function makes it an important component in helping you recompose your body to a healthier, leaner state. Sufficient chromium will help you build lean muscle pounds and, through interaction with the thyroid hormone system, help you burn fat more efficiently.

If you've got a sweet tooth, chromium deficiency may be at the root of the problem. Because chromium deficiency intensifies sugar cravings, it can spur a vicious cycle: chromium deficiency stimulates your sweet tooth and drives you to eat sugary foods, which further depletes your chromium, which aggravates your sugar cravings, and on and on. By following our macronutrient prescription and supplementing with chelated or niacin-bound chromium, you should begin to find your intense craving for sweet foods diminishing in the first few weeks.

You may add supplemental chromium to your vitamin regimen if your multivitamin and mineral does not contain at least 200 micrograms. Although you will have replenished depleted chromium stores in a few weeks or months, you should continue to take this mineral every day to keep your stores full, especially if you exercise.

Calcium and Magnesium: More Than Just Bone Builders

You may think of calcium as a bone-building mineral, and indeed 99 percent of your body's calcium is stored in your skeletal framework. What you may not know, though, is that calcium and its mineral partner, magnesium, also play important roles in the transmission of nerve signals and in the contraction of muscle fibers and are involved in the development of high blood pressure. Deficiencies of these two minerals can contribute to elevating pressure, and correcting those deficiencies can bring the pressure down. Our program encourages you to eat foods that will provide plenty of dietary calcium and magnesium: nuts, legumes, green vegetables, seafood, liver, beef, egg yolks, cabbage, cauliflower, and dairy products. Especially if you do not regularly eat these foods, you should supplement calcium and magnesium in your diet as described in the list of general vitamin and mineral supplement products at the end of this chapter.

Eating a diet richer in protein and fat increases your ability to absorb calcium and to some extent magnesium, and that is fortunate; as you exercise on this nutritional regimen to build your lean body mass, your demand for these minerals will increase.

Selenium: Powerful Immune Booster

This mineral antioxidant works in conjunction with the antioxidant vitamin E to produce the body's own natural free-radical scavenger and potent protective antioxidant, glutathione. This body chemical promotes a healthy immune system to defend you from infection, may protect you from the development of cancers, and helps to slow down the aging process. Deficiency of selenium may also contribute to elevated cholesterol.

Our program provides you with the opportunity to eat plenty of the best dietary sources of selenium: seafood, organ meats, and muscle meats. Seeds may contain selenium, but it depends on the selenium content of the soil where they grew. Fruits and vegetables contain little of it. And that means, again, that vegetarians using our program to correct their insulin-related disorders (especially elevated cholesterol) will have to rely on supplemental selenium.

Potassium: Another Balancing Act

When you begin our program, your insulin will fall quickly, and perhaps the first corrective phenomenon you will notice is water loss. The metabolic changes will send a strong signal to your kidneys to release excess sodium and water. Although sodium release is the main goal, another salt, potassium, gets caught in the cross fire. During the initial phases—especially the first few weeks and especially on Phase I—your loss of potassium in urine will accelerate dramatically. If you engage in vigorous physical exercise and sweat profusely, you will lose additional potassium. If your potassium levels fall too low, you can suffer from weakness, muscle cramping, fatigue, and breathlessness.

The potassium level in your blood must stay within a fairly narrow range for potassium to play its crucial role in the passage of nerve impulses, in muscle contraction, and in maintaining normal blood pressure. It exists mainly inside the cells of your body, and this huge reservoir acts as a buffer to keep the amount in your blood relatively constant under normal circumstances. But the rapid loss of excess fluid you will experience during the early phase of the program is not a normal circumstance. Even eating foods rich in potassium—such as cantaloupe, avocado, broccoli, liver, dairy products, and citrus fruits—may not sufficiently replace your losses. For this reason we ask that you take one or two capsules of any of the products in the following list or any commercially available product that will provide at least 90 mg of potassium salts. You can also use the over-the-counter salt substitutes (Morton's Lite Salt or NoSalt brand, both of which are potassium salts) to ensure you get plenty.

If you currently take medication for high blood pressure or fluid retention, be certain to check with your physician or pharmacist before you supplement potassium. Certain of the newer medications on the market for these conditions actually prevent potassium loss and could cause your potassium level to rise too much. Just as too low a potassium level can cause problems, so can a level that's too high. Once the program does its work, you may not have to take blood pressure medication any longer, but wait until your physician tells you it's safe to stop. And remember to check for a possible interaction.

Acceptable Products Include:

Twinlab—Potassium Aspartate (99 mg)
Twinlab—Liquid K Plus (99 mg)
Source Naturals K-Mag Aspartate (99 mg)
Alacer—The K Factors (92 mg)
KAL—KCL (99 mg)

In Search of an Excellent Vitamin and Mineral Supplement

When we looked for a high-quality complete multiple vitamin and mineral supplement to recommend to our patients, we wanted a supplement combination that would—even in the face of finicky eating, unusual taste preferences, or philosophical or religious restrictions—provide sufficiently for all of our patients' micronutrient needs. If you're searching for one on your own, look for one that approximates this list:

The Vitamins

Beta-carotene (for vitamin A)	25,000 IU
Vitamin D_3	50 IU
Ascorbic acid (vitamin C)	1,000 mg
Thiamine (vitamin B_1)	100 mg
Riboflavin (vitamin B_2)	10 mg
Niacin (vitamin B_3)	30 mg
Niacinamide	130 mg
Pantothenic acid (vitamin B_5)	450 mg
Pyridoxine (vitamin B_6)	15 mg
Cobalamin (vitamin B_{12})	250 mcg*
Folic acid	2 mg
D-alpha tocopherol (vitamin E)	200 IU

---

* Micrograms (1/1,000 of a milligram)

The Minerals

(These should be as amino acid chelates; look for the minerals bound to picolinate, citrate-maleate, aspartate, etc.) A typical example might look as follows:

Calcium (citrate-maleate)	500 mg
Magnesium (citrate-maleate)	250 mg
Potassium (citrate-maleate)	90 mg
Zinc (picolinate)	15 mg
Manganese (picolinate)	15 mg
Boron (picolinate)	3 mg
Copper (picolinate)	1 mg

Chromium (niacin bound)	200 mcg*
Selenium (picolinate)	200 mcg
Molybdenum (picolinate)	100 mcg
Vanadium (picolinate)	100 mcg

* Micrograms (1/1,000 of a milligram)

Acceptable Products Include:

KAL—High Potency Soft Multiple Vitamin

Twinlab—Dual Tab Sustained Release Mega Vitamin and Mineral Formula

Mega Food Multiple Vitamin and Mineral

Thorne Research Laboratories—Basic Nutrients V capsules (available only through medical professionals)

The Bottom Line

Your body relies on certain vitamins and minerals to work properly, to lose fat and build muscle effectively, and to remain healthy. To ensure that your diet always meets or exceeds these requirements, we encourage you to take a vitamin and chelated mineral supplement similar to the products we described here every day.

Chapter 9

Assessing Your Risk

Middle age is when your age starts to show around the middle.

BOB HOPE

Now that you've seen the scientific and historical evidence to support it, you may be saying, "Okay, I'm convinced—hyperinsulinemia and insulin resistance are at the root of the major diseases of Western civilization, but what's that mean to me?" Good question. How can you know if it applies to you? How do you determine your risk for these disorders? You can begin in just the way we begin when a patient comes to us for help in losing weight, controlling cholesterol or triglycerides, or treating diabetic problems: by looking into your own and your family's medical history. Simply knowing the kinds of problems you or members of your family have suffered will shed light on your risk for insulin-related disorders.

Take this medical history quiz to find out more:

Score 20 points if you:

• have adult-onset diabetes or developed diabetes during pregnancy

Score 10 points for each *yes* response if you:

• have elevated triglycerides
• have a *low* level of HDL ("good") cholesterol
• are overweight mainly around your middle

Score 5 points for each *yes* response if you:

• have high blood pressure
• are overweight mostly in your legs and hips

- have elevated cholesterol
- retain fluid
- crave sugar and starchy foods

Score 3 points for each parent with a *yes* response:

- has/had high blood pressure
- has/had heart disease
- has/had adult-onset diabetes

Check your scores against the following totals to assess your risk:

- Less than 10: low risk for developing insulin problems
- 10 to 15: moderate risk for insulin problems
- 15 to 20: high risk for insulin problems
- 20 or more: you very likely *have* an insulin disorder

While your history points up your risk, laboratory tests confirm these suspicions and assess the extent of your metabolic disturbance and your overall state of health. Blood tests and other such measurements also give you a benchmark against which to track your progress as you heal yourself nutritionally. What kind of testing do we recommend?

The Laboratory Evaluation of Risk

With the help of your physician you should have a battery of fasting laboratory tests performed. In preparation for your blood tests, you should eat no solid food and drink no liquids other than water for a minimum of eight to ten hours beforehand. If you take medications, please check with your physician for instructions on which medicines to take prior to your tests. The easiest time to have your blood work done is first thing in the morning after an overnight fast, rather than trying to fast throughout the day. Ask your doctor to perform the following tests:

SERUM INSULIN

The handling of this test is very important. The specimen should be kept frozen and the test completed within 24 hours of the blood draw. Be sure that the test is performed by a national reference laboratory, such as

Smith-Kline, Roche Biomedical, or Nichols, or by a research laboratory accustomed to doing this test. Results can vary widely—even from the same specimen—if it's not handled properly. Remember that even though most laboratories will set values of over 25 to 30 as abnormally high, the "normal" samples include many people with insulin resistance who have not yet developed diabetes. General clinical evaluation of insulin levels as a marker for disease is still in its infancy. In our clinic, as in many research settings, we use the fasting insulin normal values of healthy young people as the standard against which we should measure ourselves. If your insulin reading is over 10 mU/ml you can consider yourself to have developed some degree of insulin resistance. The more over 10 your reading, the greater your disturbance. With 10 as the upper end of normal, a reading of 25 would mean that it's taking $2^1/2$ times the normal amount of insulin to control blood sugar at its current level. A reading of 48 would mean it's taking over $4^1/2$ times more insulin to keep blood sugar at its current level. If your insulin reading is high, repeat the test at eight weeks and at eight-week intervals thereafter during your intervention regimen until normal.

SMA-24 OR CHEMISTRY PROFILE

This battery of tests goes by a variety of names but usually includes blood glucose, the electrolytes (sodium, potassium, chloride, bicarbonate), measures of heart, liver, and kidney function, uric acid, cholesterol, and sometimes triglycerides. Important points to note:

1. *Your blood sugar level:* If your fasting level is greater than 115 mg/dl, you are already starting to lose blood sugar control. It's also important to note how much insulin it's taking to keep your blood sugar at its current level. The ratio of blood sugar (measured in mg/dl) divided by insulin should be greater than 7. If your ratio is less than 7, you are developing or have developed insulin resistance. (A level of over 7 doesn't clear you, however.) To assess your progress, repeat this test at eight weeks and every eight weeks thereafter until normal.

2. *Your potassium level:* If it's at or below the bottom of the normal range, you must be very aware of the need to supplement your diet with extra potassium unless you take blood pressure medications that could interact with it. (Ask your doctor or pharmacist.) If your level was low initially, repeat after one week of extra supplementation to see if your level has returned to normal. If still low, double your supplementation and repeat weekly until your level is normal again.

3. Your kidney function tests: If normal, you should have no problem handling any protein intake level. If your tests show kidney damage, you probably already know that you suffer from kidney problems. In that case you should not eat more protein than your minimum daily protein requirement. If your values were abnormal, repeat this test in six to eight weeks. You should see improvement in these values, or at least they should be no worse. If they are worse, discontinue the program.

4. Your liver function tests: Often people with an unrecognized insulin-related disorder will show mild to moderate elevations in some of their liver enzymes. This elevation usually occurs because of fat deposits' being laid down within the liver itself. If this is the case for you, you should see these test numbers return to normal as you proceed through your nutritional program. If your liver tests were abnormal, your physician should repeat them after you've been on the program for about eight weeks and at eight-week intervals until they are normal again. If your alkaline phosphatase (one of the liver tests) was abnormal, it could be a sign of gallbladder disease, which often occurs in people with insulin-related problems. If you still have your gallbladder and this test result is elevated, you should have a gallbladder ultrasound to be certain you don't have gallstones.

5. Cholesterol and triglycerides: See "Lipid Profile," below.

6. Uric acid: This test helps to assess your risk for gout, which frequently afflicts people with insulin-related problems. If this value is high and you do not currently suffer from gout, count yourself lucky. The reading should improve as you progress through the diet. Repeat the test at eight weeks for high readings.

LIPID PROFILE

This test subdivides the blood fats into their various components of total cholesterol, triglycerides, VLDL cholesterol, LDL cholesterol, and HDL cholesterol. The most telling indicators of insulin-related problems are elevation of triglycerides and a low HDL cholesterol, but you may also discover elevated VLDL and LDL cholesterol as well. Whatever the actual cholesterol numbers, as stated in Chapter 7, what's most important in assessment of heart disease risk is the ratio of your total cholesterol to the HDL "good" cholesterol. If you divide your total cholesterol number (in mg/dl) by the HDL number, your ratio should be 4 or less. If your ratio is above 4, you should consider yourself at increased risk for heart disease. As you progress through our nutritional program, these readings should improve. You should see a sharp, rapid drop in triglycerides, accompanied by a decrease in your total cholesterol–to–HDL ratio. Reevaluate these readings at eight weeks if they were elevated. If you are on medication to lower cholesterol or triglycerides, your doctor will need to evaluate them sooner (at about three or four weeks) and will probably need to reduce the doses of your medication. Following the readings at three- to four-week intervals, your doctor will most likely be able to wean you slowly off your medication as you regain metabolic control. Repeat the lipid tests after you've been off your medication for eight weeks and stable on your diet during that time and then every six months to one year thereafter.

Hemoglobin A_1c

This test measures the amount of the red blood cell pigment hemoglobin that has been bound to blood sugar. The reaction that binds these two together is irreversible and depends on how much sugar is in the blood. Because red blood cells remain in circulation for about 90 to 120 days before they are removed and recycled, this test gives us a way to measure what your blood sugar has been *on average* for the last 30 to 60 days. In this test the lower your number, the better. Even if your reading falls within what the laboratory deems as "normal," you must remember that these normals include many people with insulin resistance, which shifts the levels upward. If your reading is outside the laboratory's normal, consider yourself already very insulin resistant. If you fall within the normal range, assess yourself according to the scale that follows.

Take note of the top and bottom of the normal range for Hgb A_1c for the laboratory your physician used. Determine the average value for that lab by adding the high value and the low value and dividing by 2. The middle of the range (this average number) represents an average blood sugar reading of 100. Each tenth of a point above that average correlates with 4 additional blood sugar points in mg/dl. In our lab, a reading of 5 is the average Hgb A_1c reading. Based on that average, the following scale would apply:

4.0 = 60	4.5 = 80	5.0 = 100	5.5 = 120
4.1 = 64	4.6 = 84	5.1 = 104	5.6 = 124
4.2 = 68	4.7 = 88	5.2 = 108	5.7 = 128
4.3 = 72	4.8 = 92	5.3 = 112	5.8 = 132
4.4 = 76	4.9 = 96	5.4 = 116	5.9 = 136

6.0 = 140	6.5 = 160	7.0 = 180	7.5 = 200
6.1 = 144	6.6 = 164	7.1 = 184	7.6 = 204
6.2 = 148	6.7 = 168	7.2 = 188	7.7 = 208
6.3 = 152	6.8 = 172	7.3 = 192	7.8 = 212
6.4 = 156	6.9 = 176	7.4 - 196	7.9 = 216

12-LEAD ELECTROCARDIOGRAM

Any dietary change, but especially this regimen, will result in a sometimes dramatic loss of water and electrolytes such as sodium and potassium. In people who have certain abnormal heart rhythm patterns such an abrupt change could be dangerous.[1] Although most people don't have these problems, it's wise to check first. Your physician can determine if your heart rhythm and the heart's electrical function are normal by checking the heart tracings of a standard electrocardiogram (EKG). A normal electrocardiogram within the last year or two, unless you've had any heart problems in the meantime, should be sufficient to assure you're not at risk for this kind of rhythm problem.

URINALYSIS

This test checks for sugar in your urine—a strong indicator of diabetes—but also to make certain that you don't have any blood or protein (signs of possible kidney damage) or signs of urinary infection that might blossom under the stress of a dietary change.

COMPLETE BLOOD COUNT (CBC)

This test evaluates your red blood cells for number, size, and shape to uncover anemias and your white blood cells for number and type to assess your immune function. Some nutritional clues from the CBC include (1) large, pale red blood cells indicate a need for more B vitamins, especially B_{12}; and (2) small, pale red blood cells may indicate iron deficiency. If you are anemic or your white blood count is abnormal, your physician needs to evaluate these problems fully before you make any nutritional changes.

---

[1] If your heart rhythm is abnormal, you will need to approach this program with great care, slowly reducing your carbohydrate intake in 20-gram/day drops from your current level to the level recommended in the phases described in Chapter 10 over a period of several weeks instead of making the dramatic drop we normally suggest. This method, while more difficult, will allow you to slowly waste your excess body fluid. You must stay in close contact with your physician during this time.

THYROID PANEL

Evaluation of your thyroid gland activity is important if you're over-weight, have high cholesterol, retain fluid, or have no energy. Trying to correct these problems in the face of low thyroid function is quite diffi-cult. Your evaluation should include levels for thyroid hormone (at least T_3, free T_4) and a high-sensitivity TSH, the brain stimulator that signals to the thyroid gland that it needs to make more hormone. Even in the face of normal thyroid hormone levels, if your TSH is elevated, your brain is saying you need more thyroid activity. If this is the case, your physician will need to prescribe supplemental thyroid hormone in a dose adequate to normalize your readings. Repeated testing at eight-week in-tervals will help your doctor know what the "right" level is for you and to adjust your dose accordingly.

If you currently take medication for any of the insulin-related disor-ders, you may want to take the following note to your doctor.

To Our Physician Colleagues:

Your patient has brought this note to your attention after reading our book, *Protein Power*, about how to control insulin-related disorders by nutritional means. We have used these methods to successfully treat these conditions in our own clinical practice for nearly a decade.

Hypertension: Using these dietary guidelines, your hypertensive patients will rapidly reduce blood pressure, so quickly in fact that if they currently take di-uretic medications you will need to taper and discontinue these medications quickly when the patients begin the intervention protocol. You can taper and withdraw other classes of antihypertensives, such as ACE inhibitors, calcium channel blockers, or beta blockers more slowly, monitoring their blood pressure response weekly over a three- to four-week period. In rare cases diet alone will not control their blood pressure, and in these cases your best choice is a small dose of ACE inhibitor, calcium channel blocker, or alpha agonist. None of these medications elevate insulin, whereas the beta blockers and thiazide diuretics do.

If blood pressure fails to normalize, or if it normalizes and then returns to an elevated level (this is more common in very overweight people), the cause may be an excess of arachidonic acid coming into circulation from fat breakdown. If the patient can take aspirin, place him or her on low-dose aspirin therapy to block the production of series two prostaglandins from arachidonic acid. One-half aspirin per day is enough.

Fluid Retention: Usually fluid retention disappears quickly. If it remains, however, and you need to diurese the patient, choose a loop diuretic, such as Bumex or Lasix in tiny doses, taken along with an extra potassium supplement (such as Micro-K 10). Again, because the thiazides cause elevation of insulin, their use in fluid retention would be counterproductive.

Hyperlipidemias: Because of insulin's stimulation in cholesterol synthesis (stimulation of HMG CoA Reductase in the rate-limiting step), correction of insulin resistance through dietary reduction of carbohydrates will quickly bring elevated LDL, VLDL, and total cholesterol back to normal. With the regimen and exercise, HDL remains unchanged or often rises. Triglycerides fall sharply and quickly. If your patients are on lipid-lowering agents, you will likely be able to taper them over the next several weeks and in all probability discontinue them in compliant patients. Reduce the doses incrementally (we usually halve them) and after three to four weeks check lipid levels and drop again if indicated. We've seen this regimen return cholesterol readings of over 600 and triglyceride readings of over 3,000 to normal in three weeks. The metabolic power of the right nutritional regimen for this condition is startling.

Adult-Onset Diabetes Mellitus: In patients on no medications, the regimen will return their blood sugar readings to normal in a few weeks. In patients taking oral hypoglycemic agents, you will need to keep in close contact to help taper their medication doses during the first week or two. In most cases by three weeks they will be off all oral agents for sugar control if they carefully follow the intervention protocol. We usually halve their dose the first full day on the plan, then halve it again the next. The patient should be well versed in the use of a glucometer and should take his or her blood sugar readings frequently during this period. Some patients respond so rapidly that we can totally eliminate their medication in a few days if they comply with the regimen.

You will need to watch your adult-onset patients who take insulin very closely. Before these patients can begin the protocol, we always check a C peptide level (not a fasting insulin since that would measure what they inject as well as any beta cell production) to see just how much native insulin they're making. If they've got a good solid amount of C peptide, then the problem is truly one of insulin resistance; they will respond quite well, and you will very likely be able to work their insulin dose down to zero in time as long as they adhere to the regimen.

In patients who make little C peptide, the regimen will definitely improve their health, help to restore balance to their metabolic hormones, and you will be able to reduce their doses of insulin significantly. But you won't be able to eliminate insulin entirely, since their beta cells have "burned out" or been otherwise damaged. This regimen works so dramatically to improve sugar control that you must be close at hand to interpret blood sugar changes and help your diabetic patients adjust their insulin doses accordingly.

If you have questions about managing your patients with insulin-related disorders on this regimen, please feel free to contact us at our office: 11025 Anderson Road, Suite 130, Little Rock, AR 72212.

Michael R. Eades, M.D., and Mary Dan Eades, M.D.

The Other Half of the Risk Factor: Are You an Apple or a Pear?

We don't care what you weigh! That may seem like a strange statement for two doctors who devote their clinical time to health, nutrition, weight loss, and fitness. But in fact what you weigh is not as important as what your weight is made of—how much is lean and how much fat. So we'll give you an easy method to determine your body composition. You'll be able to calculate how many of your pounds are active lean tissue (muscle, organs, hair, skin, nails, skeleton, and water) and how many pounds are fat so that you can assess your nutritional requirements and have a realistic estimate of where you're beginning as well as a good tool to track your progress. We'll also give you some guidelines to help you set a healthy goal for recomposing your body to new lean, healthy fat-to-muscle percentages.

Although being overfat is an important health risk, *where* you carry your fat is even more important. If you likened your shape to that of a fruit, would you call yourself an apple, with most of your weight around your middle? Or are you more like a pear, with the weight aggregated mostly in your hips and thighs?

When your body stores fat in the abdominal region—the apple distribution—it doesn't lay the fat down just under the skin around the abdomen and waist but also inside the abdominal cavity, around the heart, liver, kidneys, and intestine and even within these organs. This apple-shaped fat pattern occurs most frequently in men, and for that reason you may have heard it referred to as an android or male fat distribution. But since this pattern is not exclusive to men, we prefer to use the more accurately descriptive term *abdominal fat*. Although many women also develop this apple shape, more often women store their excess body fat in the pear-shaped pattern: slimmer in the chest and upper body, with the main accumulation of fat around their hips and thighs—what's been called the female or gynoid pattern. And again, since some men take on this pear shape, too, we'll simply call it *hip and leg fat* for the sake of clarity.

Insulin has a much greater influence on the fat cells in the abdominal area, and for this reason people who suffer from faulty insulin metabolism and who develop insulin resistance are more likely to store abdominal fat and take on the apple shape. Because excess insulin strongly drives the storage here, excess abdominal fat carries with it a greater risk for all the insulin-related metabolic problems: high blood pressure, elevated cholesterol, heart disease, and diabetes. Recognize that storing the fat in the abdominal region doesn't *cause* these problems; it's simply another symptom of the underlying metabolic disorder, insulin resistance.

Hip and leg fat, on the other hand, is less a consequence of underlying metabolic disorder. That is not to say there is no connection; fat cells throughout the body respond to insulin's signal to store fat. But the storage here is deposited primarily underneath the skin (subcutaneous fat) and marbles the muscles of the hips and legs. In these areas, which are outside the major body cavities, there are no vital organs for fat deposits to surround and infiltrate. For these reasons excess fat accumulation that stays confined to the hip and leg region doesn't carry with it the increased risk to health that comes with excess abdominal fat. Usually, however, if the fat accumulation continues long enough, the pear-shaped body will finally begin to store abdominal fat, too, and then the same host of insulin-related metabolic problems begins to arise. Often blood pressure goes up a little, then cholesterol, triglycerides, and finally blood sugar. For many women who have carried hip and leg fat for much of their lives and seemed perfectly healthy otherwise, these additional health problems may not occur until after the child-bearing years but then come on with a vengeance as menopause approaches.

The Waist-to-Hip Ratio

Sometimes just looking at your shape in silhouette will tell you volumes about where you store your fat, but it's not always so straightforward. Modern technological wizardry has given us a tool to look within—computerized tomography, the CAT scan—that enables researchers to see in pictures where the fat deposits accumulate and how deceptive external appearances can be. But CAT scans are very expensive, so they're not a practical tool for gauging fat distribution in the general public. Although there is no method more accurate, there are many less costly, and later in this chapter, we give you a method that doesn't require expensive equipment or physician interpretation and doesn't carry the $1000 price tag of a CAT scan. For the purpose of illustration, however, we can use representative CAT scanning studies to help you better understand the various ways that fat can deposit. Refer to Figure 9.1. These figures are photo reproductions of four CAT photographs that show us what we would see if we could cut a person in half and look end on at the fat, the muscle, the bone, and the organs. Figure A represents an "average" healthy subject, figure B is a very lean trained athlete, figure

C an apple-shaped person who stores fat inside the abdominal cavity, and figure D a pear-shaped person who lays down fat mainly in the hips and legs. In these instances the total body weight might be the same in subjects A and B and in subjects C and D, but as you can see, what makes up the weight can be vastly different. The body fat percentages may be identical in subjects C and D, but the location of the excess means that subject C, with the abdominal pattern, will have a higher risk for developing elevated blood pressure, cholesterol, triglycerides, and blood sugar.

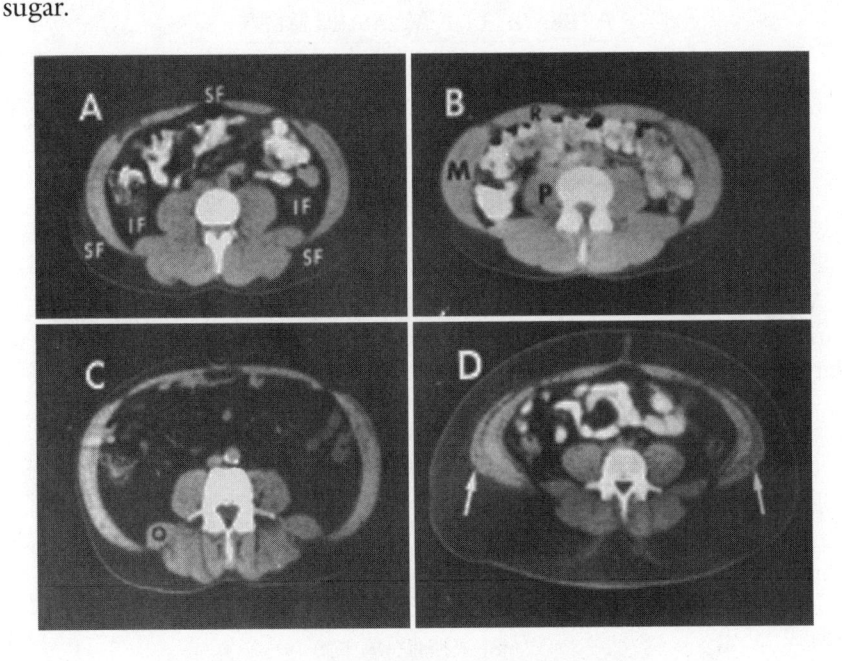

FIGURE 9. 1 DIFFERENCES IN FAT DISTRIBUTION

(IF = intra-abdominal fat   SF = fat beneath the skin   M = muscles.)

To determine your own waist-to-hip ratio—a good estimate of storage pattern—you will need only a standard cloth tape measure, a pencil, and paper. Measure your waist at the level of your navel and your hips at their widest point. To ensure accuracy in measuring, measure directly on your skin, not over clothing. Also keep the tape level and snug, but not pinching your skin. Take each measurement three times and average the numbers. Hang on to these numbers; you'll need the measurements and averages again later, when you compute your body composition.

AVERAGE WAIST MEASUREMENT

Waist #1 _____ inches

Waist #2 _____

Waist #3 _____

Total ÷ 3 = _____ inches

AVERAGE HIP MEASUREMENT

Hip #1 _____ inches

Hip #2 _____

Hip #3 _____

Total ÷ 3 = _____ inches

With these two numbers you can easily determine your waist-to-hip ratio by dividing the average waist measurement by the average hip measurement.

avg. waist measurement ÷ avg. hip measurement = _____

Refer to the following waist-to-hip ratio chart to determine your pattern.

WAIST-TO-HIP RATIOS		
Male	less than 1	hip and leg pattern
	1 or greater	abdominal pattern
Female	0.8 or less	hip and leg pattern
	greater than 0.8	abdominal pattern

If you find yourself (or your loved ones) among the apples, storing fat in the abdominal region, even if you are not currently excessively overweight and do not yet suffer from high blood pressure, elevated cholesterol or triglycerides, or blood sugar problems, you should consider yourself at risk for these insulin-related disorders. Following this program now will help to ensure that you preserve your health. If you already suffer from one or more of these disorders, then reducing abdominal fat stores becomes even more important.

You can use this measurement tool to track your progress as you proceed through the intervention phase. Men should strive to bring their waist-to-hip ratio to 1 or less, and women with apple shapes should aim for 0.8 or less. If your shape is pearlike, while you will still want to strive for a properly composed body to optimize your health, your risk of serious metabolic disorders is lower. Now that you've determined your pattern of storage, let's take a look at an equally simple method for assessing what your weight is made of—the lean and fat of you. This method requires the pencil and cloth tape measure you used before, a reasonably accurate scale, and the charts and worksheets provided.

What's Your Body Composition?

Determining Your Body Fat

The first step in determining your composition is to calculate your body fat as a percentage of your total weight. Refer now to the worksheet for computing your percentage of body fat. (The calculations vary with gender, so make sure you're using the appropriate one for you and follow the instructions. We'll take each gender in turn.)

For Women:

1. Measure your height in inches without shoes.

2. Using the measurements you made before, record your height, waist, and hip measurements in the labeled spaces on the worksheet on page 140.

3. Turn to the conversion constants chart for women and find each of these average measurements in the appropriate column. Record the adjacent constants (A for hips, B for abdomen, and C for height) on the worksheet where indicated. These constants have been derived experimentally and allow you to convert your measurements into a form that can be used to compute your body fat percentage.

WOMEN:
COMPUTING YOUR BODY FAT PERCENTAGE

First, find your average measurements IN INCHES:

	Hips	Abdomen	Height
Measurement #1	_____	_____	_____
+			
Measurement #2	_____	_____	
+			
Measurement #3	_____	_____	
Total =	_____	_____	
Divide by 3 =	_____	_____	_____

4. Using the chart that follows, look up each of these average measurements and your height in the appropriate column. The numbers listed beside them will be constant A (hips), constant B (abdomen), and constant C (height). Use these constants below. Add constants A and B, then subtract constant C from their sum. Round your answer to the nearest whole number. This figure is your percentage of body fat.

Add together _____ Constant A (hips)

+_____ Constant B (abdomen)

Total_____

Subtract − _____ Constant C (height)

_____ = your percentage of body fat

CONVERSION CONSTANTS TO PREDICT PERCENTAGE OF BODY FAT—
WOMEN

HIPS		ABDOMEN		HEIGHT	
INCHES	CONSTANT A	INCHES	CONSTANT B	INCHES	CONSTANT C
30	33.48	20	14.22	55	33.52
30.5	33.83	20.5	14.40	55.5	33.67
31	34.87	21	14.93	56	34.13
31.5	35.22	21.5	15.11	56.5	34.28
32	36.27	22	15.64	57	34.74
32.5	36.62	22.5	15.82	57.5	34.89
33	37.67	23	16.35	58	35.35
33.5	38.02	23.5	16.53	58.5	35.50
34	39.06	24	17.06	59	35.96
34.5	39.41	24.5	17.24	59.5	36.11
35	40.46	25	17.78	60	36.57
35.5	40.81	25.5	17.96	60.5	36.72
36	41.86	26	18.49	61	37.18
36.5	42.21	26.5	18.67	61.5	37.33
37	43.25	27	19.20	62	37.79
37.5	43.60	27.5	19.38	62.5	37.94
38	44.65	28	19.91	63	38.40
38.5	45.00	28.5	20.09	63.5	38.55
39	46.05	29	20.62	64	39.01
39.5	46.40	29.5	20.80	64.5	39.16
40	47.44	30	21.33	65	39.62
40.5	47.79	30.5	21.51	65.5	39.77
41	48.84	31	22.04	66	40.23
41.5	49.19	31.5	22.22	66.5	40.38
42	50.24	32	22.75	67	40.84
42.5	50.59	32.5	22.93	67.5	40.99
43	51.64	33	23.46	68	41.45
43.5	51.99	33.5	23.64	68.5	41.60
44	53.03	34	24.18	69	42.06
44.5	53.41	34.5	24.36	69.5	42.21
45	54.53	35	24.89	70	42.67
45.5	54.86	35.5	25.07	70.5	42.82
46	55.83	36	25.60	71	43.28
46.5	56.18	36.5	25.78	71.5	43.43
47	57.22	37	26.31	72	43.89
47.5	57.57	37.5	26.49	72.5	44.04
48	58.62	38	27.02	73	44.50
48.5	58.97	38.5	27.20	73.5	44.65
49	60.02	39	27.73	74	45.11
49.5	60.37	39.5	27.91	74.5	45.26
50	61.42	40	28.44	75	45.72
50.5	61.77	40.5	28.62	75.5	45.87
51	62.81	41	29.15	76	46.32
51.5	63.16	41.5	29.33	76.5	46.47
52	64.21	42	29.87	77	46.93
52.5	64.56	42.5	30.05	77.5	47.08
53	65.61	43	30.58	78	47.54
53.5	65.96	43.5	30.76	78.5	47.69
54	67.00	44	31.29	79	48.15
54.5	67.35	44.5	31.47	79.5	48.30
55	68.40	45	32.00	80	48.76
55.5	68.75	45.5	32.18	80.5	48.91
56	69.80	46	32.71	81	49.37
56.5	70.15	46.5	32.89	81.5	49.52
57	71.19	47	33.42	82	49.98
57.5	71.54	47.5	33.60	82.5	50.13
58	72.59	48	34.13	83	50.59
58.5	72.94	48.5	34.31	83.5	50.74
59	73.99	49	34.84	84	51.20
59.5	74.34	49.5	35.02	84.5	51.35
60	75.39	50	35.56	85	51.81

Let's look at how one patient computed her body fat percentage. Lisa is 5'6" and weighs 157 pounds. She measured her hips at 38.5", 38", and 38.5". Her average hip measurement is 38.3 inches. (Calculate as follows: 38.5 + 38 + 38.5 = 115, and 115 ÷ 3 = 38.3.) Lisa should round the hip measurement down to 38. Her abdomen measurements are 27", 26.5", and 27.75" for an average abdominal measurement of 27.08", rounded to 27. Turning to the conversion constants chart, she will find her hip measurement (38) and to its right constant A (44.65), then her abdominal measurement (27) and to its right constant B (19.20), and finally her height (66 inches) and to its right constant C (40.23). Following the worksheet, she will now add constants A and B (44.65 + 19.20 = 63.85), and from that number she will subtract constant C (63.85 − 40.23 = 23.62). Lisa's body fat is 23.6 percent.

FOR MEN:

1. Measure your wrist at the space between your hand and your wrist bone, where your wrist bends. Keep the tape snug, but do not compress the skin. Take three measurements for your wrist, record them on the worksheet, and compute the average.

2. Weigh yourself on a scale in pounds and record the weight in the appropriate space on the worksheet. Record the waist measurement you made earlier for the waist-to-hip ratio.

3. Subtract your average wrist measurement from your average waist measurement. Find this number listed as waist-minus-wrist across the top of the body fat calculation chart for men. On the left side of this table, find your weight. Follow across from your weight and down from your waist-minus-wrist measurement. Where these two columns intersect, you will find your body fat percentage. Let's work through an example using these worksheets and charts.

Mark weighs 200 pounds. He takes the following wrist measurements: 6.5", 6.75", and 6.75" for an average wrist measurement of 6.67". (Calculate as follows: 6.5 + 6.75 + 6.75 = 6.7.) His waist (abdomen) measurements are 38", 37.75", and 38.25" for an average of 38 inches. (Compute as follows: 38 + 37.75 + 38.25 = 114, and 114 ÷ 3 = 38.) Mark will subtract his wrist measure from his waist (38 − 6.7 = 31.3) and round to the nearest one-half. Then he will find his waist-minus-wrist number (31) across the top of the conversion constants chart. Tracking down the left side of the chart, he will find his weight (200 pounds), and he will follow across to the column under his measure of 31 to find the number 22. Mark has a body fat percentage of 22 percent.

MEN:
COMPUTING YOUR BODY FAT PERCENTAGE

First, find your average measurements IN INCHES or POUNDS:

	Wrist	Waist	Weight
Measurement #1	_____	_____	_____
Measurement #2	_____	_____	
Measurement #3	_____	_____	
Total =	_____	_____	
Divide by 3 =	_____	_____	
Waist measurement	_____		
Minus wrist measurement –	_____		
	_____ = "waist minus wrist"		

Using the waist-minus-wrist chart, find your weight in pounds in the left column. Find your "waist minus wrist" number across the top of the chart. Going across from the left and down from the top, find the point at which these two readings intersect. This figure represents your percentage of body fat:

_____ = percentage of body fat

Calculating Your Lean Body Weight

Now that you've got a good estimate of your body fat percentage, you can use this number to compute your lean body weight. Because the body is made of two basic segments—fat weight and lean weight—if you know how much you weigh and what percent of your weight is fat, you can determine how much your lean tissue weighs.

First, take your weight in pounds and multiply it by your percentage

WAIST MINUS WRIST (IN INCHES) Weight in lbs.	22	22.5	23	23.5	24	24.5	25	25.5	26	26.5	27	27.5	28	28.5	29	29.5	30	30.5	31
120 :	4	6	8	10	12	14	16	18	20	21	23	25	27	29	31	33	35	37	39
125 :	4	6	7	9	11	13	15	17	19	20	22	24	26	28	30	32	33	35	37
130 :	3	5	7	9	11	12	14	16	18	20	21	23	25	27	28	30	32	34	36
135 :	3	5	7	8	10	12	14	15	17	19	20	22	24	26	27	29	31	32	34
140 :	3	5	6	8	10	11	13	15	16	18	19	21	22	24	26	28	29	31	33
145 :	3	4	6	7	9	11	12	14	15	17	19	20	22	23	25	27	28	30	31
150 :	2	4	6	7	9	10	12	13	15	16	18	19	21	23	24	26	27	29	30
155 :	2	4	5	6	8	10	11	13	14	16	17	19	20	22	23	25	26	28	29
160 :	2	4	5	6	8	9	11	12	14	15	17	18	19	21	22	24	25	27	28
165 :	2	3	5	6	8	9	10	12	13	15	16	17	19	20	22	23	24	26	27
170 :	2	3	4	6	7	9	10	11	13	14	16	17	18	20	21	22	24	25	26
175 :	2	3	4	6	7	8	10	11	12	14	15	16	17	19	20	21	23	24	25
180 :	1	3	4	5	7	8	9	10	12	13	14	16	17	18	19	21	22	23	25
185 :	1	3	3	5	6	8	9	10	11	13	14	15	16	18	19	20	21	23	24
190 :	1	2	3	5	6	7	8	10	11	12	13	15	16	17	19	20	21	22	23
195 :	1	2	3	4	5	7	8	9	11	12	13	14	15	16	18	19	20	21	22
200 :	1	2	3	4	6	7	8	9	10	11	12	14	15	16	17	18	19	21	22

WAIST MINUS WRIST : (IN INCHES)

Weight in lbs.	22	22.5	23	23.5	24	24.5	25	25.5	26	26.5	27	27.5	28	28.5	29	29.5	30	30.5	31
205	1	2	3	4	5	6	8	9	10	11	12	13	15	16	17	18	19	20	21
210	1	2	3	4	5	6	8	9	10	11	12	13	14	15	16	17	18	19	21
215	1	2	3	4	5	6	7	8	9	10	11	12	13	15	16	17	18	19	20
220	0	2	3	4	5	6	7	8	9	10	11	12	13	14	15	16	17	18	20
225	0	2	3	4	5	6	7	8	9	10	11	12	13	14	15	16	17	18	19
230	0	1	2	3	4	5	6	7	9	10	11	12	13	14	15	16	17	18	19
235	0	1	2	3	4	5	6	7	8	10	11	12	13	14	15	16	16	17	18
240	0	1	2	3	4	5	6	7	8	9	10	11	12	13	14	15	16	17	18
245	0	1	2	3	4	5	6	7	8	9	10	11	12	13	14	15	16	16	17
250	0	1	2	3	4	5	6	7	8	9	10	11	12	13	14	14	15	16	17
255	0	1	2	3	3	5	6	6	7	8	9	11	12	13	13	14	15	16	17
260	0	1	2	3	4	4	5	6	7	8	9	10	11	12	13	14	15	15	16
265	0	1	2	3	4	4	5	6	7	8	9	10	11	12	13	13	14	15	16
270	0	1	1	2	3	4	5	6	7	7	8	9	10	11	12	13	13	14	15
275	0	0	1	2	3	4	5	5	6	7	8	9	10	11	11	12	13	14	15
280	0	0	1	2	3	4	4	5	6	7	8	9	9	10	11	12	13	14	14
285	0	0	1	2	3	3	4	5	6	7	7	8	9	10	11	12	13	13	14
290	0	0	1	2	2	3	4	5	6	6	7	8	9	10	11	12	12	13	14
295	0	0	1	2	2	3	4	5	5	6	7	8	9	10	10	11	12	13	14
300	0	0	1	2	3	3	4	5	6	6	7	8	9	9	10	11	12	12	13

WAIST-MINUS-WRIST
BODY FAT CALCULATION—MALE

WAIST MINUS WRIST (IN INCHES)

Weight in lbs.

Weight :	31.5	32	32.5	33	33.5	34	34.5	35	35.5	36	36.5	37	37.5	38	38.5	39	39.5	40	40.5
120 :	41	43	45	47	49	50	52	54	56	58	60	62	64	66	68	70	72	74	76
125 :	39	41	43	45	46	48	50	52	54	56	58	59	61	63	65	67	69	71	72
130 :	37	39	41	43	44	46	48	50	51	53	55	57	59	61	63	64	66	68	69
135 :	36	38	39	41	43	44	46	48	50	51	53	55	56	58	60	62	63	66	67
140 :	34	36	38	39	41	43	44	46	48	49	51	53	54	56	58	59	61	63	64
145 :	33	35	36	38	39	41	43	44	46	47	49	51	52	54	55	57	59	60	62
150 :	32	33	35	36	38	40	41	43	44	46	47	49	50	52	53	55	57	58	60
155 :	31	32	34	35	37	38	40	41	43	44	46	47	49	50	52	53	55	56	58
160 :	30	31	33	34	35	37	38	40	41	43	44	46	47	48	50	51	53	54	56
165 :	29	30	31	33	34	36	37	39	40	41	43	44	45	47	48	50	51	52	54
170 :	28	29	30	32	33	34	36	37	39	40	41	43	44	45	47	48	49	51	52
175 :	27	28	29	31	32	33	35	36	37	39	40	41	43	44	45	47	48	49	51
180 :	26	27	28	30	31	32	34	35	36	37	39	40	41	43	44	45	47	48	49
185 :	25	26	27	28	30	31	33	34	35	36	38	39	40	41	43	44	45	46	48
190 :	24	26	27	28	29	30	31	33	34	35	37	38	39	40	41	43	44	45	46
195 :	24	25	26	27	28	30	31	32	33	34	36	37	38	39	40	41	43	44	45
200 :	23	24	25	26	28	30	31	32	33	35	36	37	38	39	40	41	43	44	44

WAIST MINUS WRIST : 31.5 32 32.5 33 33.5 34 34.5 35 35.5 36 36.5 37 37.5 38 38.5 39 39.5 40 40.5
(IN INCHES)

Weight in lbs.

Weight in lbs.	31.5	32	32.5	33	33.5	34	34.5	35	35.5	36	36.5	37	37.5	38	38.5	39	39.5	40	40.5
205	22	23	25	26	27	28	29	30	31	32	34	35	36	37	38	39	40	41	43
210	22	23	24	25	26	27	28	29	30	32	33	34	35	36	37	38	39	40	42
215	21	22	23	24	25	26	27	28	30	31	32	33	34	35	36	37	38	39	40
220	20	22	23	24	25	26	27	28	29	30	31	32	33	34	35	36	37	38	39
225	20	21	22	23	24	25	26	27	28	29	30	31	32	33	34	35	36	37	38
230	19	20	21	22	23	24	25	26	27	28	30	31	32	33	34	35	36	37	38
235	19	20	21	22	23	24	25	26	27	28	29	30	31	32	33	34	35	36	37
240	18	19	20	21	22	23	24	25	26	27	28	29	30	31	32	33	34	35	36
245	18	19	20	21	22	23	23	24	25	26	27	28	29	30	31	32	33	34	35
250	18	19	19	20	21	22	23	24	25	26	27	27	28	29	30	31	32	33	34
255	17	18	18	19	20	21	22	23	24	25	26	27	28	28	29	30	31	32	33
260	17	18	18	19	20	21	22	23	24	25	26	26	27	28	29	30	31	31	32
265	16	17	18	18	19	20	21	22	23	24	25	26	26	27	28	29	29	30	31
270	16	17	17	18	19	20	20	21	22	23	24	25	26	27	27	28	29	30	31
275	16	16	17	18	18	19	20	21	22	23	24	25	25	26	27	28	29	30	30
280	15	16	17	17	18	19	20	20	21	22	23	24	25	26	27	27	28	29	30
285	15	15	16	17	18	18	19	20	21	22	23	24	24	25	26	27	28	28	29
290	15	15	16	16	17	18	19	19	20	21	22	23	24	25	25	26	27	28	29
295	14	15	15	16	17	18	18	19	20	21	22	23	24	25	25	26	27	28	28
300	14	15	16	16	17	17	18	19	20	20	21	22	23	24	25	26	26	27	28

WAIST-MINUS-WRIST BODY FAT CALCULATION—MALE

Weight in lbs.	WAIST MINUS WRIST (IN INCHES)																		
	41	41.5	42	42.5	43	43.5	44	44.5	45	45.5	46	46.5	47	47.5	48	48.5	49	49.5	50
120	77	79	81	83	85	87	89	91	93	95	97	99	99	99	99	99	99	99	99
125	74	76	78	80	82	84	87	89	91	93	95	98	99	99	99	99	99	99	99
130	71	73	75	77	78	80	82	84	86	87	89	91	93	94	96	98	99	99	99
135	68	70	72	74	75	77	79	80	82	84	86	87	89	91	92	94	96	98	99
140	66	68	69	71	72	74	76	77	79	81	82	84	86	87	89	91	92	94	96
145	63	65	67	68	70	71	73	75	76	78	79	81	83	84	86	87	89	91	92
150	61	63	64	66	67	69	70	72	74	75	77	78	80	81	83	84	86	87	89
155	59	61	62	64	65	67	68	70	71	73	74	76	77	79	80	82	83	85	86
160	57	59	60	61	63	64	66	67	69	71	72	74	75	77	79	80	82	83	86
165	55	57	58	60	61	62	64	65	67	68	69	71	72	74	75	76	78	79	81
170	54	55	56	58	59	60	62	63	64	66	67	69	70	71	72	74	75	77	78
175	52	53	55	56	57	59	60	61	63	64	65	66	68	69	70	72	73	74	76
180	50	52	53	54	56	57	58	59	61	62	63	65	66	67	68	70	71	72	74
185	49	50	51	53	54	55	56	58	59	60	61	63	64	65	66	68	69	70	71
190	48	49	50	51	52	54	55	56	57	58	60	61	62	63	65	66	67	68	69
195	46	47	49	50	51	52	53	55	56	57	58	59	60	62	63	64	65	66	68
200	45	46	47	48	50	51	52	53	54	55	57	58	59	60	61	62	63	65	66

WAIST MINUS WRIST (IN INCHES)

Weight in lbs.	41	41.5	42	42.5	43	43.5	44	44.5	45	45.5	46	46.5	47	47.5	48	48.5	49	49.5	50
205	44	45	46	47	48	49	51	52	53	54	55	56	57	58	60	61	62	63	64
210	43	44	45	46	47	48	49	50	51	53	54	55	56	57	58	59	60	61	62
215	42	43	44	45	46	47	48	49	50	51	52	53	54	56	57	58	60	61	
220	41	42	43	44	45	46	47	48	49	50	51	52	53	54	56	57	58	59	
225	40	41	42	43	44	45	46	47	48	49	50	51	52	53	54	55	56	57	58
230	39	40	41	42	43	44	45	46	47	48	49	50	51	52	53	54	55	56	57
235	38	39	40	41	42	43	44	45	46	47	48	49	50	51	52	53	54	55	
240	37	38	39	40	41	42	43	44	45	46	47	48	49	50	51	52	53	54	
245	36	37	38	39	40	41	42	43	44	45	46	46	48	49	50	51	52	53	
250	35	36	37	38	39	40	41	42	43	44	44	45	46	48	49	50	51	52	
255	34	35	36	37	38	39	40	41	42	43	44	44	46	47	48	49	50	51	52
260	34	35	36	37	38	39	40	41	42	43	43	44	45	46	47	48	49	50	
265	33	34	35	36	37	38	39	40	41	42	43	43	44	45	46	47	48	49	
270	32	33	34	35	36	37	38	38	39	40	41	42	43	44	45	46	47	48	49
275	32	32	33	34	35	36	37	38	38	39	40	41	42	43	43	44	45	46	47
280	31	32	33	33	34	35	37	38	38	38	39	39	41	42	43	43	44	45	46
285	30	31	31	32	33	34	35	36	37	38	39	39	40	41	42	43	43	44	45
290	30	31	31	32	33	34	35	35	36	37	38	39	39	40	41	42	43	43	44
295	29	30	31	32	32	33	34	35	36	36	37	38	39	39	40	41	42	43	43
300	29	29	30	31	32	33	34	34	36	36	37	37	38	39	39	40	41	42	43

of body fat as a decimal (for example, if your body fat is 42 percent, you would multiply by 0.42 to get your answer):

total weight × % body fat = weight of fat in pounds

Once you know the weight of your body fat, you can subtract it from your total weight to get your lean body weight:

total weight − fat weight = lean body weight

For Lisa in our earlier example, the calculation would look like this: Her weight (157 pounds) times her body fat percentage as a decimal (23.6 percent becomes 0.236) equals the total number of pounds of fat she carries (157 × 0.236 = 37 pounds of fat). Her total weight (157) minus her fat weight (37) equals her lean weight (120 pounds).

Mark would figure his lean weight the same way. His weight (200 pounds) times his body fat percentage as a decimal (22 percent becomes 0.22) equals the total pounds of fat he carries (200 × 0.22 = 44 pounds of fat). His total weight (200) minus his fat weight (44) equals his lean weight (156 pounds).

Knowing your lean body weight is important for two reasons: it's the basis for determining your daily protein requirement (which you'll do in Chapter 10), and it allows you to calculate a *realistic* goal weight for yourself. Even though we stress to our patients as we have to you that we don't care what you weigh as long as it's composed properly, if you're like most people, you have an "ideal" weight in your head that you'd like to reach and maintain. Based on how many pounds of lean body tissue you currently have, that may or may not be an attainable weight for you. If you have to sacrifice lean muscle weight to reach it, we encourage you to revise your goal. So what is a realistic "ideal" goal weight for you?

Your Ideal Body Weight

Refer to the next chart to find the body fat percentage range that is appropriate for your age and gender. Take the numbers at each end of the range and subtract each from 100 percent as we show with the following example. We'll need to use another subject, because Lisa is already within her ideal weight range.

Example: Missy, age 35
         Lean body weight = 96 pounds
         Ideal body fat percentage = 21–27
         percent
Step 1: Subtract each of the ideal range numbers from 100.
         100% – 21% = 79% and 100% – 27% = 73%
Step 2: Divide lean body weight by these numbers.
         96 ÷ 79 = 1.22 and 96 ÷ 73 = 1.32
Step 3: Multiply these numbers by 100.
         1.22 × 100 = 122 and 1.32 × 100 = 132

This calculation gives an ideal body weight range of 122 to 132 pounds for Missy. These numbers are actually those of a patient in our practice. She is 5'3" tall, and the "ideal" weight charts doctors usually follow tell her she should weigh about 115 pounds. She has not weighed 115 since junior high school, and it's easy to see why she isn't likely ever to weigh so little. Were she to attempt to do so, she would have to dwindle her body fat percentage down below 16 percent (which is unlikely for a woman of her age unless she were a trained athlete, and from a hormonal standpoint would not be particularly healthy even if she could manage to do it). Or she would have to lose pounds of lean body mass from the 96 she currently carries, also not advisable. A better option is to keep every pound of metabolically active lean tissue she has, carry an appropriate amount of body fat for good health, and forget about what she weighs, because **what she weighs doesn't matter!** At 125 pounds, she's tight and lean and strong and healthy. To force herself toward an "ideal" of 115 is lunacy.

IDEAL BODY FAT PERCENTAGES

AGE	MALES	FEMALES
10–30	12–18%	20–26%
31–40	13–19%	21–27%
41–50	14–20%	22–28%
51–60	16–20%	22–30%
61 and older	17–21%	22–31%

Now it's your turn. Using the Ideal Body Weight Worksheet, on page 153, calculate your realistic ideal body weight. This weight will be the target that you aim for. Every pound of lost body fat takes you closer to it. Every inch lost in the waist reduces your apple shape and your risk for metabolic disorder. Great motivators will say that unless you know where you're going, you can't hope to get there. Now you've got a clear picture of your destination, and that will help you focus your efforts toward a specific goal.

The Well-Composed Body

Unless, like Lisa, you already fall well within the guidelines for a well-composed body, you're about to begin on a journey of self-improvement. After completing the worksheets, you may—like Missy—have found that you had an unrealistically low target weight in mind. Or you may have found that the 20 pounds you've been saying you needed to shed is really more like 40. Wherever you begin, keep reminding yourself that you're not out to lose weight. Your real goal is to develop a properly composed body—one supported by a lean healthy muscle mass, strong and vigorous, with enough fat for good health. Whatever weight that turns out to be is a perfect weight for you. We stress to our clinic patients that our program is not just a weight-loss diet—it's a prescription for reclaiming your health. Fat loss is only a small part of the overall benefit. That's why, when you've completed your intervention and you're ready to maintain your fitness for life, we want you to begin that new lifestyle fitter, leaner, and healthier, not just lighter.

IDEAL BODY WEIGHT WORKSHEET

Your calculated lean body weight = _____

Ideal body fat range percentage for your age and sex from charts on pages 141 and 144–49

_____% to _____%

Step 1: Subtract each of these percentages from 100:

100% – _____% = _____ and 100% – _____% = _____

Step 2: Divide your lean body weight by each of the numbers from step 1:

_____ / _____ = _____ and _____ / _____ = _____

Step 3: Multiply each of these answers from step 2 by 100:

_____ × 100 = _____

your ideal weight is
in this range

_____ × 100 = _____

Chapter 10

Putting It All Together: Designing Your Food Plan

So it may be true after all; eating pasta makes you fat.

The New York Times
February 8, 1995

If you've been struggling with your weight, your blood pressure, your cholesterol, or your blood sugar on a diet of pasta and whole grains, living the fat-free, low-fat, no-fat way and failing, *stop blaming yourself!* You haven't failed; you've just been on the wrong diet. If you've been feeling discouraged because your doctor said, "Cut the fat to 30 grams a day or less and your weight will come down," and you did, but it didn't, don't despair. Help is here. If you suffer from elevated cholesterol and you've forgotten what it's like to eat a juicy steak for dinner and can't remember the last time you ate an egg, and your levels remain elevated, take heart. Changing your diet can and will help you regain control over these metabolic disorders. You can lose fat, you can reduce your cholesterol and triglycerides, you can lower your blood pressure, you can normalize your blood sugar by changing the way you eat—and you can maintain these benefits for a lifetime. Good health is within your grasp—all you need is the right information. This chapter will provide that information. Join us now, and we'll show you how to eat your way to good health and fitness, from the two-stage intervention process through transition and into maintenance.

Before you begin a word of medical caution: if you are pregnant or are currently taking medications to control cholesterol, blood pressure, fluid retention, or blood sugar, do not begin this regimen without a physician's guidance.

The Program in a Nutshell

• Determine your protein needs (page 156) and plan your meals around the right number of grams of protein. Choose fish, poultry, red meat, low-fat cheese (cottage cheese, feta, mozzarella, muenster), eggs, tofu. Be sure you get enough protein (your body can't store it); if you're hungry, it's fine to go beyond your requirement. 1 ounce of protein = 7 grams.

• Add 30 carbohydrate grams or less divided throughout the day for Phase I Intervention—(if you need to lose a lot of fat and/or correct a health problem)—or 55 grams or less per day for Phase II—if you want to lose a little fat, recompose your body (your lean to fat ratio), or improve your general health. If you're taking medication for a serious health problem or you're more than 20 percent overweight, you should have medical supervision. Remember, you can subtract the fiber grams from the carbohydrate grams in commercial foods (check the labels) which means you can eat more carbs. The subtracting has already been done for you in the food charts in the book. Choose green leafy vegetables, tomatoes, peppers, avocados (yes!), broccoli, eggplant, zucchini, green beans, asparagus, celery, cucumber, mushrooms, and salads. Check the carb bargain lists on pages 168, 169, and 170.

• Aim for 25 grams of fiber each day.

• Don't worry about fat, but choose healthy fats: olive oil, nut oils, avocado, and butter (yes!). Your body can and will use incoming fat as fuel.

• Never let yourself get hungry—keep snacks on hand and eat regular meals.

• Drink at least 8 glasses of water a day.

- A glass of wine (3 grams of carbohydrate) or a Miller Lite beer (slightly over 3) is fine, but count the carbs.
- Take a high-quality vitamin supplement (page 161) plus at least 90 mg of potassium.
- Artificial sweeteners and diet sodas are fine, in moderation.
- You'll be (temporarily) cutting out sugar and starches, even potates and beans (except green beans) and corn. Dessert can be a low-carb fruit—berries, peaches, melon—or sugar-free Jell-O.
- If you snack, remember to subtract those carb grams from your next meal.
- Exercise!—resistance training (with weights) is best, but any activity that makes you sweat is fine.
- When in doubt, eat lean meat, fish, or fowl and salad.

How Much Protein Do You Need?

The cornerstone of any good nutritional program is an adequate amount of high-quality protein. Whatever stage of our nutritional program you're in, it is of paramount importance that you get adequate daily protein.

In Chapter 9 you learned how to calculate your lean body mass and percentage of body fat. If you have not already done so, do this now. Your lean body mass (LBM) is the metabolically active part of you, consuming most of the energy, repairing the daily wear and tear on vital body structures, and replacing vital fluids and body chemicals—in short, doing all the work of living. It's what gives you a reason to eat. Ideally, you want to keep all of it, every glorious pound, so you must feed it, love it, water it, exercise it, and be thankful for it.[1] On typical low-calorie, high-carbohy-

---

[1] We say ideally you hope to keep every pound, but in point of fact, if you are significantly overweight, you will probably lose some lean body mass as your declining weight reduces the demand on those muscles that get you from place to place. If you are currently more than 40 percent above your ideal weight, your weight-bearing muscles do more than their share of work and they beef up to meet the demand placed on them. As your weight declines, the demand goes down, and the muscles can taper too. When this happens, they can weigh less because their work is less. That's fine. We just don't want you to lose pounds of muscle because you starved the muscle to death.

drate, low-fat diets, protein intake is often marginal, and as a result as much as 50 percent of weight lost can be muscle weight. Each pound of active muscle mass lost reduces your rate of metabolism. (You can offset this loss by exercising your muscle mass against resistance—weight training, resistance stair stepping, etc. See Chapter 12.)

The proper care of a lean body mass requires that every day you provide it with enough high-quality complete protein to carry out all its vital functions. Specifically, each and every pound of your LBM needs six-tenths of 1 gram (0.6 gram) of protein every day if you are a person of moderate physical activity and fitness—that is, you do modest exercise for 20 to 30 minutes a couple of times a week. That means 60 grams of protein per day for a person with a 100-pound LBM, 72 grams per day for a person with a 120-pound LBM, 90 grams for a 150-pound LBM, and 108 grams per day for someone with a 180-pound LBM. Your specific daily protein need will depend on how many pounds of LBM you have and how active you are. If you are 40 percent or more above your ideal weight, you should rate yourself one activity category higher (more active) than you actually are to account for the increased work you must do when you walk, run, climb stairs, etc., carrying the excess pounds along.

The activity categories are as follows:

1. *Sedentary.* If you get no physical activity whatsoever, your protein need will be 0.5 gram per pound of lean mass. Sedentary = 0.5

2. *Moderately Active.* If you are average in physical activity, devoting 20 or 30 minutes to exercise two or three times per week, your protein need is 0.6 gram per pound of lean mass. Moderately active = 0.6

3. *Active.* If you participate in organized physical activity for more than 30 minutes three to five times per week, your protein need is 0.7 gram per pound of lean mass. Active = 0.7

4. *Very Active.* If you engage in vigorous physical activity lasting an hour or more five or more times per week, your lean mass requires 0.8 gram per pound. Very active = 0.8

5. *Athlete.* If you are a competitive athlete in training, doing twice-daily heavy physical workouts for an hour or more, your protein need is 0.9 gram per pound of lean mass. Athlete = 0.9

To figure your own daily protein need, simply take your LBM (in pounds) and multiply it by the activity category number that most closely describes your current level.

_____ pound of lean body mass
× _____ activity category number
_____ = daily minimum protein need

The answer will be your minimum protein requirement in grams per day. Divide this number by three to discover your own minimum protein intake per meal, based on three meals per day.

_____ ÷ 3 = _____ grams per meal

Ideally, each of your three meals per day should contain *at least* this amount of high-quality complete protein, no matter which phase of the program you're following. You can use any standard guide of food contents (*The Complete Book of Food Counts*, Corinne T. Netzer, Dell, 1994, is a good one) to select foods that will fulfill your protein requirement.

We've made this plan even easier to follow; we've done the calculations for you by breaking down the protein intake per meal into four general categories with serving sizes for the main food sources of lean protein in various combinations. Refer now to the protein equivalency charts at the end of this chapter (starting on page 199), where you will find these four basic levels of protein intake providing 20 grams per meal, 27 grams per meal, 34 grams per meal, and 40 grams per meal. Select the equivalency chart that meets *and exceeds* your protein need, and you will find the serving sizes of these foods alone and in combination sufficient to meet your needs. Don't worry about getting too much protein; concern yourself with making sure you don't get too little.

Let's run through an example of how to use these charts. Imagine your protein need is 70 grams per day. Your protein requirement per meal is 70 divided by 3, or 23 grams per meal. Now turn to the protein equivalency charts. Chart A, the 20-gram-per-meal level, would not provide enough protein for you, so you would have to step up to Chart B, the 27-gram-per-meal level. Scan down the left-hand side of the table and across the bottom to find entries for each of the major sources of complete protein: meat, eggs, hard cheese, soft cheese, curd cheese, and tofu or soy. Select a protein source from the left side and one from the bottom (note that they could be the same source or you could combine different sources). Follow the table across from the left choice and up from the bottom choice, and where the two intersect you will find the serving size for that source or combination of sources. For example, if you wanted to eat an omelet made of eggs and soft cheese, you would find egg on the bottom and soft cheese on the left and follow them to their intersection, where you would find that you would require 2 whole eggs plus 2 egg whites plus 2 ounces of soft cheese to fulfill your needs at that meal.

You should also note that 1 ounce of lean "meat" and 1 ounce of hard cheese are equivalent in protein content. Therefore, if you wanted to prepare your omelet with smoked turkey and Gouda cheese, you could substitute turkey for half the cheese and create a delicious egg dish with 2 whole eggs plus 2 egg whites plus $1/2$ ounce of smoked turkey and $1/2$ ounce of shredded Gouda cheese.

You will also note that with regard to its protein content any "meat" source provides very close to 7 grams of protein to the ounce. Whenever we refer to "meat" in our discussions of the protein equivalent listing labeled "meat, fish, or poultry," we mean beef, chicken, tuna, pork, salmon, shrimp, scallops, herring, turkey, rabbit, alligator, rattlesnake, wild boar, bass, lobster, gazelle . . . you get the idea—all protein from animal sources is "meat" to us. And that means that in conjunction with any of a wide variety of cheeses, tofu, and egg protein, and within the boundaries of what you can and will eat, you can create endless combinations of protein varieties to meet your daily needs.

I *CAN* EAT RED MEAT AND EGGS?

Yes, you can. And no, your cholesterol will not go up because you eat red meat and egg yolk. Because you'll be carefully controlling your metabolic hormones, your liver will not take the incoming saturated fats and dietary cholesterol from these (or any) foods and turn them into excess blood cholesterol. (See Chapter 7 for details.) Does that mean you could have steak and eggs for breakfast again? Sure. Or pork ribs for lunch? Yes. What you absolutely *cannot* do, however, is eat all the red meat and egg yolks you want and at the same time load up on starch and sugar. That means you can't have biscuits and gravy and hash brown potatoes with your steak and eggs.

If you suffer from elevated blood pressure, elevated cholesterol, marked fluid retention, or inflammatory conditions such as arthritis, bursitis, asthma, allergies, or skin rashes, you may want to limit your intake of red meat and egg yolk somewhat. We suggest this not because of the cholesterol content but because these foods are also rich in arachidonic acid, one of the fatty acids that leads directly to the production of the "bad" eicosanoids that promote or worsen these conditions. (See Chapter 6.) If you suffer from these problems, eliminate red meat and egg yolk entirely from your regimen for a full three weeks to see if your symptoms improve. Then eat a hearty serving of them for a meal or two and see if your symptoms return or worsen. If so, you are a person sensitive to the arachidonic acid content of foods and should take care to indulge only occasionally in these foods—especially egg yolk, the most concentrated source of arachidonic acid. And when you choose to eat beef, follow the guidelines for preparation from Chapter 6.

BUT WHAT IF I'M A VEGETARIAN?

Strict vegetarianism can create a little monotony in protein provisioning since the only adequate sources not overly laden with carbohydrate come in the form of soy (as tofu or tempeh) and the algae spirulina. You may find you have to get very creative, because you'll need to eat quite a lot of these to meet your protein need. The most serious deficiency that vegetarians face is protein malnourishment. Your choice of an animal-free diet doesn't alter your human need for enough good-quality protein to nourish your lean body mass, nor does it spare you from the consequences of getting too little.*

For example, our patient Kathy, a strict vegetarian, came to us complaining that she was always tired. Upon examining her, we found her triglycerides and blood pressure mildly elevated and her blood count a little low. Kathy had been active in running and sports until chronic foot pain and fatigue caused her to quit running; as a result, she began to gain a little weight. Although Kathy occasionally ate tofu, she primarily followed a nearly all-carbohydrate, low-fat to no-fat diet of whole grains, pasta, potatoes, rice, salads, fruits, and juices. Our first order of business was to increase her protein and fat intake and then reduce her reliance on starches. With an 88-pound lean body mass, Kathy needed at least 60 grams of protein per day, which meant a $1/2$-cup serving of firm tofu or about 3 ounces of tempeh at every meal along with some olive oil in such dishes as tofu stir-fry or tempeh burgers—a much larger quantity than she had been consuming. Within a few weeks she not only began to feel more energetic, but her triglycerides and blood pressure quickly normalized and she began to feel like running again.

Ovolactovegetarians will enjoy much greater variety in their diets since an endless variety of cheeses, eggs, a little yogurt, and other milk products can augment the tofu, tempeh, and spirulina. Take note on the protein equivalency charts that firm tofu provides a generous 10 grams of protein per $1/4$ cup with only about 2 grams of carbohydrate, whereas tempeh is slightly lower in protein content and higher in carbohydrate. Like animal "meats," tempeh provides 7 grams of protein to the ounce or $1/4$ cup but also contains 7 grams of carbohydrate. And spirulina, in

---

*See Appendix for information on *The Soya Bluebook*.

dried form, is very protein rich, providing about 15 grams per ounce, but also contains 7 grams of carbohydrate.

NOT JUST THREE MEALS A DAY

Whether you're vegetarian or omnivorous, you must eat breakfast, lunch, and dinner each day to ensure that you meet the minimum amount of protein required to protect and provide for your lean body mass and that you spread out your intake throughout the day. *But remember that these three servings provide your minimum intake.* You may add additional protein in several snacks (more about snacks a little later on) during the day if you're hungry. A good rule of thumb for portion size in protein snacking is an amount equal to about half a protein meal serving. And although this is the ideal to which you aspire, because protein has a balancing effect on the hormones of metabolism, you needn't limit your protein intake to these amounts. If you're hungry—especially in the early part of your nutritional rehabilitation—eat lean protein to your heart's content. Additional lean protein won't disrupt the metabolic harmony you're striving to achieve. Later, when you've moved into a dynamic phase of correction, instead of cravings and hunger haunting you, you will more often have to remind yourself to eat all your meals.

The other major component in constructing your new nutritional regimen will be to set your carbohydrate limits, but before we do, let's go over the other components: fluid intake, fat, and vitamin, mineral, and electrolyte needs. None of these plays a role in driving or disrupting the metabolic apple cart, but they're still important, and you need to understand how they fit into your plan.

Don't Forget Your Vitamins, Minerals, and Electrolytes

As we pointed out in Chapter 8, optimal metabolic function depends on your getting adequate amounts of all the important vitamins and minerals regularly. If you eat all the kinds of fruits, vegetables, meats, cheeses, and grains that are available to you—even at the most restrictive stages of this diet—you will get adequate amounts of every necessary vitamin and mineral. Unfortunately, most of us have food likes and dislikes. We eat the things we like in quantity and usually make little effort to eat those foods we're not so fond of, even though they might contain important micronutrients. For that reason we ask that you supplement your food intake with a daily complete multiple vitamin and chelated mineral supplement—for good measure. You will find a number of good complete ones listed in Chapter 8.

Even if there is no food that you don't like and eat regularly, the power of insulin control to signal your kidney to waste excess fluid will result in potassium loss in urine. You will need to replace potassium in the first few weeks of your intervention to keep your body from becoming depleted. You can augment your potassium intake through the regular use of Morton's Lite Salt or NoSalt brand salt substitute, which are pure potassium salts, or by taking any of the supplemental potassium replacements listed in Chapter 8. *Remember! If you are currently taking blood pressure medication, ask your physician before you take extra potassium. Some of these medications prevent potassium loss, and your potassium level could become dangerously high from supplementing potassium while you are on the medication.*

So How Much Fat Can I Eat?

In Chapter 6 you learned which fats are best and why. Here they are in brief.

The Good Fats and Oils

Olive oil: extra-virgin, virgin, or pure
Nut oils: walnut, macadamia, hazelnut
Peanut oil
Sesame seed oil (light)
Avocado and avocado oil
Unsalted butter or clarified butter (saturated source)

More important, however, you learned why *fat doesn't make you fat.* Don't worry about eating high-quality monounsaturated and naturally saturated fats as long as you follow the plan guideline with regard to carbohydrate intake. Most of the problems associated with "dieting"—dry skin, brittle nails, dull hair, hair loss, the development of gallstones, menstrual irregularities, susceptibility to colds and other infections—occur because the fat content of the diet is too low. Because humans need fat and use it quite well as fuel, we don't limit fat in our clinic patients. We allow them to set their own intake need, because fat intake is self-regulating. By that we mean that people have a built-in "off" switch for fat consumption. Few people would sit and eat a stick of butter, consume lard by the spoonful, or swig olive oil by the cup. Without carbohydrate to wrap the fat around, it's not very appealing. When you don't eat chips, french fries, baked potatoes, doughnuts, cakes, pies, pastries, cookies, and chocolate, you avoid a huge amount of incoming fat, even when you get a moderate amount in lean meats. Select fats from the "good fat" list and eat them responsibly as you feel the need.

Unless your body fat storage signal has been turned on—i.e., excess dietary carbohydrate has elevated your insulin level—*your body can and will use incoming dietary fat as fuel to burn to meet its energy needs.*[2] You must remember, however, that if the fat storage system *has* been turned on by excess insulin driven by too much dietary carbohydrate, the fat coming in via your diet will know right where to go to find a good home—straight to your fat cells to be stored or to your liver to be turned into cholesterol. If you hope to correct the metabolic disturbance from which you suffer—be it excess body fat, elevated blood pressure, deranged blood sugar, excessive cholesterol production, or some combination of these—you cannot eat a diet that is both high in carbohydrate *and* full of fat.

However, if you carefully follow the guidelines of this plan—which means keeping a weather eye on your carbohydrate intake—*don't worry about counting fat grams.*

Drink Till You Float

We tell our patients to drink till they float, and for two very important reasons we want you to do the same thing. When you burn body fat or dietary fat for fuel in the absence of an abundance of carbohydrate, some of the fat may be burned incompletely. These partially burned fat by-products are called *ketones*. Far from being the dangerous or detrimental substance some nutritional authorities would have you think, ketones are nothing more than the natural by-product of fat breakdown. Your body can and will burn them for energy, or, if there are too many to use, it will dispose of them in your breath or by passing them out in the stool or in the urine. And this is where water drinking becomes important: the more water you drink, the more urine you make, the more ketones will pass out in the urine, and the more fat you lose. So drink up!

A second reason for increasing your water intake is exercise. Because your body in its hormonally balanced state will not retain excess fluid, the increased water loss in exercise can leave you dehydrated. Especially if you engage in vigorous athletic competition, *you must increase your water intake by as much as 50 percent!*

---

[2] If you are trying to lose weight—especially if you are a small person—you may have to curb your fat intake somewhat. Otherwise you may have too much food coming in, so your body won't need to dip into your fat stores—see the questions and answers at the end of this chapter.

And although we've said "water" here, in truth any water-based fluid will work (as long as it doesn't have carbohydrate or calories). You need to drink *at least* 2 quarts of noncaloric fluid daily. Your fluid intake could be water, mineral water, diet soda, coffee, tea, or herbal tea. Your coffee or tea can be artificially sweetened or unsweetened, and you can lighten it with a small amount of whole milk or half-and-half. Both these lighteners have fewer carbohydrates than skim milk or nondairy creamers.

You may drink your coffee, tea, or diet cola caffeinated or decaffeinated. Most people don't have any trouble with caffeine use. But a few people will be sensitive enough to insulin output that the caffeine in beverages will keep their insulin levels somewhat elevated. If you are doing everything else right, and you find yourself still hungry between meals, still retaining fluid, or not losing weight at the rate you would predict, you may be one of those caffeine-sensitive people, and you should try to decaffeinate yourself.

Most of your daily intake should occur between and before meals. What difference could it make to your nutritional well-being *when* you drink your daily fluid requirement? Why not drink it with meals?

Although some people say drinking with meals slows them down, we've come to the conclusion that the only function cold beverages serve during a meal is to allow you to eat much faster and consume larger quantities of food than you otherwise would. Without water or a big glass of iced tea, we eat more slowly, chew the food better, enjoy the meal more, and eat a lot less than before. Now, we'll frequently have just a glass of wine with our meal. Try it yourself, and see if you don't eat much less when your meal isn't accompanied by a large cold beverage. Even though you're eating less, you don't feel deprived.

Instead, *precede* every meal, even breakfast, with the large beverage. Research suggests that drinking a large glass of cold water 15 to 30 minutes before a meal tends to reduce hunger, and as a result you will eat less. You'll also get a head start on drinking enough water; it's sometimes easy to forget to drink the full amount during the day. So our best advice is that you drink, drink, drink—before meals, in between meals, but not while you eat. Limit your mealtime beverage to $1/2$ to 1 cup in sips, not gulps!

Bottoms Up: Wine and Spirits

If you like, have a glass of *dry,* not sweet, white or red wine with one of your meals. Several recent studies have shown wine (particularly red wine) to be an effective agent for increasing the body's sensitivity to insulin—the main goal of this program. Since we are shooting for lower insulin levels, it not only doesn't hurt to add the wine to our regimen; it actually helps. In our research files we have the report of an old study done by a New York physician back in the early sixties in which he divided his dieting patients into three groups—wine drinkers, hard-liquor drinkers, and nondrinkers. He kept all groups on the same reducing diet and found that the wine drinkers lost the most weight. He had no idea why; he just reported his results. They make sense now because we understand that wine improves insulin sensitivity. Many researchers believe the disparity between the levels of heart disease found in France and other southern European countries and those of the United States and Britain—the so-called French paradox—can be laid at the doorstep of increased wine consumption. And so, like the French, Italians, and others living around the Mediterranean, we can increase our insulin sensitivity, decrease our insulin levels, and enjoy life more by adding a moderate amount of wine to our program.

Moderate means a glass of wine or two—no more—with one meal. Wine does have some carbohydrate content left in it after the fermentation process, so the drier the wine, the fewer grams of carbohydrate it will contain. A good rule of thumb is that *dry* white and red wines contain about 1 to 1.5 grams of carbohydrate per ounce; sweet dessert wines or sherries contain significantly more, too many more to enjoy them in the intervention phases of this program. If you choose to drink wine with your meals, remember to include these grams as a part of your daily carbohydrate allotment. More on that in the next section.

Distilled spirits, while they contain scant to no carbohydrates—it's all been turned to alcohol—tend to *raise* insulin and to impair insulin sensitivity if consumed in more than modest quantities. In general, avoid distilled alcohol during your intervention, except for an occasional cocktail containing a single ounce of distilled liquor, straight, on the rocks, or in a mixed drink (no sweet mixers allowed). An occasional margarita is okay if you make your own without the sugar syrup most bars use. Forget about beer, except Miller Lite (3.2 grams of carbohydrate per can).

Controlling the Starches and Sugars

To achieve metabolic control, your tasks are simple—reduce the amount of insulin circulating in your blood during the day and restore the sensitivity of your tissues to insulin. The quickest—and actually the only—way to achieve metabolic control is to restrict the amount of metabolically active carbohydrate you put into the system. Does this mean that you can never enjoy fruit or bread or pasta again? No. But it does mean that you will at first need to lean toward the carbohydrate bargains in these food categories and exert some control over your intake. How much control? That depends on how out of kilter your system currently is, based on your medical history and/or laboratory evaluations. For that reason we have provided two levels of intervention. Select the protocol that most closely describes your own condition and begin there.

PHASE I INTERVENTION—30 GRAMS CARBOHYDRATE OR LESS PER DAY

If you are overfat by 20 percent or more, have high blood pressure, elevated cholesterol and/or triglycerides, low HDL cholesterol, type II diabetes or glucose intolerance, or have any combination of these disorders, you need strong corrective action and must begin with this protocol. Phase I places the strongest rein on insulin output and will help you gain control of your insulin production quickly.

PHASE II INTERVENTION—55 GRAMS OF CARBOHYDRATE PER DAY

This phase also lowers insulin production but allows for a slightly richer carbohydrate intake. We offer this phase for people who need to reduce their body weight by less than 20 percent to reach ideal weight and have none of the metabolic conditions just mentioned, for people who are happy at their current weight but wish to reduce body fat and build lean muscle, and as an intermediate step for people who began with Phase I and have now normalized their blood pressure, blood lipids, and blood sugars.

COUNTING CARBS THE SMART WAY

You may refer to one of the standard reference guides such as *The Complete Book of Food Counts* to develop your own portions of vegetables, salads, fruits, and cereal grains to meet your carbohydrate quota. But remember in calculating your carbohydrate intake for these foods that the actual usable carbohydrate content of a given food is the total carbohydrate content minus the dietary fiber—what we call the *effective carbohydrate content* or *ECC* (see pages 203-213). In a nutshell, this means that you don't have to count the fiber grams in your daily carbohydrate total because the fiber doesn't act metabolically as a carbohydrate. *The usable carbohydrate per serving as given on a standard nutrition label for a food will be the total carbohydrate content listed, minus any dietary fiber listed.*

You don't have to calculate any portions if you don't want to. We've developed a list of the effective carbohydrate content for a wide range of everyday foods. Refer to the effective carbohydrate content charts, where we've given you specific tables listing the ECC for fruits, vegetables, and breads and cereal grains in usable portion sizes. The values are arranged in 5-gram increments, so you will find a 5-gram portion, a 10-gram portion, a 15-gram portion, a 20-gram portion, and a 25-gram portion for each food listed. All you have to do is decide what food you want to eat, and the list will automatically tell you how much of it you can have at that carbohydrate level. Next to the serving size you will see the actual number of grams of carbohydrate the serving contains (in most cases it will be equal to that gram level or slightly below it). You will see that the standard portion of some foods is actually considerably less than 5 grams—these entries represent real carbohydrate bargains. See our bargain boxes on pages 168–170.

For example, on a Phase I diet, at breakfast you might choose to spend your 7 to 10 grams of carbohydrate as 1 cup of sliced strawberries or as a slice of buttered "light" wheat toast. Or at lunch you might like five saltine crackers with your tuna salad, or perhaps you'd prefer half an apple. For 7 grams in a carbohydrate meal or snack, you *could* eat any of the items in the box. Remember that once it is digested, your body turns all carbohydrate to sugar, so from that standpoint all these entries are equivalent. However, what's missing from the junk choices are the fiber, the vitamins and minerals, and the cancer-fighting phytochemicals found in the fresh fruits and vegetables. The choice of what you eat is always yours, but so are the consequences of that choice. Choose wisely.

Carbohydrate Comparisons

7 Skittles = 1 marshmallow = 1 medium raw carrot = $^1/_3$ medium banana = $^1/_4$ very small potato = 1 caramel = $^1/_7$ Milky Way bar = $^1/_2$ Reese's peanut butter cup = 14 Reese's Pieces = 7 jelly beans = $^1/_3$ Hershey Bar = $^1/_2$ cup grapes = $^1/_2$ orange = $^1/_2$ cup melon = $^1/_2$ cup fresh berries = 1 Starburst fruit chew = 7 cups mushrooms = 14 cups fresh lettuce = $3^1/_2$ cups fresh broccoli = 3 french fries

You'll quickly see that most of your foods at this level will be in their natural state.

You will also note that at the higher levels of carbohydrate per portion—where you will be in maintenance—a number of foods are listed as "unlimited." This means that reaching that carbohydrate level in a single serving would give you an amount too large for anyone to consume. In these cases, refer to the lower carbohydrate levels for that food to see how many grams a more realistically sized portion contains.

The ECC charts make it easy for you to ferret out those foods lowest in carbohydrate for Phase I, when your per-meal carbohydrate intake will be small, as well as to assemble combinations of carbohydrate foods when your per-meal carbohydrate intake increases as you move to Phase II or into maintenance. For example, in Phase II your total carbohydrate intake per meal will be 15 grams. That means you could have one serving from the 15-gram-portion column for a single food or that you could have three servings from the 5-gram-portion column for three different foods—or one from the 10-gram-portion column and one from the 5-gram one. By the time you get to maintenance—where in a later section you will learn that your per-meal carbohydrate intake may be 20, 25, or more grams—you might be able to select five different carbohydrate foods and have the 5-gram portion for all of them at one meal! Or you could choose any combination—the total must simply add up to the amount you need at your meal or snack.

Carbohydrate Bargains Under 1 Gram of Carbohydrate

1 cup alfalfa sprouts (0.4)
$^1/_2$ cup arugula (0.4)
1 cup sliced bok choy (0.8)
1 celery rib (0.9)
1 tablespoon minced chives (0.1)
$^1/_2$ cup sliced endive (0.8)
1 cup shredded lettuce (0.4)
1 tablespoon chopped canned pimiento (0.6)
$^1/_2$ cup sliced raw radicchio (0.9)
5 radishes (0.8)
1 cup fresh spinach (0.6)

The ECC charts will take you effortlessly from early intervention all the way through maintenance and beyond, so make copies of these lists and tape them to the front of your refrigerator.

Carbohydrate Bargains of 3 or Fewer Grams of Carbohydrate

$1/4$ cup blackberries (2.9)
6 fresh asparagus spears (2.4)
$1/2$ cup canned asparagus (2.8)
4 frozen asparagus spears (2.9)
$1/2$ cup canned bamboo shoots (2.3)
1 cup chopped raw broccoli (2.2)
$1/2$ cup frozen broccoli/cauliflower florets (2.7)
$3/4$ cup frozen broccoli/pearl onions/red peppers (2.6)
$1/4$ cup cooked sliced carrots (3.0)
1 cup cauliflower florets (2.6)
$1/2$ medium cucumber (3)
$1/4$ cup chopped leeks (2)
$1/2$ cup raw mushroom pieces (1.1)
$1/2$ cup cooked mushroom pieces (2.3)
5 whole enoki mushrooms (2)
$1/2$ cup chopped raw scallions (2.5)
$1/2$ cup chopped parsley (1.9)
$1/2$ cup chopped sweet pepper (2.4)
1 tablespoon chopped raw shallot (1.7)
$1/2$ cup boiled sliced summer squash (2.6)
1 medium tomatillo (2)
1 cup turnip greens (1.8)

To Snack or Not to Snack?

If that is the question, in America the answer is usually "Snack!" But before you get the wrong idea, by *snack* we don't mean cupcakes and chips. We mean a well-composed small meal or a little meal on the run.

The crux of controlling your metabolism lies in controlling your metabolic hormones: insulin and glucagon. When you eat a meal (or snack) made up of the proper composition of protein and carbohydrate, you set the hormonal tone in your body for the next several hours. After that time you need to fine-tune the system again. In the course of a normal day that will mean eating four or more times a day, and for most of us that translates into breakfast, lunch, dinner, and a snack or two.

Carbohydrate Bargains of 5 or Fewer Grams of Carbohydrate

$1/2$ medium avocado (3.7)
$1/4$ cup blueberries (4.3)
$1/2$ cup strawberries (3.3)
$1/2$ cup beet greens (3.9)
$1/2$ cup frozen Pillsbury broccoli/carrots (3.1)
4 brussels sprouts (3.4)
1 cup red or green cabbage (3.6)
1 medium carrot (5)
$1/2$ cup chopped Swiss chard (3.6)
$1/2$ cup chopped dandelion greens (3.3)
$1/2$ cup diced eggplant (3.2)
$1/2$ cup chopped fresh fennel (3.1)
$1/2$ cup sliced snap beans (3.8)
$1/4$ cup frozen Japanese-style vegetables (3.7)
1 cup mustard greens (4)
1 whole hot chili pepper (4.3)
$1/2$ cup chopped jalapeño peppers (4.2)
$1/2$ cup boiled unsweetened rhubarb (3.5)
1 cup frozen spinach (3.1)
$1/2$ cup spaghetti squash (5)
1 cup raw diced summer squash (4)
1 medium tomato (4.3)
1 cup boiled turnip pieces (4.4)
4 whole water chestnuts (4)
$1/2$ cup canned sliced water chestnuts (4.5)
$1/2$ cup sliced wax beans (4.5)

Quick snacks on the run should still ideally provide high-quality protein (a good rule of thumb is an amount equal to one-half your regular protein meal) with a controlled amount of carbohydrate. *Snack* is not a euphemism for junk, although as a country we've come to think so. Now you have to work a little to find commercially available snack foods that are not composed mainly of carbohydrate, but there are a few out there. Be patient. Remember how the food manufacturing industry quickly hopped on the low-fat bandwagon to bring us fat-free pretzels, fat-free cookies, fat-free coffee cake, ice cream, and potato chips? Well, as the tide of nutrition turns—and believe us, it is turning—we'll all soon be bob-

Snack Possibilities

SNACK	PORTION	PROTEIN	CARB
Sunflower seeds	1 oz.	5	4
Walnuts	1 oz.	4	5
Macadamia nuts	1 oz.	3	4
Peanuts	1 oz.	7	5
Pork rinds	1 oz.	17	0
Lean meat slices	1 oz.	7	0–1
String cheese	1 oz.	6	1
Meat/cheese/cracker	1/2 oz each on 2 crackers	7	4
Homemade peanut butter crackers	1 T./2 crackers	4	5
Hard-cooked egg	1 large	6	0.6
Cottage cheese	1/4 cup	7	2
Apple/cheddar slices	1/4 apple/1 oz.	7	6
Jerky	1 oz.	7	1
Sandwich (light bread, 1 oz. meat)	1/2	7	7

bing about in a sea of commercially packaged carbohydrate-restricted snacks. Until then, good snacks could include those in the box.

Remember that your three regular meals will provide your minimum daily protein need, so you don't absolutely have to snack—it's optional. But if you choose to do so, especially during the first few weeks of the diet, while you're gaining corrective momentum (see the questions and answers at the end of this chapter for an explanation), you should stick carefully to the guidelines.

Phase I Intervention

BREAKFAST

1 protein meal serving*
7–10 grams carbohydrate†
2 cups noncaloric fluid
(1–1^1/$_2$ cups before meal, ^{1}/$_2$–1 cup during)
Multivitamin and mineral supplement
Potassium supplement or added potassium

OPTIONAL MORNING SNACK

^{1}/$_2$ protein meal serving
5 grams carbohydrate
1 cup noncaloric fluid

LUNCH

1 protein meal serving
7–10 grams carbohydrate†
2 cups noncaloric fluid
(1–1^1/$_2$ cups before meal, ^{1}/$_2$–1 cup during)
Potassium supplement or added potassium

OPTIONAL AFTERNOON OR BEDTIME SNACK

^{1}/$_2$ protein meal serving
5 grams carbohydrate
1 cup noncaloric fluid

DINNER

1 protein meal serving
7–10 grams carbohydrate†
2 cups noncaloric fluid
(1–1^1/$_2$ cups before meal, ^{1}/$_2$–1 cup during)
Potassium supplement or added potassium

---

* You must calculate *your* protein requirement, page 156.
† You should reduce your carbohydrate intake per meal to 7 grams if you choose to eat the optional snacks—unless they contain zero carbohydrate. You may combine the contents of one snack with a meal or have wine with dinner; however, *do not allow the total carbohydrate content of any meal to exceed 12 grams or the total for the day to exceed 30 grams.*

Phase I Worksheet

Record your values below:

Lean Body Mass = _____ pounds.

Protein requirement per day = _____ grams.

Protein requirement per meal = _____ grams.

    As ounces of lean meat = _____ ounces.

    As egg protein = _____ eggs + _____ egg whites.

    As curd cheese = _____ cup(s).

    As tofu = _____ ounce(s).

    Combined sources = _____

_____

_____

_____

Daily carbohydrate total = 30 grams.

Carbohydrate per meal = 7–10 grams.

Carbohydrate per snack = 5 or fewer grams.

Portion sizes for your favorite carbohydrate choices:_____

_____

_____

_____

_____

_____

_____

_____

Phase II Intervention

BREAKFAST

1 protein meal serving*
15 grams carbohydrate†
2 cups noncaloric fluid
(1–1^1/$_2$ cups before meal, ^{1}/$_2$–1 cup during)
Multivitamin and mineral supplement

OPTIONAL MORNING SNACK

^{1}/$_2$ protein meal serving
5 grams carbohydrate
1 cup noncaloric fluid

LUNCH

1 protein meal serving
15 grams carbohydrate
2 cups noncaloric fluid
(1–1^1/$_2$ cups before meal, ^{1}/$_2$–1 cup during)

OPTIONAL AFTERNOON OR BEDTIME SNACK

^{1}/$_2$ protein meal serving
5 grams carbohydrate
1 cup noncaloric fluid

DINNER

1 protein meal serving
15 grams carbohydrate
2 cups noncaloric fluid
(1–1^1/$_2$ cups before meal, ^{1}/$_2$–1 cup during)
Potassium supplement or added potassium

---

* You must calculate *your* protein requirement, page 156.
† You may combine the two snacks to make a single larger one if you so desire, you may drop them entirely, you may use them following the meals as a dessert, or you may add the snacks to any two of the other three meals to make them slightly larger meals. *In no event should you allow your carbohydrate intake for any one meal or snack to exceed 20 grams or your daily total to exceed 55 grams.*

Phase II Worksheet

Record your values below:

Lean Body Mass = _____ pounds.

Protein requirement per day = _____ grams.

Protein requirement per meal = _____ grams.

    As ounces of lean meat = _____ ounces.

    As egg protein = _____ eggs + _____ egg whites.

    As tofu = _____ ounce(s).

    As curd cheese = _____ cup(s).

    Combined sources = _____

_____

_____

_____

Daily carbohydrate total = 55 grams.

Carbohydrate per meal = 15 grams.

Carbohydrate per snack = 5 grams.

Portion sizes for favorite carbohydrate choices: _____

_____

_____

_____

_____

_____

_____

_____

Following the Plan

Now that you're acquainted with the diet plans, let us explain how to use them to reclaim your health, fitness, and vitality.

If your current state of health dictates that you should begin with Phase I—i.e., you need to lose more than 20 percent of your weight, you suffer from elevated blood pressure, cholesterol, or triglycerides or disturbances in blood sugar, or your laboratory evaluation (see Chapter 9 for complete recommendations) uncovered abnormalities such as elevation of your insulin or hemoglobin A_1c—you should remain in Phase I, adhering as strictly to the plan as you possibly can, until your abnormal laboratory values and/or blood pressure readings have stabilized in the normal range and have remained so for at least four weeks. By that time you should have developed a corrective momentum and the metabolic changes that have taken place should now permit you to slide up to Phase II and a slightly higher carbohydrate intake. If you are more than 20 percent above your ideal body weight remain on Phase II until you are near your goal.

If you are currently on medication to lower your blood pressure, blood sugar, or cholesterol, you should remain at Phase I, adhering as strictly as possible to the plan, until your medication doses are significantly reduced or eliminated *by your physician* and your readings have remained normal for at least four weeks. *This plan is so powerful in lowering blood pressure, blood sugar, and blood fats that you must under no circumstances attempt it without close supervision by a physician. You will not be able to remain on your current medications at your current doses safely. Your physician will need to taper and in all probability discontinue your medications for these problems once you begin Phase I. Do not make these changes on your own.* Once your medications have been tapered and your readings have remained stable for at least four weeks, you may move to the Phase II plan for the duration of your diet, just as we've described.

If you are not overweight and have used the diet only to reduce elevated blood fats, blood pressure, or blood sugar, when all your readings are stable you should move to Phase II for three to four weeks and then begin your transition to maintenance.

If you are overweight but have no other metabolic disturbances and are using the plan as a tool to reduce excess body fat and/or recompose your weight, begin on Phase I for four to six weeks, then move to the Phase II plan and remain there until you are near your goal.[3] Your goal should be to work toward an ideal body composition of under 20 percent body fat if you are an average male and approximately 20 to 25 percent if you are an average female.[4] We give you these ideal percentages as targets. Aim for them, and if you hit them, fantastic! Depending on where you've begun this journey toward fitness, getting there may take some time, but every percentage point closer that you come to that ideal is travel in the right direction—toward a leaner, healthier you. Take your time; you can safely stay on this plan as long as it takes to reach your health and fitness goals. How long is that? Read on.

Recomposing Your Body

If a part of your goal is to lose excess body fat—and for most people who suffer from insulin resistance, it is—this plan offers you the easiest and most effective system available for doing that quickly, safely, and permanently. The two questions most often asked by our clinic patients are "How fast can I lose and how long will it take me to get to my goal?" and "How many calories can I eat a day?" We've spent nearly a decade taking care of thousands of overweight people, and we have found that you don't usually have to worry about calories on this program.[5] The metabolic alterations that take place as your insulin falls and your sensitivity to it improves will increase the rate at which you use calories, and you will find that the standard calorie rules simply don't apply in predicting weight loss.

Fat Loss vs. Weight Loss

You will note that we specifically said *fat loss,* not *weight loss.* From this moment forward, we ask that you divorce yourself from the notion that

---

[3] If you choose to remain in Phase I, you may do so. Some of our patients have found that remaining on the more restrictive plan lessens their cravings for carbohydrate foods. If you find that by moving to Phase II you seem hungrier, drop back to Phase I and remain there until you approach your goal.

[4] Competitive athletes will be leaner: 8 to 12 percent fat for men and low to mid-teens in percentage for women. We do not advise women to push their body fat percentages lower than this because of the increased risk for menstrual changes and infertility.

[5] When you're eating a diet structured to keep the metabolic hormones in balance, your caloric intake will pretty much take care of itself. Eat all your meals and snacks every day, and even if you're not especially hungry (this happens more often than you would imagine), be sure that your intake never falls below about 850 to 1,000 calories a day.

you want to lose **weight**. You don't. You want to lose **fat** and **size** and become lean and healthy again. You want to recompose your body by losing excess fat and maintaining your lean mass as closely as you can. And that's a very different proposition from merely losing weight. Weight includes everything. It's water; it's what's in your stomach or intestine or bladder; it's fat; it's muscle.

This plan is designed to help you lose fat and not muscle. When you follow it diligently, you will lose fat steadily. And remember, when fat is what you lose, size changes occur very quickly, because six pounds of fat takes up almost a gallon of space in volume!

Your weight on the scale may not always reflect an accurate loss of fat from week to week, again because everything has weight. Fluctuations in rate of scale weight loss occur especially with women who regularly experience fluid gains and losses with menstrual cycling. In a given week a woman might have lost 2 pounds of fat but retained 3 pounds of water. When she steps on the scale, all she sees is a 1-pound gain. For that reason we encourage our patients not to rely on the scale as a measure of progress except over the long haul. A much more reliable measure is your volume. Select an article of clothing—a pair of pants or jeans, a fitted skirt or dress—that you cannot currently wear. Each week, attempt to put it on and chart how close you come. Maybe the pants will come only to mid-thigh level. Fine. But in a few weeks you'll find that you can pull them all the way up. Not zip them, mind you, but get them on. Then the zipper gets closer to meeting week by week, until one day it will actually zip if you lie down across the bed and wrestle with it. Finally, it will zip easily.

That's how it was for our patient Wayne, who began his corrective regimen under our care at a weight of 326 pounds, suffering from high blood pressure and sleep apnea,[6] with a 56-inch waist. (Wayne had actually begun his own attempt to reduce at 340 pounds using a low-fat diet and heavy exercise. After a year, he'd lost only 14 pounds!) Wayne used his 56-inch belt as his gauge, making a new hole every inch along the way, until his waist measured 36 inches. Now—eight months since he began our diet—he's working to get back into his 34-waist blue jeans. Of course, he has also been able to track his progress in other ways: he no longer needs to take blood pressure medication, and the machine that he once depended on to help him breathe during sleep is gathering dust on a shelf. Wayne and his belt appear on the back cover.

---

[6] Many excessively overweight people suffer from sleep apnea, which means that they quit breathing in their sleep many times during the night, rousing themselves almost awake but not quite. They sleep fitfully, restlessly, usually snore loudly, and toss about. They awaken fatigued and fall asleep easily during the day.

This volume-measuring technique really gives you a true reflection of your progress—nothing has changed about the clothing; what's changed is your size. It also helps to take your focus away from the scale as an indication of how poorly or how well you've done. It helps to reinforce the important message that it's not what you weigh, but what your weight is made of that counts.

Put It in Writing

Make copies of the following worksheet entitled Daily Meal Outline and use it to design your daily meal plans. We encourage you to use it every day to plan for and think about what you are going to eat and where: Will you be eating breakfast at home? On the way to work? Grabbing something on the run? Sitting down with family? Will you dine at your desk at lunch, or do you need to meet with clients or friends and dine out? What will you eat? Where? When you plan ahead, you will find you won't very often get caught in that well-known spot where there's simply nothing for you to eat but a honey bun and a soft drink!

Try to be as honest with your records as you can. A common finding by garbologists is that most Americans eat much more junk food than they admit to, and they admit to a fair amount. One such study in Arizona a few years ago reported that residents ate 20 times more chocolate and 15 times more pastries than they reported having eaten in a consumer survey.

Try to make it a habit to keep good records of what you're eating, how much you exercise, and how you feel. Having an accurate written record also gives you some hard data to look at if you hit a plateau (see Questions Commonly Asked About the Program, page 188) or don't lose fat at your predicted rate. Are you simply eating too much? Have you missed exercising regularly? Are you drinking your fluid and taking your vitamins? Drinking a lot of caffeine? Eating more carbohydrate than you realized? Having a journal to review will help you answer those questions honestly.

Make the commitment that if it goes into your mouth it goes into your journal. Studies have shown that people who will commit to keeping an honest and accurate diary of nutrition and exercise are as much as four times more successful than people who will not. So plan for success and you will succeed!

Daily Meal Outline

BREAKFAST

(Protein source) _____

(Carb source) _____

_____

(Fluid) _____

MORNING SNACK (?)

(Protein source) _____

(Carb source) _____

(Fluid) _____

LUNCH

(Protein source) _____

_____

(Carb source) _____

_____

(Fluid) _____

AFTERNOON OR BEDTIME SNACK (?)

(Protein source) _____

(Carb source) _____

(Fluid) _____

DINNER

(Protein source) _____

_____

(Carb source) _____

_____

(Fluid) _____

Restaurant Dining Guide

For those of you who eat out often and get most of your nutrition either on the run or on the road, this dining guide will help you make selections in keeping with your *Protein Power* prescription. Even if you don't own a skillet, you can successfully restore your health, fitness, and metabolism dining out.

*Alcohol: A single 3-ounce glass of dry red or white wine or a Miller Lite will add 3 to 4 grams of carbohydrate to your meal.

*Beverages: diet soda, water, mineral water, tea or coffee without sugar.

*Desserts: Fresh berries or fresh fruit salad will work. Avoid cakes, cookies, custards, pies, pastries, and ice cream.

American Grill or Bistro

*Grilled meat, fish, or fowl, a large green salad with ranch, blue cheese, or olive oil vinaigrette dressing; steamed or sauteed vegetables in place of the usual potatoes, pasta, or rice. Hold the bread and crackers.

*Chef's salad or grilled chicken Caesar salad. Beware the croutons and crackers—limit to four or five of either on maintenance.

*Quiche and green salad or small fresh fruit salad. Eat only the quiche filling, scooping it out of the crust.

*Tomato stuffed with chicken, tuna, or crab salad, or cottage cheese. Keep crackers to a limit of three or four, none on intervention.

Barbecue Joint

*Sliced beef, pork, chicken, or dry rub ribs with cole slaw and tossed salad. Deviled eggs are fine. Ask for barbecue sauce on the side and limit it to a tablespoon, none on intervention. Hold the beans, fries, or other potatoes and Texas toast, bread, or biscuits.

Fast Foods/Burger Joints

*Grilled chicken sandwich or burger (with cheese and bacon if you like) along with a side salad, ranch, blue cheese, or Italian dressing. Remove one or both buns and eat with a knife and fork. Avoid the fries, baked potatoes, pasta bar, pies, and sundaes.

*Grilled chicken salad with ranch or Italian dressing.

*Sub-sandwich-style (but no bread), deli meats and cheeses on salad greens with ranch or Italian dressing.

Chinese Restaurant
   *Soups: Egg drop or hot and sour soup.
   *Appetizers: Skewered beef or chicken.
   *Beef, chicken, pork, shrimp (or combinations) with broccoli or assorted mixed Chinese vegetables.
   Avoid: Egg roll, noodles, mu shu pancakes, and limit rice to about $1/8$ to $1/4$ cup. Read your fortune, give away the cookie!
French Restaurant
   *Clear soups and fresh green salads.
   *Medallions of beef or pork finished with butter sauces, green peppercorn sauce, or Choron sauce.
   *Roasted lamb, duck, quail, game hen.
   *Grilled or poached fish.
   *Sauté of vegetables (squashes, carrots, onion, cauliflower, asparagus).
   Avoid: bread, potatoes, rice, and heavy cream sauces which may contain significant carbohydrate from flour.
Indian Restaurant
   *Tandoori chicken or lamb; chicken, beef, or lamb curry; chicken tikka or chicken masala.
   *Tossed green salad, tomato and cucumber salad, pickled onion, *zukeni bhaghi* (stewed zucchini and yellow squash), *saag panir* (creamy spinach).
   Avoid: The breads, breaded and fried vegetables, potato dishes, and limit rice to a tablespoon or two.
Italian Restaurant
   *Sautéed (not breaded) calamari or antipasto appetizers.
   *Chicken or veal piccata, grilled fish or pork cutlet, or rotisserie or grilled chicken with tossed salad and any sautéed or steamed vegetables available to substitute for pasta.
   Avoid: The pasta dishes and bread. Even a single piece of garlic bread can contain 14 or more grams of carbohydrate.
Japanese Sushi/Teriyaki Restaurant
   *Sushi or sashimi. Beware of overeating the rice.
   *Miso soup (seaweed, broth, and bean curd).
   *Teriyaki chicken, beef, or fish with salad. Avoid tempura, which is breaded and fried.

Mexican Restaurant
*Chicken or beef fajitas, minus the tortilla wrappers. Eat the garnishes: lettuce, chopped tomato, guacamole, sour cream, pico de gallo.
*Grilled chicken, fish, beef, beef or pork medallions, or shredded beef, pork, or chicken with *insalata mista* (tossed salad).
*Taco salad—but leave the taco uneaten.
Avoid (for intervention) or strictly limit: rice and beans (no more than 1 tablespoon of either), tortilla wrappers (one half), shells (one half), or chips (3 or 4).

Pizza Parlor
*Pizza and a tossed salad with ranch, blue cheese, or Italian dressing. Load up the toppings you like: the trick is to eat only the toppings and leave the crust uneaten.
Avoid: breadsticks, garlic toast, spaghetti or other pasta dishes.

Transition and Maintenance

When are you ready to make the transition from intervention to maintenance?

1. When you have reduced or eliminated any medicines you took to lower blood pressure, blood sugar, or blood fats with Phase I and normalized your readings for at least four weeks and these values have remained stable in Phase II for an additional three to four weeks.

2. When you have recomposed your weight to your desired lean and fat percentages on Phase II.

3. When you are within 5 percent of your ideal body weight if you're using the plan to lose body fat.

4. When you must leave the plan for some reason—such as surgery, pregnancy, severe injury, or illness. You should not place yourself in a reduced-calorie state in any of these circumstances, and you should, if they arise, quickly move to controlled maintenance at sufficient calories to meet their high energy demands even if you have not reached your ultimate goal. Because these kinds of situations often occur without warning, you will need to hasten your transition to a maintenance level. If you have even a few days, follow the step-by-step instructions outlined here

as day-by-day increases in intake instead of week by week. It's not the best solution, but it will suffice in an emergency. Once the situation resolves and you have healed completely, you can resume your Phase I or Phase II diet as before—with all the same caveats.

THE SMOOTH TRANSITION

The next several weeks are the most important of the entire regimen, so take great care to follow the guidelines strictly. For some time your body has been in a controlled slide, a state of corrective momentum. It's now time to gently slow and then stop the momentum of those changes and equilibrate and stabilize at your new leaner, healthier level.

The changes that you've wrought occurred because you harnessed your rampaging insulin and kept it under tight rein. Your job now is to slowly and carefully let out some slack. You will accomplish this by gradually increasing your per-meal carbohydrate level until you reach a daily total carbohydrate gram intake roughly equal to or slightly more than your daily protein intake. It's important that you make this transition to maintenance slowly and methodically (except in the face of emergencies). Moving in one big leap from the controlled carbohydrate level that's kept you in a state of hormonal balance to your maintenance level will stimulate a sudden big release of insulin with all the attendant potential for adverse consequences.

Move from Phase II to maintenance according to the following guidelines: Increase your daily carbohydrate intake in 10-gram increments until you reach an amount approximately equal to your daily protein intake—e.g., if your daily protein intake is 75 grams, increase your daily carbohydrate gram total from 55 grams (the Phase II level) to 65 grams and finally to 75 grams. Remain at each new higher intake level for five to seven days to stabilize your insulin production before advancing again. This slow upward climb will allow you to ease the reins on your insulin production and prevent rebound weight gain, fluid retention, or blood pressure increases that could occur by turning insulin loose all at once.

If you are active or very active physically, or if you continue to lose weight while consuming protein and carbohydrate in equal amounts, you may continue to increase your carbohydrate grams in 10-gram jumps (again, stabilizing after each jump for five to seven days) until your carbohydrate intake exceeds your protein intake by 30 percent. For a daily protein intake of 75 grams, you would multiply 75 by 1.3 for a total carbohydrate intake of 97.5 grams (which you could round up to 100 grams) per day. A few people might even be able to go to a little higher carbohydrate intake, but in general your maintenance carbohydrate level should be equal to or up to about 30 percent more than your protein intake.

If weight reduction was a part of your goal, *slowly* increase your carbohydrate intake as outlined until your carbohydrate intake equals your protein intake or until you stop losing weight. Remain at that daily total carbohydrate level for two months to allow your fat cell activity to stabilize.[7] Then slowly—in 10-gram jumps followed each time by a five- to seven-day stabilization period—continue to increase your daily carbohydrate intake. Weigh yourself (a poor measurement, we know, but the handiest one for this purpose) at the end of each stabilization period, and when you first see a gain, drop back to the last carbohydrate gram intake at which your weight remained stable and stay there.[8]

Refer to your ECC charts for fruits, vegetables, and bread and cereal grains. You can enjoy these 10-gram jumps by selecting servings of those higher-carbohydrate goodies you've been missing. For example, you might add a peach at breakfast if you love fruit; an extra half pita pocket at lunch, a small serving of pasta, or a small biscuit with your dinner if you've missed starches; or a small frozen yogurt as a snack to satisfy your sweet tooth. Ideally, try to spread your added carbohydrate intake throughout the day instead of piling it all onto one meal, because *the more carbohydrate you eat at a sitting, the bigger insulin response you'll stir up.* (Although it's better not to do so, if you do plan to bank your carbohydrates to eat a bigger serving—for example, you've planned a "night on the town"—scale back the carbohydrate portion of the remaining meals or snacks throughout the day so that your total intake doesn't exceed your allotment. And remember, it's better *not* to do this!)

In our years of practice we've seen people who would begin to lose their metabolic control on fewer than 60 grams per day and others who had to push their carbohydrate intake above 150 grams per day to stop weight loss. Each of us is a little different, and what you will discover through your diligent upward creep in making this transition from intervention to maintenance is your own tolerance level for carbohydrate in-

---

[7] The very act of weight loss causes your fat cells to *want* to store fat. This heightened storage activity falls back to normal after several months. This is another reason why it's in your best interest to get focused on the program and lose all your excess at once, not stop-start.

[8] Your weight will be a reflection of appropriate carbohydrate intake only if you've actually adhered to that daily gram total. If you intentionally or inadvertently exceed your prescribed carbohydrate total, you will retain fluid quickly, which will cause a gain in scale weight. It's important that you be very careful to follow your plan during this period.

take. The key to maintaining your correction is keeping your daily intake of carbohydrate at or very near this level most of the time. Now we'll show you how to develop a realistic strategy for maintaining your achievement and still enjoying your life.

YOU *CAN* MAINTAIN FOR LIFE

You've worked hard to reclaim your health, to reduce or recompose your weight, and to restore your body to balance. Now the work of living within the system begins. With your new understanding of how food influences the hormones of metabolism you have the key to maintaining your health and fitness for the rest of your life. The choice of whether to eat a well-composed meal or a poorly composed one will always be yours, and therefore the responsibility for maintaining your balance and health is yours alone. You've got the tools and information to do so, and you should endeavor to do so *most of the time.*

Good things have happened to you metabolically that will help you maintain more easily. One of the benefits of going through Phases I and II of this plan is that you restore your insulin receptors to a level of better sensitivity, which allows you to *occasionally* "blow it out" dietarily on foods you love without suffering long-term damage.

In our clinical practice this is the advice we give to our patients as they go into the phase of maintenance: there is no food you can't have—in some quantity at some time. There will be foods, however, that are so rich in sugars and starches, such potent unbalancers of your metabolic hormones, that you cannot have unlimited amounts of them anytime you want unless you are willing to accept the consequences of that action. The inescapable consequences of a return to your old dietary habits will be to disrupt your metabolic balance and send you hurtling pell-mell back to your previous weight and beyond, back to taking daily medications to lower your blood pressure, cholesterol, or blood sugar to curb the skyrocketing values.

Nutritional maintenance of your health requires vigilance and effort most of the time interspersed with occasional brief vacations from the straight and narrow. Let's see how this works.

The Nutritional Vacation

Our society—like most—celebrates by feasting. Think of any joyous holiday celebration, and the first thing that will likely come to your mind is some favorite or traditional family dish associated with it. In our family, Thanksgiving just wouldn't be complete without a turkey stuffed with Granny Eades's cornmeal stuffing. And we wouldn't recognize Christmas Eve without homemade eggnog and decorated sugar cookies or Christmas dinner without mincemeat pie. And a Fourth of July picnic without traditional strawberry shortcake? Not at our picnic table. Celebration by feasting traces its origins as far back as mankind has kept written records, and as long as humans gather together in joy or thanks, food will play a big role. It does in our family, and it will in yours.

The fact that you have inherited a tendency for metabolic disturbance doesn't mean you must forever forfeit your right to join in the celebrations. We urge you to take a look at the celebrations and food traditions that are most meaningful in your life, whatever they may be. Select several times a year—perhaps your birthday, anniversary, holidays traditionally celebrated in your family or faith, a romantic getaway, a long-planned trip, or those once-in-a-lifetime events, such as weddings or class reunions—and *plan to enjoy them*. The key is to plan for it, look forward to it, enjoy it, and then, using the Recovery Guidelines outlined in the next section, recover from it and return to maintenance until the next planned vacation. Knowing that you have planned a vacation from maintenance somehow makes the idea of maintaining more tolerable and the small sacrifices you make day by day less burdensome. By choosing when and how you vary, you free yourself from anxiety and guilt that you might otherwise associate with breaking from your maintenance plan. You planned it, you knew in advance what the short-term consequences would be, and you had a prearranged plan of action to get back on the track immediately. It's not uncommon for a day or two of dietary debauchery to leave you four, five, six, even seven pounds heavier with retained fluid—and feeling lousy. So the purpose of this brief phase of recovery is to quickly drop your elevated insulin levels that the vacation inspired, waste off that fluid excess, get your eicosanoids flowing back in the right direction, get you feeling chipper again, and slide you back onto your maintenance intake.

Recovery Guidelines

1. Return to Phase I for three days or until you have lost any weight you gained during your vacation (most of which will be from fluid retention).
2. Move to Phase II for the remainder of the week.
3. Return to your maintenance level and keep on living in metabolic equilibrium.

Although we want you to live happily and enjoy life to the fullest in your maintenance, we'd be remiss in not reminding you that the fewer variances the better. Our own experience—personally and with thousands of our patients—is that the longer you adhere to this biochemically correct lifestyle, the less appealing dietary indiscretion becomes. When you're in balance, you feel so good—mentally sharp, physically strong and well, emotionally stable—and when you vary from balance you feel so lousy that you will ask yourself, as we often have, "Why did I eat that?"

Questions Commonly Asked About the Program

Q. *Won't eating all this protein harm my kidneys?*

A. No, not if your kidneys are normal to begin with. People who restrict their carbohydrate intake seem to believe they are following a "high-protein" diet. On this program you calculate your *minimum* protein requirements—the amount of protein you would need no matter what kind of diet you followed. Even if you exceed this amount substantially—as long as your kidneys function normally—you should have no ill effects. A number of researchers have studied this exact question and, in fact, an impeccable 1995 study from Germany demonstrated that kidney function actually improved with increased protein consumption.

Q. *What should I do if I feel dizzy or light-headed?*

A. If you feel like you're going to pass out, or especially if you feel this sensation immediately upon standing up from a chair or bed, you probably need to increase your salt intake. This regime packs a potent diuretic force. As you progress on the program, your lowered insulin begins to allow your kidneys to release their retained fluid. You will notice how much more time you spend in the rest room as you rid yourself of this excess fluid. Unfortunately the kidneys also get rid of sodium and potassium along with this excess fluid, often leading to a sodium and/or potassium deficit and a little dehydration. The lowered sodium along with the dehydration causes the light-headedness. Increase your salt intake by adding regular table salt to your foods, eating a dill pickle, or drinking bouillon, and you should find your problem solved in short order.

Q. *I used to be able to lose weight easily, but now I have a difficult time even getting the first few pounds off. Why?*

A. Because you must first overcome what we call the inertia of weight loss. If you have dieted repeatedly, you are going to have more trouble getting into gear than someone who has never dieted. With repeated dieting your body gets more adept at squeezing out every ounce of energy from each bit of food as it is given smaller and smaller amounts. Your metabolism has an internal computer that has served our species well over eons of evolutionary time that resets your metabolic response to food depending on how much it gets. If you are used to eating large amounts of food, your metabolic rate is probably pretty high because the computer knows your body has fuel to waste. When you diet—or if you were somehow stranded in the Arctic or suffered a famine—your metabolic computer rapidly decreases your metabolic rate to conserve stored energy (fat) and wring the last dollop of energy out of any food coming in (all for survival reasons; your computer doesn't know you're dieting—it thinks you're starving, and it wants you to survive the lean time ahead). Not only is this computer exquisitely sensitive, but unfortunately for repeat dieters, it has a memory. If you have been through Jenny Craig twice, the Diet Center several times, Nutri/System and Optifast a time or two, not to mention Weight Watchers every other year, your computer has it all stored. And when you start on the next diet, it immediately adopts a bunker mentality and signals the entire metabolic system to go into conserve mode, making it progressively more and more difficult to lose. One of the nicest features of this program is that the large amount of food it provides begins to reprogram the computer and gradually brings it out of the fear-of-famine mode that is such an obstacle to weight loss. It will take a few weeks of diligent work, but you'll finally break free and begin to lose easily—a phase we call *dynamic weight loss* in which the fat reduction takes on a life of its own.

Q. *I have hit a plateau. What can I do to get things going?*

A. Plateaus are the purgatory of dieting. Everyone seems to experience them, hate them, and become frustrated by them. There are a few things you can do to get beyond the plateau, but before you do them, make sure you're on a true plateau. If you are just monitoring your weight on the scales and you seem stuck, you may be recomposing your body by gaining muscle weight as you lose fat. If you gain several pounds of muscle because you're exercising while at the same time you lose several pounds of fat, your weight on the scales doesn't change, but your size sure does. People who have been on a low-fat diet for a long time and who are protein deficient sometimes gain a few pounds of muscle simply from the decent amounts of protein they begin eating. If either of these situations describes you, you're not on a plateau; you're simply building muscle and/or rebuilding your lean body mass. You should notice a significant decrease in size even though you're not losing any scale weight.

If you truly are on a plateau, you can try several things. First, make absolutely certain you're following the program correctly. The most common mistake we see in our clinic with patients on plateaus is that they are not following their plan. That's one reason we have patients keep diaries and recommend that you keep a diary. Go back and *count* the number of grams of carbohydrate consumed—don't guess. It takes a while to get used to counting carbohydrates, and it can be disastrous to your success to assume or to guess. Until you get it down pat, always look it up before you eat it. We can't tell you how many patients we have who, when we discuss their "plateaus" with them, tell us, "Well, I did just like you told me except I ate a bagel on this day, and I had a banana on that day, and . . ." A bagel can contain anywhere from 30 to 50 grams of carbohydrate, a banana about 30. Fifty grams of carbohydrate—from whatever source—is the equivalent of $1/4$ cup of pure sugar. If you add this to your regimen every day or so, we can guarantee that you'll have plenty of plateaus.

If you absolutely are sticking to the plan and are still plateauing, try reducing your overall intake of food. Keep your protein intake at the minimum for your lean body mass, keep your carbohydrates at the level recommended for your phase, and lower your fat intake a little. That should do the trick, and when your weight loss starts picking back up, you can start increasing your intake a little. You can also cut your carbohydrate intake down to about 10 to 20 grams per day for a few days to get things going. Another thing you can do is to try some of the pre-packaged nutritional products we've used in our clinic for years with great success. (See Appendix.)

Finally, make sure your fluid intake is sufficient. We have found often that a simple increase in fluids gets the weight coming off again in a hurry.

Q. *I've read a lot lately about "good" carbohydrates and "bad" carbohydrates, and I don't really understand the difference. Should I try to eat only the good ones? Or does it matter?*

A. The notion of "good" versus "bad" carbohydrates stems from the concept of the glycemic index developed by researcher David A. Jenkins and his group in Toronto in the early 1980s. Dr. Jenkins gave subjects 100 grams of pure glucose, then measured the amount of blood sugar rise this glucose produced. He then gave the same subjects various kinds of food containing the same 100 grams of carbohydrate, measured their blood sugar responses, and compared them with the blood sugar rise stimulated by the pure glucose. If the blood sugar rise was the same as glucose, then the food in question was said to have a glycemic index of 100. The lower the glycemic index, the less blood sugar response the particular food caused. Dr. Jenkins and others have continued to refine and improve on his early work, and the idea that low glycemic index foods are good carbohydrates and high glycemic index foods are bad has taken root.

The only problem with the whole concept is that the glycemic index doesn't compare apples to apples. It compares apples to glucose. Apples contain the whole complicated mélange of pectins, lignins, celluloses, hemicelluloses, and all the other substances that are collectively known as fiber along with the pure carbohydrate. Fiber slows the absorption of the pure carbohydrate, causing a lower blood sugar response, and probably has other independent actions on blood sugar and insulin as well. So the glycemic index of the apple is a function not of the specific carbohydrate it contains, but of the actions on this carbohydrate by the rest of the apple. In developing our ECC charts, we have removed the fiber component and left only the pure, *metabolically* active carbohydrate for you to count so that the whole concept of good and bad carbohydrates becomes meaningless *metabolically*. We emphasize the word *metabolically* because we're talking only about the blood sugar and insulin response to the food in question, not its overall nutritional worth.

For example, if you eat 5 grams of carbohydrate in a piece of candy, you will get about the same insulin response as you would if you ate 5 grams of carbohydrate in broccoli—not much. But what a difference nutritionally, not to mention in volume. The broccoli would be much more filling. The beauty of the ECC charts is that by using them you tend to gravitate toward foods that are more nutritionally dense and filling, and you never really have to worry about what is a good or a bad carbohydrate. Simply stay within your carbohydrate limits, select them from the ECC charts, and you will find that you probably have more food than you can eat.

Once you're on maintenance, you may want to remember that rice causes a lower blood sugar rise than potatoes, corn, and wheat. Next in line are beans and oats. But in the end the body receives it all as glucose—sugar—and you'll always need to watch your carbs.

Q. *Will I be constipated on this program, and if so, what can I do about it?*

A. You shouldn't be constipated for a number of reasons. First, if you select your carbohydrates from the ECC charts, you will tend to select foods with a high fiber content, which will help prevent constipation. Second, by reducing your insulin levels you will begin to make more good eicosanoids, which will increase the water content of your colon contents and prevent constipation. If you do experience a little constipation, it should be short-lived, but until it resolves you may want to use some of the fiber supplements described in the box at the end of Chapter 7, increase your fluid intake, and perhaps add one or two capsules of fish oil. (One good choice is MaxEPA-1000; another is Eico Marine from Eicotec, Inc., 21 Tioga Way, Marblehead, MA 01945.)

Q. *What if I have diarrhea?*

A. Surprisingly, this is a more common complaint on this regime than constipation. Usually loose stools, and occasionally diarrhea, start a few days into the program and resolve a few days later as the body adjusts to its new diet. If it doesn't resolve, you need to be checked for an infection—nothing to do with your new diet, just a possible coincidence. If that test is negative, reduce your intake of fish oil capsules, if you're taking them, reduce your intake of high-fiber foods, and, finally, make sure you don't have an allergy or sensitivity to one or more of the new foods you're consuming.

Q. *I've just started the program, and I feel extremely fatigued. Why?*

A. This is a common experience with our new patients. All of life is catalyzed by enzymes. If it weren't for enzymes, we would just be piles of nonreactive chemicals instead of the living, breathing beings we are. Our DNA codes for millions of enzymes, but we make and have circulating at any given time only those we need. If you have been on a low-fat, high-complex-carbohydrate diet, you have all the enzymes circulating around that deal with storing, breaking down, and retrieving carbohydrates as needed for energy. When you drastically change your diet, all these enzymes are then running around with nothing to do because they're so specific to their function that they can't work on your new diet. It takes a few days for your body to produce the new enzymes to deal with the composition of your new diet. After a couple of days of a little tiredness, however, your energy levels should rise considerably, and you should actually end up with a lot more energy than you had before you started the diet.

Q. *I have been on the diet for a couple of weeks now. I felt a little tired at first, then I felt fabulous, and now, all of a sudden, I feel exhausted, and my legs ache.*

A. You have described a textbook case of hypokalemia, or low blood potassium. Because the diet has such a diuretic effect on the kidneys, it often gets rid of enough potassium along with the excess fluid that some people become potassium deficient. Low potassium can cause all kinds of different symptoms such as tingling, light-headedness, fatigue, muscle aches, and especially deep muscle fatigue and cramps. We recommended that you use Morton's Lite Salt or NoSalt because these are pure potassium salts and usually will compensate for the potassium lost through the kidneys. If you aren't using these, start now. If you are, then get one of the potassium supplements listed on page 124 and start taking it. If your symptoms are from potassium deficiency, they should resolve in a matter of hours after beginning potassium supplementation. *If you are taking blood pressure medicines or diuretics, you must check with your physician or pharmacist before taking potassium supplements because some of these medicines prevent the body's release of potassium, and taking extra can cause serious problems.* If you are not taking any of these medications and have normal kidney function, it is virtually impossible to overdose on potassium taken as the salt substitute or as a supplement from a health food store.

Q. *Do I have to spread my carbohydrates around throughout the day, or can I save them up and eat them all at once?*

A. You will do better if you divide your carbohydrates into approximately equal portions and eat them throughout the day. If you have a special occasion coming up and you know you will overindulge, then save your carbohydrates and eat them all at once. We have had several patients who found some sort of carbohydrate treat they enjoyed immensely that they would save up for and eat once during the day. One patient was losing weight by leaps and bounds and lowering his dangerously elevated cholesterol on the Phase I Intervention when he found a candy he liked that contained 17 grams of carbohydrate. He would eat one of these candies every afternoon. He then spread his remaining 13 grams of carbohydrate around the rest of his meals. He continued to lose and told us that the pleasure he got from that one piece of candy more than offset the reduction in carbohydrate the rest of the day. If you decide to pursue this line of dieting, remember to cut back during the rest of the day, or your progress will slow.

Q. *I have suffered with indigestion and reflux for years and take medication every day to stop the burning. Since I've been on this diet, I've forgotten to take my medicine several times and I've had no indigestion. Could the diet have done this?*

A. Yes. In fact the disappearance of gastritis, reflux, and indigestion on our Protein Power plan is one of its most predictable beneficial effects. This diet improves the quality of protective mucous in the stomach lining and normalizes muscular control of the esophageal sphincter to prevent reflux and spasm. Eicosanoid modulation is the reason (see Chapter 6) for this dramatic response, working in the same way as the newest ulcer and reflux medications, but without the considerable expense and unpleasant side effects.

Q. *I've heard that diets high in protein can cause osteoporosis. Is this true?*

A. No. In the first place this diet is *not* a high protein diet, it is an *adequate* protein diet. Second, even a high protein diet doesn't cause an overall loss of calcium. The notion that high protein diets cause calcium loss is a persistent rumor—even among those who should know better—that no amount of scientific research (and there's plenty) seems to be able to dispel. Diets high in meat protein have been consumed for millennia by people the world over without harm, so don't worry about osteoporosis.

Q. *If I make some of the changes you recommend—for example, cutting back some on my carbohydrate intake—will I see improvement, or do I need to follow the program exactly to get results?*

A. If you are overweight or have any of the other problems we have been discussing, cutting back a little on your carbohydrates won't accomplish much. If you indeed have one of these disorders, you have damaged insulin receptors. The only way to repair them is to get your insulin level down and let them heal. A little bit of carbohydrate cutting won't do that—it has to be fairly drastic, as in the Phase I Intervention. Only then can you expect the long-term benefits you really want.

Q. *Will I lose weight faster if I cut out all carbohydrates? Would it be dangerous?*

A. Cutting your carbohydrate below the level of Phase I (7 to 10 grams per meal) probably won't speed your loss, so there's little point in going lower. Each gram of carbohydrate provides only about 4 calories, so you can see that you're saving only about 100 calories in the day (eating three meals each containing 28 to 40 calories in carbohydrate). As to the danger of it, traditional Eskimos, living above the Arctic Circle, eat virtually no carbohydrate and do fine. Refer to the study undertaken by Vilhjalmur Stefansson (see footnote 2, Chapter 1) for more details.

Q. *Won't this diet put me into ketosis?*

A. If you're very much overweight, Phase I will almost certainly put you into ketosis, but there's nothing wrong with that. It simply tells you that you're burning fat. If you're not much overweight, the diet will probably put you right on the cusp of ketosis, which is where you want to be. Ketosis is a much-misunderstood subject, so let's go into it in a little detail. Ketones (ketone bodies, the actual scientific name) are made when fat breaks down. As you read the words on this page you are producing ketones, but unless you're on this diet or have been fasting, you're probably not in ketosis—the state of having a measurable level of ketones in your blood. Ketones are an intermediate stage of fat breakdown, and not only are they not poison as described by several health writers, but they're used as fuel by most of the body's tissues including the brain. The heart, in fact, prefers ketones to all other fuel. The body must have sufficient carbohydrate to completely burn for energy all the ketones produced. The diet causes the breakdown of fat, producing an abundance of ketones—especially in the overweight person—but the intervention diets don't provide enough carbohydrate to burn all of them. These excess ketones circulate in the blood and must be gotten rid of in other ways. The body releases them via the urine, the stool, and the breath. Since ketones are incompletely burned fat, any that you get rid of without actually using them for energy means you are ditching unwanted fat without having to actually burn it off.

Q. *But aren't ketones and ketosis dangerous?*

A. Unless you're a type I diabetic, not at all. You might think so, however, because some health writers such as Jane Brody of *The New York*

Times, a major proponent of the low-fat, high-complex-carbohydrate diet, say that ketones are "toxic compounds that can damage the brain and cause nausea, fatigue, and apathy." She goes on to tell you that ketones are "fat waste products" that "pollute" the blood. But Dr. Lubert Stryer, Professor of Biochemistry at Stanford University and the author of the biochemistry textbook used in most medical schools, says ketones are "normal fuels of respiration and are quantitatively important as sources of energy." "Indeed," Dr. Stryer continues, "heart muscle, and the renal cortex [kidney] use [ketones] in preference to glucose." Drs. Donald and Judith Voet, authors of another popular medical biochemistry textbook, say that ketones "serve as important metabolic fuels for many peripheral tissues, particularly heart and skeletal muscle." So if you believe Ms. Brody, you would think that ketones poison you; if you trust the consensus among medical experts and scientists, you will understand that ketones are a perfectly normal fuel used preferentially by most of the tissues in the body for their energy needs. In fact—except for type I diabetics—there is no evidence for the opinion that ketones are dangerous.

Q. *Why do I sometimes get a funny taste in my mouth or bad breath on this diet?*

A. Ketones released through the lungs can cause an unpleasant odor (acetone breath) and/or a funny taste in the mouth. The best thing to do for this is to drink plenty of fluids. If you make a lot of urine, most of the ketones will escape that way. If not, about the only way out they have is through the breath. Breath sprays and sugar-free gum can help, but beware of overusing the gum. Sugar-free means *sucrose* (table sugar) free, not necessarily carbohydrate free.

Q. *Why have I had trouble sleeping since starting the diet?*

A. Heavy ketosis can cause sleeplessness. If you are producing and releasing a lot of ketones,[9] you may be able to increase your carbohydrates a little or move ahead to Phase II Intervention.

Q. *I don't have any trouble getting to sleep, but I wake up in the middle of the night starving. I raid the refrigerator and eat whatever is at hand before I can get back to sleep. Will the diet do anything to stop these cravings?*

---

[9]You can check your ketone production status by purchasing Ketostix from any drugstore. These little coated plastic sticks, when dipped into a sample of your urine, will change color. By comparing the color on the stick to the chart on the jar they came in, you can determine your ketone status.

A. Yes. This is not the typical description of a food craving but sounds more like an ulcer or gastritis problem—both of which are common to insulin-resistant people on high-carbohydrate diets. The body naturally releases a surge of stomach acid in the wee hours of the morning that doesn't bother anyone with a normal stomach lining. But in people who have either ulcers or gastritis (inflammation of the stomach lining), this surge of acid often produces enough pain and discomfort to awaken them. They typically don't have a sense of actual stomach pain but instead feel a kind of gnawing hunger that begs to be relieved. Consuming a large portion of food neutralizes this excess acid, they feel better, and they go back to sleep. On our program the reduction in carbohydrate intake begins immediately to allow most ulcers and gastritis to heal. Most of these problems are caused by an eicosanoid imbalance that is quickly normalized as soon as insulin levels fall. A few days after starting the program these episodes should begin to become much less frequent and finally go away. If you do awaken, however, make sure you eat according to your intervention plan, and *don't overeat carbohydrates* or you will perpetuate the problem.

Q. *What about artificial sweeteners? Aren't they dangerous?*

A. Our own preference is to avoid artificial sweeteners as much as possible simply because no one knows the very long-term effects of them. We try to eat as few unnatural products as possible, but we don't completely avoid artificial sweeteners because they are found in too many good low-carbohydrate foods. Are they dangerous? That depends. Compared to what? Compared to an equivalent sweetening amount of sugar, they are innocuous. If all you consumed was 1 teaspoon of sugar per day in your morning coffee, we would say go ahead and use the sugar. But, if you're talking about a soft drink, that's a different story. A 12-ounce can of most soft drinks contains about 4 tablespoons of pure sugar, $1/4$ cup, which calculates to 48 grams, more than your whole day's allotment on Phase I. In the case of soft drinks the sugar poses much more of a health risk than the artificial sweetener that replaces it in the diet version.

Aspartame, the artificial sweetener in NutraSweet, passed more than one hundred FDA tests before it was approved. On the horizon is left-handed sugar, a molecular manipulation of real sugar that is not metabolized by the body—no calories, almost no carbohydrates. The FDA is still testing, but this sugar is available in Canada, where it's called Splenda and has been in general use for more than six years.

You can ruin your diet by overindulging in artificial sweeteners, as

one of our patients did. It turned out she was using some 50 teaspoons of Equal a day—and those little fractions of carbohydrate
added up to big trouble.

Q. *What about my "sweet tooth"? Because of the carbohydrate restriction,
this program doesn't have any really sweet foods, so I can't indulge my
cravings for sweets.*

A. Believe it or not, your craving for sweets will diminish with time. Just
as insulin receptors become resistant to the stimulation of insulin over
time, requiring much more insulin to make them work, your sweet receptors (taste buds) do the same. With chronic stimulation by a sweet,
sugary diet your taste buds become resistant to the stimulation of
sweets, requiring more and more to give you the pleasant sensation
you desire. As you destimulate them by removing the refined carbohydrate from your diet, your sweet receptors will regain their sensitivity. At that point foods that you previously would have eaten by the
plateful to get your sweet fix will provide the same sensation in much
smaller amounts. In fact, if you try to eat the amounts you did before,
you will pay the price in the way you feel later. A few such experiences
and your sweet-consumption habits will have changed for good.

Q. *I understand about calculating protein, carbohydrate, and all that, but
what does that mean in real food? What would a day of eating look like?*

A. Let's suppose your protein need is 27 grams per meal and set up a
typical day on Phase I.

For breakfast, you might enjoy a ham and cheese omelet, a slice of
"light" sourdough toast with a pat of sweet butter, half a cup of
sliced fresh strawberries with cream, and a cup of coffee.

At lunch, you might dine with friends at a local restaurant, where
you could have a grilled chicken Caesar salad (hold the croutons)
with sliced fresh peaches and cream for dessert, with coffee. Or if
you're on the run, and the only thing available is the local burger
joint, you could dash in for a double cheeseburger with everything—
hold the buns—a salad, and a big glass of iced tea—remember to
drink most of the tea *before* you eat.

In the afternoon, for a snack, you might eat some slices of hard salami
with sharp cheddar cheese and a glass of mineral water or a diet soda.

For dinner you could grill a juicy steak, with sautéed mushrooms,
fresh asparagus in a vinaigrette dressing, sliced fresh tomatoes, and a
large green salad. Accompany the meal with a glass of dry red wine
if you like, or just have a little water and coffee or tea, and save room
for a little sliced melon.

PROTEIN EQUIVALENCY CHART A

TOTAL PROTEIN INTAKE ≤60 GRAMS PER DAY (20 GRAMS PER MEAL)

	Meat, fish, poultry	Egg	Hard cheeses	Soft cheeses	Curd cheeses	Tofu
Meat, fish, poultry	3 oz.					
Eggs	1 egg + 2 whites + 1 oz. "meat"	2 eggs + 2 whites	Unacceptable*	Unacceptable		
Hard cheeses	2 oz. "meat" + 1 oz. cheese	1 egg + 2 whites + 1 oz. cheese				
Soft cheeses	2 oz. "meat" + 2 oz. cheese	1 egg + 2 whites + 2 oz. cheese	Unacceptable	Unacceptable		
Curd cheeses	2 oz. "meat" + 1/4 cup cheese	1 egg + 1 white + 1/4 cup cheese	1/2 cup curd + 1 oz. hard cheese	1/2 cup curd + 2 oz. soft cheese	3/4 cup curd	
Tofu	1/4 cup tofu + 1.5 oz. "meat"	1 egg + 1 white + 1/4 cup tofu	1/4 cup tofu + 1 oz. cheese	1/4 cup tofu + 2 oz. cheese	1/4 cup curd + 1/4 cup tofu	1/2 cup tofu

"Meat" = 7 grams per ounce
Eggs = 6 grams whole, 4 grams white
Hard Cheese = 6–7 grams per ounce
Soft Cheese = 3–4 grams per ounce
Curd Cheese = 7 grams per 1/4 cup
Tofu = 10 grams per 1/4 cup

*Because of the high fat content, the number of calories consumed to make these an adequate sole protein source would be too high for most people.

PROTEIN EQUIVALENCY CHART B

TOTAL PROTEIN INTAKE 61–80 GRAMS PER DAY (27 GRAMS PER MEAL)

	Meat, fish, poultry	Egg	Hard cheeses	Soft cheeses	Curd cheeses	Tofu
Meat, fish, poultry	4 oz.					
Eggs	2 eggs + 2 whites + 1 oz. "meat"	2 eggs + 4 whites				
Hard cheeses	3 oz. "meat" + 1 oz. cheese	2 eggs + 2 whites + 1 oz. cheese	Unacceptable*			
Soft cheeses	3 oz. "meat" + 2 oz. cheese	2 eggs + 2 whites + 2 oz. cheese	Unacceptable	Unacceptable		
Curd cheeses	3 oz. "meat" + 1/4 cup cheese	2 eggs + 1/2 cup cheese	3/4 cup curd + 1 oz. hard cheese	3/4 cup curd + 2 oz. soft cheese	1 cup curd	
Tofu	1/2 cup tofu + 1 oz. "meat"	1 egg + 3 whites + 1/4 cup tofu	1/2 cup tofu + 1 oz. cheese	1/2 cup tofu + 2 oz. cheese	1/2 cup tofu + 1/4 cup curd	3/4 cup tofu

"Meat" = 7 grams per ounce
Eggs = 6 grams whole, 4 grams white
Hard Cheese = 6–7 grams per ounce
Soft Cheese = 3–4 grams per ounce
Curd Cheese = 7 grams per 1/4 cup
Tofu = 10 grams per 1/4 cup

*Because of the high fat content, the number of calories consumed to make these an adequate sole protein source would be too high for most people.

PROTEIN EQUIVALENCY CHART C

TOTAL PROTEIN INTAKE 81–100 GRAMS PER DAY (34 GRAMS PER MEAL)

	Meat, fish, poultry	Egg	Hard cheeses	Soft cheeses	Curd cheeses	Tofu
Meat, fish, poultry	5 oz.					
Eggs	2 eggs + 2 whites + 2 oz. "meat"	3 eggs + 4 whites				
Hard cheeses	4 oz. "meat" + 1 oz. cheese	2 eggs + 4 whites + 1 oz. cheese	Unacceptable*			
Soft cheeses	4 oz. "meat" + 2 oz. cheese	2 eggs + 4 whites + 2 oz. cheese	Unacceptable	Unacceptable		
Curd cheeses	3 oz. tofu + 1/2 cup cheese	2 eggs + 2 whites + 1/2 cup cheese	1 cup curd + 1 oz. hard cheese	1 cup curd + 2 oz. soft cheese	1¼ cups curd	
Tofu	1/2 cup tofu + 2 oz. "meat"	2 eggs + 1/2 cup tofu	scant 3/4 cup + 1 oz. cheese	3/4 cup + 1 oz. cheese	1/2 cup tofu + 1/2 cup curd	heaping 3/4 cup tofu

"Meat" = 7 grams per ounce
Eggs = 6 grams whole, 4 grams white
Hard Cheese = 6–7 grams per ounce
Soft Cheese = 3–4 grams per ounce
Curd Cheese = 7 grams per 1/4 cup
Tofu = 10 grams per 1/4 cup

*Because of the high fat content, the number of calories consumed to make these an adequate sole protein source would be too high for most people.

PROTEIN EQUIVALENCY CHART D

TOTAL PROTEIN INTAKE 101–120 GRAMS PER DAY (40 GRAMS PER MEAL)

		Meat, fish, poultry	Egg	Hard cheeses	Soft cheeses	Curd cheeses	Tofu
Meat, fish, poultry	6 oz.						
Eggs	3 eggs + 6 whites	2 eggs + 4 white + 2 oz. "meat"					
Hard cheeses	Unacceptable*	2 eggs + 5 whites + 1 oz. cheese	5 oz. "meat" + 1 oz. cheese				
Soft cheeses	Unacceptable	2 eggs + 5 whites + 2 oz. cheese	Unacceptable	5 oz. "meat" + 2 oz. cheese			
Curd cheeses		2 eggs + 3 whites + 1/2 cup cheese	1 1/4 cups curd + 1 oz. hard cheese	1 1/4 cups curd + 2 oz. soft cheese	4 oz. "meat" + 1/2 cup cheese		
Tofu		2 eggs + 2 whites + 1/2 cup tofu	3/4 cup tofu + 1 oz. cheese	3/4 cup tofu + 2 oz. cheese	3/4 cup tofu + 1/2 cup curd	1/2 cup tofu + 3 oz. "meat"	
		Egg	Hard cheeses	Soft cheeses	Curd cheeses	Tofu	
				1 1/2 cups curd		1 cup tofu	1 cup tofu

"Meat" = 7 grams per ounce
Eggs = 6 grams whole, 4 grams white
Hard Cheese = 6–7 grams per ounce
Soft Cheese = 3–4 grams per ounce
Curd Cheese = 7 grams per 1/4 cup
Tofu = 10 grams per 1/4 cup

*Because of the high fat content, the number of calories consumed to make these an adequate sole protein source would be too high for most people.

EFFECTIVE CARBOHYDRATE CONTENT OF FRUITS

FOOD	5-GRAM PORTION	10-GRAM PORTION	15-GRAM PORTION	20-GRAM PORTION	25-GRAM PORTION
Apple—Raw	1/4 apple (4.5)	1/2 apple (9)	3/4 apple (13.5)	1 apple (18)	1 1/4 apples (22.5)
Microwave-cooked	1/4 cup (5)	1/2 cup (10)	3/4 cup (15)	1 cup (20)	1 1/4 cups (25)
Applesauce—unsweetened	1/8 cup (3)	1/4 cup (6)	1/2 cup (12)	3/4 cup (18)	1 cup (24)
Apricots—raw	1 1/2 med.	3 med. (10.4)	4 med. (14)	5 med. (17.5)	7 med. (24.5)
canned (water)	4 halves (5)	8 halves (10)	12 halves (15)	16 halves (20)	20 halves (25)
Avocado (California)	3/4 med. (5.4)	1 med. (7.3)	2 med. (14.6)	2 1/2 med. (18.3)	3 med. (21.9)
Banana—raw	*	1/3 med. (8.3)	1/2 med. (12.5)	2/3 med. (16.7)	1 med. (25)
Blackberries—raw	1/2 cup (5.9)	3/4 cup (8.9)	1 1/4 cups (14.7)	1 1/2 cups (17.8)	2 cups (23.6)
Blueberries—raw	1/3 cup (5.7)	1/2 cup (8.6)	3/4 cup (13)	1 cup (17.2)	1 1/2 cups (25.8)
Boysenberries—frzn/unsweet	1/4 cup (4)	1/2 cup (8)	1 cup (16)	1 1/4 cups (20)	1 1/2 cups (24)
Cantaloupe—raw pieces	1/2 cup (5.7)	3/4 cup (8.6)	1 cup (11.4)	1 3/4 cups (20)	2 cups (22.8)
Cherries—sour canned (water)	1/4 cup (5.4)	1/2 cup (10.9)	3/4 cup (15.7)	1 cup (21)	1 1/4 cups (26.4)
—sweet raw	5 whole (5.1)	10 whole (10.2)	15 whole (15.3)	20 whole (20.4)	25 whole (25.5)
—sweet canned (water)	*	1/4 cup (7.3)	1/2 cup (14.6)	2/3 cup (19.5)	3/4 cup (22)
Crabapples—raw slices	*	1/4 cup (8.3)	1/2 cup (11)	3/4 cup (16.5)	1 cup (22)
Cranberries—raw	1/3 cup (4)	3/4 cup (8)	1 cup (12)	1 1/2 cups (16)	2 cups (24)
Cranberry sauce, jellied	2 tsp (4.6)	1 Tblsp (7)	2 Tblsp (14)	*	*
Currants—black raw	1/2 cup (5.6)	3/4 cup (8.4)	1 cup (11.2)	1 1/2 cups (16.8)	2 cups (22.4)
Dates—dried whole	*	1 whole (6)	2 whole (12)	3 whole (18)	4 whole (24)
Figs—raw whole	1/2 med. (4.8)	1 med. (9.6)	1 1/2 med. (14.4)	2 med. (19.2)	2 1/2 med. (24)
—dried whole	*	*	1 whole (12.2)	1 1/2 whole (18.3)	2 whole (24.4)
Fruit cocktail—canned, water	1/4 cup (5.2)	1/2 cup (10.4)	3/4 cup (15.6)	1 cup (20.8)	1 1/4 cups (26)
Fruit salad—canned, juice	*	1/3 cup (10.6)	1/2 cup (16)	1 cup (16)	3/4 cup (24)
Grapefruit—raw	1/4 whole (4.4)	1/2 whole (8.8)	3/4 whole (12.4)	1 whole (17.6)	1 1/2 whole (26.4)
—canned, juice	1/4 cup (5.5)	1/3 cup (7.4)	2/3 cup (14.8)	3/4 cup (16.7)	1 cup (22.2)
Grapes—seedless	1/3 cup (5.3)	1/2 cup (7.6)	1 cup (15.8)	1 1/3 cups (21.1)	1 1/2 cups (23.4)
Guava—raw	1/2 med. (5.3)	1 med. (10.7)	1 1/2 med. (16)	2 med. (21.4)	2 1/2 med. (25.7)

EFFECTIVE CARBOHYDRATE CONTENT OF FRUITS

FOOD	5-GRAM PORTION	10-GRAM PORTION	15-GRAM PORTION	20-GRAM PORTION	25-GRAM PORTION
Honeydew—raw, pieces	1/4 cup (3.9)	1/2 cup (7.8)	1 cup (15.6)	1 1/4 cups (19.5)	1 1/2 cups (26.5)
Kiwifruit—raw	1/2 med. (4.4)	1 med. (8.7)	1 1/2 med. (13)	2 med. (17.4)	2 1/2 med. (21.7)
Lemon peel	*	*	*	*	*
Lemon—raw	1 med. (5.4)	2 med. (10.8)	3 med. (16.2)	4 med. (21.6)	5 med. (27)
Lime—raw	1/2 med. (3.5)	1 med. (7.1)	2 med. (14.2)	*	*
Mandarin orange—juice-packed	*	1/3 cup (8)	1/2 cup (11.9)	3/4 cup (17.9)	1 cup (23.8)
Mango—raw, pieces	*	1/4 cup (8)	1/2 cup (16.5)	2/3 cup (21.1)	3/4 cup (24.8)
Nectarine—raw	1/2 med. (5.5)	3/4 med. (8.6)	1 med. (13.8)	1 1/2 med. (20.7)	2 med. (23)
Orange, Valencia or navel—raw	*	1/2 med. (6.9)	1 med. (11.5)	1 1/2 med. (17)	2 med. (23)
Papaya—raw	*	1/4 med. (6.8)	1/2 med. (13.5)	3/4 med. (20)	1 med. (27)
Passionfruit, purple—raw	1 med. (4.2)	2 med. (8.4)	3 med. (12.5)	5 med. (21)	6 med. (25.2)
Peach—raw	1/2 med. (4.2)	1 med. (8.3)	1 1/2 med. (12.5)	2 med. (16.6)	3 med. (25)
—canned, water	1/3 cup (5)	3/4 cup (11.1)	1 cup (14.9)	1 1/3 cups (20)	1 3/4 cups (26)
—dried, halves	*	1 half (8)	1 1/2 halves (12)	2 halves (16)	3 halves (24)
Pear—raw	1/4 med. (5.2)	1/2 med. (10.4)	3/4 med. (15.6)	1 med. (20.8)	1 1/4 med. (26.4)
—canned, water	1/4 cup (4.8)	1/2 cup (9.5)	3/4 cup (14.3)	1 cup (19.1)	1 1/4 cups (23.8)
—dried, halves	*	1/2 half (6.1)	1 half (12.2)	1 1/2 halves (18)	2 halves (24.4)
—Asian	1/4 med. (3.3)	3/4 med. (9.9)	1 med. (13.1)	1 1/2 med. (19.6)	2 med. (26.2)
Persimmon—raw	*	1/2 med. (8.4)	3/4 med. (12.6)	1 med. (16.8)	1 1/2 med. (25.2)
Pineapple—raw, pieces	1/4 cup (4.3)	1/2 cup (8.7)	3/4 cup (13)	1 cup (17.3)	1 1/2 cups (26)
—canned, juice	*	1/4 cup (9.3)	1/3 cup (12.4)	1/2 cup (18.6)	2/3 cup (24.8)
Plum—raw	1/2 med. (4.3)	1 med. (8.6)	1 1/2 med. (12.9)	2 med. (17.2)	3 med. (25.8)
Pomegranate—raw	*	1/4 med. (6.6)	1/2 med. (13.2)	3/4 med. (19.8)	1 med. (26.4)
Prunes—dried	1 whole (5.3)	2 whole (10.6)	3 whole (15.9)	4 whole (21.2)	5 whole (26.5)
Quince	*	1/2 med. (7)	1 med. (14)	1 1/2 med. (21)	1 3/4 med. (24.5)
Raisins	*	*	1/8 cup (13.9)	*	1/4 cup (27.8)
Raspberries—raw	1/2 cup (4.2)	1 1/4 cups (10.5)	1 3/4 cups (14.7)	2 cups (16.8)	3 cups (25.2)
Strawberries—raw	3/4 cup (5)	1 1/2 cups (9.9)	2 cups (13.2)	3 cups (19.8)	4 cups (26.4)
—frozen, unsweet	1/3 cup (4.5)	1/2 cup (6.8)	1 cup (13.6)	1 1/2 cups (20.4)	2 cups (26.2)

FOOD	5-GRAM PORTION	10-GRAM PORTION	15-GRAM PORTION	20-GRAM PORTION	25-GRAM PORTION
Tangerine—raw	1/2 med. (4.7)	1 med. (9.4)	1 1/2 med. (14.1)	2 med. (18.8)	2 1/2 med. (23.8)
Watermelon—raw, pieces	1/2 cup (5.5)	3/4 cup (8.3)	1 cup (11)	1 1/2 cups (16.5)	2 cups (22)

EFFECTIVE CARBOHYDRATE CONTENT OF BREADS, CEREALS, AND GRAINS

FOOD	5-GRAM PORTION	10-GRAM PORTION	15-GRAM PORTION	20-GRAM PORTION	25-GRAM PORTION
Bagel	*	*	1/2 med. (15)	1/2 med. (15)	1 small (27)
Biscuit—small (3/4 oz.)	1/2 small (4.8)	1 small (9.7)	1 1/2 small (14.5)	2 small (19.4)	2 1/2 small (24.2)
—med. (1 oz.)	*	1/2 med. (6)	1 med. (12)	1 1/2 med. (18)	2 med. (24)
—large (2 oz.)	*	*	*	1/2 large (16)	1/2 large (16)
Boston brown bread—canned	*	1/2 slice (10)	3/4 slice (15)	1 slice (20)	1 slice (20)
Bread, pita pocket	*	1/2 pocket (10.1)	1/2 pocket (10.1)	1 pocket (20.3)	1 pocket (20.3)
Bread, raisin, regular—sliced	*	1/2 slice (6.3)	1 slice (12.6)	1 1/2 slices (18.9)	2 slices (25.2)
Bread, sandwich, regular—sliced	*	1/2 slice (6)	1 slice (12)	1 1/2 slices (18)	2 slices (24)
light—sliced	1/2 slice (3.5)	1 slice (7)	2 slices (14)	2 1/2 slices (17.5)	3 slices (21)
Breadstick, sesame (Keebler)	2 sticks (5.3)	4 sticks (10.6)	5 sticks (13)	7 sticks (18.2)	9 sticks (23.4)
Breadstick, soft (Pillsbury)	*	1/2 stick (8.3)	3/4 stick (12.5)	1 stick (16.6)	1 1/2 sticks (24.9)
Bun, hamburger or hot dog—regular	*	1/2 bun (10)	1/2 bun (10)	1 bun (20.1)	1 bun (20.1)
—light		1/2 bun (7)	1 bun (14)	1 1/2 buns (21)	1 1/2 buns (21)
Couscous—cooked		1/4 cup (10)	1/3 cup (13.6)	1/2 cup (20.5)	scant 2/3 cup (26)
Crackers (saltine, club, Ritz-style, melba)	2 regular (4)	4 regular (8)	6 regular (12)	10 regular (20)	12 regular (24)
(oyster type)	10 (5.3)	20 (10.6)	25 (13.3)	35 (18.6)	45 (23.9)
(Triscuits)	1 cracker (3)	3 crackers (9)	5 crackers (15)	6 crackers (18)	8 crackers (24)
(Sociables, Nabisco)	3 crackers (4.5)	6 crackers (9)	10 crackers (15)	12 crackers (18)	15 crackers (22.5)
(Wasa, Sesame Rye)	2 pieces (4)	5 pieces (10)	7 pieces (14)	10 pieces (20)	12 pieces (24)
Cheez-It (Sunshine)/ Cheese Nips (Nabisco)	8 Nips (4.8)	15 Nips (9)	25 Nips (15)	30 Nips (18)	40 Nips (24)

EFFECTIVE CARBOHYDRATE CONTENT OF BREADS, CEREALS, AND GRAINS

FOOD	5-GRAM PORTION	10-GRAM PORTION	15-GRAM PORTION	20-GRAM PORTION	25-GRAM PORTION
Flours					
cornmeal—whole-grain	*	2 Tblsp (10)	3 Tblsp (15)	4 Tblsp (20)	5 Tblsp (25)
oat bran—raw	*	4 Tblsp (11.7)	5 Tblsp (15)	6 Tblsp (18)	8 Tblsp (24)
rice flour—brown	*	1 Tblsp (7.5)	2 Tblsp (15)	2 Tblsp (15)	3 Tblsp (22.5)
rye flour	*	2 Tblsp (10)	3 Tblsp (15)	4 Tblsp (20)	5 Tblsp (25)
soy flour—roasted, full-fat	scant 1/4 cup (5.5)	1/3 cup (8.3)	1/2 cup (12.5)	2/3 cup (16.6)	1 cup (25)
wheat germ	1/8 cup (5.3)	1/4 cup (10.6)	1/3 cup (14)	1/2 cup (21.2)	scant 2/3 cup (26)
white flour—all-purpose	*	2 Tblsp (10.5)	3 Tblsp (15)	4 Tblsp (20)	5 Tblsp (25)
whole-wheat flour	*	2 Tblsp (9)	3 Tblsp (13.5)	4 Tblsp (18)	5 Tblsp (24)
Grain cakes—pressed (rice, oats, wheat, popcorn, sesame, barley)	1/2 cake (3.5)	1 cake (7)	2 cakes (14)	3 cakes (21)	3 cakes (21)
Melba toast	2 pieces (4)	5 pieces (10)	7 pieces (14)	10 pieces (20)	12 pieces (24)
Muffin—English (plain)	*	*	1/2 muffin (12.5)	3/4 muffin (19)	1 muffin (25)
—Corn (small)	*	1/2 muffin (10)	3/4 muffin (15)	1 muffin (20)	1 muffin (26.2)
—Oat bran (Estee from mix)	*	1/2 muffin (7.5)	1 muffin (15)	1 muffin (20)	1 muffin (20)
—Oat bran (General Mills from mix)	*	*	1 muffin (15)	1 1/2 muffins (22.5)	1 1/2 muffins (22.5)
Oatmeal—cooked, plain	*	*	scant 1/2 cup (15)	1/2 cup (16.5)	2/3 cup (22)
Pancake (from mix, plain, 4" diameter)	*	1/2 cake (6)	1 cake (12)	1 1/2 cakes (18)	2 cakes (24)
Pancake (frozen Aunt Jemima, plain)	*	1/2 cake (6)	1 cake (12)	1 1/2 cakes (18)	2 cakes (24)
Pancake—Fluffy (our recipe)	*	1 serving (10)	1 1/2 servings (15)	2 servings (20)	2 1/2 servings (25)
Pasta					
(egg noodles, spaghetti, macaroni—cooked)	*	1/4 cup (10)	1/3 cup (13)	1/2 cup (20)	3/4 cup (26.6)
(chow mein noodles)	*	1/3 cup (8.7)	1/2 cup (13)	3/4 cup (20)	1 cup (26)

FOOD	5-GRAM PORTION	10-GRAM PORTION	15-GRAM PORTION	20-GRAM PORTION	25-GRAM PORTION
(noodles w/rice—LaChoy)	*	1/4 cup (10)	1/3 cup (13)	1/2 cup (21)	3/4 cup (26)
(lasagne—dry uncooked)	*	1/2 oz. (10)	2/3 oz. (13)	1 oz. (20)	1 1/4 oz. (25)
Piecrust (Keebler, Pillsbury All Ready, 9" dia.)	*	*	1/8 crust (15)	1/6 crust (20)	1/5 crust (24)
Pizza crust (small, thin-crust 9" diameter)	*	*	1/8 crust (15)	1/6 crust (20)	1/5 crust (24)
Popovers—homemade, small	1/2 small (5.1)	1 small (10.3)	1 1/2 small (15.4)	2 small (20.6)	2 small (20.6)
Rice—brown, cooked	1/8 cup (5.2)	1/4 cup (10.4)	1/3 cup (13.5)	1/2 cup (20.9)	scant 2/3 cup (25)
—white, long grain, cooked	1/8 cup (5.3)	1/4 cup (10.5)	1/3 cup (14)	1/2 cup (21)	scant 2/3 cup (25)
—wild, cooked	1/8 cup (4.4)	1/4 cup (8.8)	scant 1/2 cup (15)	1/2 cup (17.5)	scant 3/4 cup (26)
Rice—fried	1/8 cup (5.2)	1/4 cup (10.5)	1/3 cup (14)	1/2 cup (21)	1/2 cup (21)
Risotto—cooked	*	1/8 cup (6)	1/4 cup (12)	1/3 cup (16)	1/2 cup (21)
Rolls—crescent (Pillsbury, canned), small	1/2 roll (5.4)	1 roll (10.8)	1 roll (10.8)	1 1/2 rolls (16.2)	2 rolls (21.6)
—dinner, small	*	1/2 roll (7)	1 roll (14)	1 1/2 rolls (21)	1 1/2 rolls (21)
Stuffing, corn bread or bread	*	1/4 cup (10.5)	1/3 cup (14)	1/2 cup (21)	1/2 cup (21)
Tortillas (corn—tostada, taco shell, small)	*	1 shell (7)	2 shells (14)	3 shells (21)	3 shells (21)
(flour—fajita, small)	*	1/2 small (7.5)	1 small (15)	1 small (15)	1 1/2 small (22)
Waffle—plain, homemade 7" diameter	*	*	1/2 waffle (13)	3/4 waffle (19.5)	1 waffle (26)
—frozen, small	*	1/2 waffle (7)	1 waffle (14)	1 1/2 waffles (21)	1 1/2 waffles (21)

EFFECTIVE CARBOHYDRATE CONTENT OF VEGETABLES

FOOD	5-GRAM PORTION	10-GRAM PORTION	15-GRAM PORTION	20-GRAM PORTION	25-GRAM PORTION
Alfalfa sprouts—raw	*	*	unlimited	unlimited	unlimited
Amaranth—boiled	1 cup (5.4)	2 cups (10.8)			
Artichoke—boiled	*	1/2 med. (6.7)	1 med. (13.4)	1 1/2 med. (20.1)	2 med. (26.8)

EFFECTIVE CARBOHYDRATE CONTENT OF VEGETABLES

FOOD	5-GRAM PORTION	10-GRAM PORTION	15-GRAM PORTION	20-GRAM PORTION	25-GRAM PORTION
Artichoke hearts—boiled	1/4 cup (4.4)	1/2 cup (8.7)	3/4 cup (13)	1 cup (17.4)	1 1/2 cups (21.7)
—marinated, oil	1/4 cup (3.5)	1/2 cup (6.9)	1 cup (13.8)	1 1/2 cups (20.7)	1 3/4 cups (24)
Arugula—raw	unlimited	unlimited	unlimited	unlimited	unlimited
Asparagus—boiled	10 spears (4)	20 spears (8)	30 spears (12)	unlimited	unlimited
—canned	1 cup (5.6)	1 1/2 cups (8.4)	2 1/2 cups (14)	3 cups (16.8)	4 cups (22.4)
—frozen, boiled	6 spears (8.2)	13 spears (9.5)	20 spears (14.6)	unlimited	unlimited
Bamboo shoots—raw	1 cup (4)	2 cups (8)	3 cups (12)	5 cups (20)	6 cups (24)
—canned	1 cup (4.6)	2 cups (9.2)	3 cups (13.8)	unlimited	unlimited
Bean salad (Pillsbury)—canned	1/8 cup (3.6)	1/4 cup (7.3)	1/2 cup (14.5)	2/3 cup (19.3)	3/4 cup (21.8)
Beans, chili (Hunt's)—canned	scant 1/4 cup (5)	1/3 cup (8)	1/2 cup (12)	3/4 cup (18)	1 cup (24)
Beans, chili (Hunt's)—canned (Joan of Arc, Caliente)	1/4 cup (5.4)	1/2 cup (10.8)	2/3 cup (14.4)	3/4 cup (16.2)	1 cup (21.6)
Beans, w/pork&tom (Joan of Arc)—can	1/8 cup (4.4)	1/4 cup (8.7)	1/3 cup (11.6)	1/2 cup (17.4)	2/3 cup (23.2)
Beans, refried (Rosarita)					
—canned	1/8 cup (3.5)	1/3 cup (9.3)	1/2 cup (14)	2/3 cup (18.7)	3/4 cup (21)
Beet greens—boiled	2/3 cup (5.2)	1 cup (7.8)	2 cups (15.6)	2 1/2 cups (19.5)	3 cups (23.4)
Beets—boiled, sliced	1/2 cup (5.7)	3/4 cup (8.5)	1 cup (11.7)	1 1/2 cups (17.1)	2 cups (23.4)
—Harvard, canned	*	1/4 cup (11.2)	1/3 cup (14.9)	1/3 cup (14.9)	1/2 cup (22.4)
—pickled, canned	1/8 cup (4.7)	1/4 cup (9.3)	1/3 cup (12.4)	1/2 cup (18.6)	2/3 cup (24.8)
Black beans—boiled	1/8 cup (4.2)	1/4 cup (8.4)	1/3 cup (11.1)	1/2 cup (16.8)	3/4 cup (25.2)
Black turtle beans—canned	1/8 cup (4.9)	1/4 cup (9.9)	1/3 cup (13.2)	1/2 cup (19.8)	2/3 cup (26.4)
Broccoli—raw, chopped	4 cups (4.4)	unlimited	unlimited	unlimited	unlimited
—boiled, chopped	1 cup (4)	2 cups (8)	3 cups (12)	5 cups (20)	unlimited
—frozen, chopped or spears	3/4 cup (4.4)	1 1/2 cups (8.7)	2 1/2 cups (14.5)	3 cups (17.4)	4 cups (23.2)
Broccoli/carrots (Pillsbury)					
—frozen	3/4 cup (4.7)	1 1/2 cups (9.3)	2 cups (12.4)	3 cups (18.6)	4 cups (24.8)
Broccoli/cauliflower—frozen	1 cup (5.4)	2 cups (10.8)	2 1/2 cups (13.5)	3 cups (16.2)	4 cups (21.6)

Food					
Broccoli/corn/red pepper—frozen	1/3 cup (5)	2/3 cup (10.1)	1 cup (15.2)	1 1/3 cups (19.8)	1 1/2 cups (22.8)
Broccoli/peppers/bamboo shoots/mushrooms—frozen	1 cup (3.5)	2 cups (7)	4 cups (14)	5 cups (17.5)	6 cups (21)
Broccoli/pearl onions/ red peppers—frozen	1 cup (3.5)	2 cups (7)	4 cups (14)	5 cups (17.5)	6 cups (21)
Brussels sprouts—boiled	5 sprouts (4.3)	11 sprouts (9.4)	15 sprouts (12.8)	17 sprouts (14.5)	25 sprouts (21.3)
—with cheese—frozen	*	*	1/2 cup (12.5)	3/4 cup (18.8)	1 cup (25)
Butter beans—canned	1/3 cup (8)	1/2 cup (12.2)	2/3 cup (16)	3/4 cup (18.8)	1 cup (24.4)
Cabbage, Chinese (bok choy)—raw	3 cups (2.4)	unlimited	unlimited	unlimited	unlimited
Cabbage, green or red—raw	1 1/2 cups (4.5)	2 cups (6)	5 cups (15)	6 cups (18)	6 cups (21.6)
—boiled	1 1/2 cups (5.4)	2 cups (7.2)	3 cups (10.8)	5 cups (18)	6 cups (21.6)
Carrots—raw	1 med. (5)	2 med. (10)	3 med. (15)	4 med. (20)	5 med. (25)
—boiled, sliced	3/4 cup (4.5)	1/2 cup (6.7)	1 cup (13.4)	1 1/2 cups (20.1)	2 cups (26.8)
—canned, slices	1/2 cup (4.7)	1 1/2 cups (9)	2 cups (12)	3 cups (18)	4 cups (24)
—frozen, slices	*	1 cup (9.4)	1 1/2 cups (14.1)	2 cups (18.8)	2 1/2 cups (23.5)
Cauliflower—raw/boiled/frozen, pieces	2 cups (5.2)	4 cups (10.4)	5 cups (13)	unlimited	unlimited
Celery—raw	4 stalks (3.6)	unlimited	unlimited	unlimited	unlimited
—boiled, diced	3/4 cup (4.5)	1 1/2 cups (9)	2 cups (12)	3 cups (18)	4 cups (24)
Chard, Swiss—boiled, chopped	3/4 cup (5.4)	1 cup (7.2)	2 cups (14.4)	2 1/2 cups (19.8)	3 cups (21.6)
Chickpeas—boiled	*	1/4 cup (10)	1/3 cup (13.3)	1/2 cup (20)	2/3 cup (26.6)
—hummus	*	*	1/4 cup (12.5)	1/3 cup (16.6)	1/2 cup (25)
Chives—raw	unlimited	unlimited	unlimited	unlimited	unlimited
Coleslaw—homemade	1/3 cup (5)	1/2 cup (7.5)	1 cup (15)	1 1/3 cups (20)	1 2/3 cups (25)
Collard greens—boiled, chopped	1/2 cup (3.9)	1 cup (7.8)	2 cups (15.6)	2 1/2 cups (19.5)	3 cups (23.4)
—frozen, chopped	1/3 cup (4)	2/3 cup (8)	1 cup (12)	1 1/2 cups (18)	2 cups (24)
Corn, white—frozen or canned	*	1/4 cup (8)	1/3 cup (10.6)	1/2 cup (16)	2/3 cup (22.6)
Corn, yellow—boiled	*	1/4 cup (8.5)	1/3 cup (11.3)	1/2 cup (17)	3/4 cup (22.6)
—frozen, boiled	*	1/2 cup (9)	1/2 cup (15.1)	2/3 cup (20)	3/4 cup (22.5)
— on the cob	*	1/2 cup (10)	1/2 ear (12)	1/2 ear (12)	1 ear (24)

EFFECTIVE CARBOHYDRATE CONTENT OF VEGETABLES

FOOD	5-GRAM PORTION	10-GRAM PORTION	15-GRAM PORTION	20-GRAM PORTION	25-GRAM PORTION
Cowpeas (black-eyed peas)					
—canned	*	1/3 cup (10.9)	1/3 cup (10.9)	1/2 cup (16.4)	2/3 cup (21.8)
—frozen, boiled	*	1/4 cup (10)	1/3 cup (13)	1/2 cup (20)	2/3 cup (26.6)
Cucumber—raw	1/2 med. (3)	1 med. (6)	2 med. (12)	3 med. (18)	4 med. (24)
Dandelion greens—raw	1 cup (5.2)	2 cups (10.4)	3 cups (15.6)	4 cups (20.8)	5 cups (26)
—boiled, chopped	1/2 cup (3.3)	1 cup (6.6)	2 cups (13.2)	3 cups (19.2)	4 cups (26.4)
Eggplant—raw pieces	1 cup (5)	2 cups (10)	3 cups (15)	4 cups (20)	5 cups (25)
—steamed, pieces	3/4 cup (4.8)	1 cup (6.4)	2 cups (12.8)	3 cups (19.2)	4 cups (25.6)
Endive, raw	2 cups (3.2)	4 cups (6.4)	unlimited	unlimited	unlimited
Fava beans—canned	1/8 cup (3.9)	1/4 cup (7.8)	1/2 cup (15.5)	2/3 cup (20.6)	3/4 cup (23.3)
Fennel—fresh	3/4 cup (4.7)	1 cup (6.3)	2 cups (12.6)	3 cups (18.9)	4 cups (25.2)
Garlic, raw	3 cloves (3)	unlimited	unlimited	unlimited	unlimited
Ginger—raw, sliced	1/4 cup (3.6)	1/2 cup (7.2)	2/3 cup (15.6)	3/4 cup (20.8)	1 cup (24)
Great Northern beans—boiled (Joan of Arc)—canned	*	1/3 cup (10.4)	1/2 cup (15.6)	2/3 cup (20.8)	3/4 cup (24)
Green beans (snap beans)					
—boiled	1/2 cup (3.8)	1 cup (7.6)	2 cups (15.2)	2 1/2 cups (19)	3 cups (22.8)
—canned	1 cup (4.4)	2 cups (8.8)	3 cups (13.2)	4 cups (17.6)	5 cups (22)
—frozen, whole	1/2 cup (4.2)	1 cup (8.4)	1 1/2 cups (12.6)	2 cups (16.8)	3 cups (25.2)
Hominy, canned	*	1/4 cup (7.5)	1/2 cup (15)	2/3 cup (20)	3/4 cup (22.5)
Italian-style vegs—frozen	1/3 cup (7.3)	1/2 cup (11)	2/3 cup (14.6)	3/4 cup (20)	1 cup (22)
Japanese-style vegs—frozen	1/3 cup (6.6)	1/2 cup (11)	3/4 cup (15)	1 cup (20)	1 1/4 cups (25)
Kale—boiled, chopped	1/2 cup (3.7)	1 cup (7.4)	2 cups (14.8)	2 1/2 cups (18.5)	3 cups (22.2)
Kelp—raw	1/2 cup (5.5)	1 cup (11)	1 1/2 cups (16.5)	1 3/4 cups (20)	2 cups (22)
Kidney beans, red—boiled	*	1/4 cup (8.4)	1/3 cup (11.2)	1/2 cup (16.5)	2/3 cup (22.4)
—canned	1/8 cup (5)	1/4 cup (10)	1/3 cup (13.3)	1/2 cup (20)	2/3 cup (26.6)
Leeks—boiled, chopped	1/2 cup (4)	1 cup (8)	1 1/2 cups (12)	2 cups (16)	3 cups (24)
Lentils—boiled	1/8 cup (4)	1/4 cup (8)	1/3 cup (10.6)	1/2 cup (16)	3/4 cup (24)

Lettuce, butterhead or iceberg—raw	unlimited	unlimited	unlimited	unlimited
romaine—shredded	unlimited	unlimited	unlimited	unlimited
Lima beans—boiled	1/8 cup (3.3)	1/3 cup (8.6)	1/2 cup (12.9)	1 cup (25.8)
—canned	1/8 cup (4.5)	1/4 cup (9)	1/3 cup (12)	2/3 cup (23.9)
Mushrooms—raw, pieces	1 cup (2.2)	unlimited	unlimited	unlimited
—steamed or canned, pieces	1 cup (4.6)	2 cups (9.2)	3 cups (13.8)	5 cups (23)
(enoki)—raw, whole	unlimited	unlimited	unlimited	unlimited
(straw)—canned	1 cup (5.6)	unlimited	unlimited	unlimited
(shiitake)—whole, broiled	2 whole (5.1)	4 whole (10.3)	6 whole (15.4)	8 whole (20.6)
—dried, whole	2 whole (5.6)	3 whole (8.4)	5 whole (14)	8 whole (22.4)
Mustard greens—boiled, chopped	1 1/2 cups (4.5)	3 cups (9)	unlimited	unlimited
—frozen, chopped	1 cup (4.6)	2 cups (9.2)	3 cups (13.8)	unlimited
Navy beans—boiled	*	1/4 cup (10.4)	1/4 cup (13.4)	1/3 cup (17.8)
—canned				
Okra—boiled, slices	1/2 cup (5.8)	3/4 cup (8.7)	1 cup (11.6)	2 cups (23.2)
—frozen, slices	1/3 cup (5)	1/2 cup (7.5)	1 cup (15)	1 1/2 cups (22.5)
Onions—raw, chopped	1/2 cup (5.6)	3/4 cup (8.4)	1 cup (11.2)	unlimited
—boiled, chopped	1/4 cup (5.3)	1/2 cup (10.7)	3/4 cup (15.9)	1 1/4 cups (26.3)
—dehydrated, flakes	1/8 cup (5.9)	1/4 cup (11.7)	1/3 cup (15.6)	1/2 cup (23.4)
Onions, green (spring)—raw, chopped	1 cup (5)	unlimited	unlimited	unlimited
Parsley—raw, chopped	unlimited	unlimited	unlimited	unlimited
—freeze-dried	unlimited	unlimited	unlimited	unlimited
Parsnips—boiled, slices	1/4 cup (5.1)	1/3 cup (8.7)	1/2 cup (13.1)	2/3 cup (17.5)
Peas, green—boiled	1/3 cup (5.2)	1/2 cup (10.3)	3/4 cup (15.5)	1 cup (20.6)
—canned		1/4 cup (10)	1 cup (15.6)	1 1/3 cups (20.8)
Peas, split—boiled	*		1/3 cup (14)	1/2 cup (21.2)
Peas, sweet—canned	1/4 cup (4.2)	1/2 cup (8.4)	3/4 cup (12.6)	1 1/2 cups (25.2)

EFFECTIVE CARBOHYDRATE CONTENT OF VEGETABLES

FOOD	5-GRAM PORTION	10-GRAM PORTION	15-GRAM PORTION	20-GRAM PORTION	25-GRAM PORTION
Peppers, hot chili—raw	1 whole (4.3)	2 whole (8.6)	3 whole (12.9)	4 whole (17.2)	6 whole (25.8)
—canned, chopped	1/2 cup (4.2)	1 cup (8.4)	1 3/4 cups (14.7)	2 cups (16.8)	unlimited
Peppers, jalapeño—canned, chopped	1/2 cup (3.3)	1 cup (6.6)	unlimited	unlimited	unlimited
Peppers, sweet—raw, chopped	1 cup (4.8)	2 cups (9.6)	unlimited	unlimited	unlimited
—freeze-dried, chopped	1 cup (4.4)	unlimited	unlimited	unlimited	unlimited
Peppers, sweet, yellow—raw, whole	1/2 large (5.9)	3/4 large (8.9)	1 large (11.8)	1 3/4 large (20.7)	2 large (23.6)
Pimientos—canned	unlimited	unlimited	unlimited	unlimited	unlimited
Pinto beans—boiled	1/8 cup (4.7)	1/4 cup (9.3)	1/3 cup (12.4)	1/2 cup (18.6)	2/3 cup (24.8)
—canned (Joan of Arc, Picante Style)	1/8 cup (4.4)	1/4 cup (8.7)	1/3 cup (11.6)	1/2 cup (17.5)	2/3 cup (23.3)
Potato, sweet—baked, skin eaten *	*	1/4 med. (6)	1/2 med. (12)	3/4 med. (18)	1 med. (24)
—boiled, mashed	1/8 cup (3.7)	1/3 cup (9.7)	1/2 cup (14.6)	2/3 cup (19.5)	3/4 cup (21.9)
Potato, white—baked, skin eaten *	*	*	1/4 med. (12.8)	1/4 med. (17)	1/3 med. (25.9)
—baked, no skin	*	1/4 med. (7.8)	1/3 med. (10.4)	1/2 med. (15.7)	1/2 med. (25.5)
—boiled, no skin	*	1/4 med. (6.3)	1/2 med. (12.5)	2/3 med. (16.7)	3/4 med. (23.4)
Potato, new—canned, whole	*	1/3 cup (10)	1/2 cup (15)	2/3 cup (20)	3/4 cup (22.5)
Potatoes—french fried, drained	*	5 fries (10)	7 fries (14)	10 fries (20)	12 fries (24)
Potatoes, white—mashed	*	1/2 cup (7.5)	1/2 cup (15)	2/3 cup (20)	3/4 cup (22.5)
Pumpkin—boiled, mashed	1/4 cup (3)	1/2 cup (6)	1 cup (12)	1 1/2 cups (18)	2 cups (24)
—canned, solid pack	1/4 cup (2.2)	1/2 cup (6.3)	1 1/2 cups (12.6)	1 1/2 cups (18.9)	2 cups (25.2)
Radicchio—raw, shredded	unlimited	unlimited	unlimited	unlimited	unlimited
Radishes—raw	unlimited	unlimited	unlimited	unlimited	unlimited
Radishes, red—raw	unlimited	unlimited	unlimited	unlimited	unlimited
Radishes, white—raw, sliced	unlimited	unlimited	unlimited	unlimited	unlimited
Red beans—canned	*	1/3 cup (8)	1/2 cup (12)	2/3 cup (16)	1 cup (24)
Rhubarb—boiled	1/2 cup (3.5)	1 cup (7)	2 cups (14)	3 cups (21)	3 1/2 cups (24.5)
Rutabaga, boiled, sliced	1/3 cup (4.4)	1/2 cup (6.6)	1 cup (13.2)	1 1/2 cups (19.8)	1 3/4 cups (23.1)
Sauerkraut—bottled or canned	1/2 cup (5.1)	3/4 cup (7.6)	1 cup (10.2)	2 cups (20.4)	2 1/2 cups (26.5)

Shallots—raw, chopped	3 Tblsp (5.1)	unlimited	unlimited	unlimited
Spinach—raw, chopped	unlimited	unlimited	unlimited	1.4 grams per cup
—frozen, boiled	1 cup (3.1)	3 cups (9.3)	5 cups (15.1)	unlimited
—canned	3 cups (3.6)	unlimited	unlimited	unlimited
Squash, summer varieties (crookneck, scallop, zucchini)				
—raw, pieces	1 cup (4)	2 cups (8)	4 cups (16)	6 cups (24)
—boiled	1 cup (5.2)	2 cups (10.4)	3 cups (15.6)	5 cups (26)
Squash, winter varieties (acorn, butternut, Hubbard)				
—raw, pieces	1/2 cup (5.1)	1 cup (10.2)	1 1/2 cups (15.3)	2 cups (20.4)
—baked	1/3 cup (4)	2/3 cup (8)	1 cup (12)	1 1/2 cups (18)
(spaghetti variety)—baked or boiled	1/2 cup (5)	1 cup (10)	1 1/2 cups (15)	2 cups (20)
Succotash—boiled	*	*	1/4 cup (11.7)	1/3 cup (15.6)
—canned or frozen	*	1/4 cup (8.5)	1/3 cup (11.3)	1/2 cup (17)
Tomatillo—raw, whole	2 med. (4)	5 med. (10)	10 med. (20)	12 med. (24)
Tomato, green—raw, whole	1 med. (4.1)	2 med. (8.2)	3 med. (12.5)	6 med. (24.6)
red—raw, whole	2 med. (4.1)	3 med. (8.2)	5 med. (20.5)	6 med. (24.6)
red—canned	1/2 cup (5)	1 cup (10)	2 cups (20)	2 1/2 cups (25)
red with green chilies—canned	1/2 cup (4.3)	1 cup (8.6)	2 cups (17.2)	2 1/2 cups (21.5)
Tomato—sun-dried	1/8 cup (3.8)	1/4 cup (7.5)	1/2 cup (15)	3/4 cup (22.5)
Turnips—boiled, pieces	1 cup (4.4)	2 cups (8.8)	4 cups (17.6)	5 cups (22)
Turnip greens—boiled, chopped	2 cups (3.6)	4 cups (7.2)	unlimited	unlimited
—canned, chopped	2 cups (5.6)	3 cups (8.4)	4 cups (13.2)	unlimited
Water chestnuts—raw, sliced	1/8 cup (3.7)	1/4 cup (7.4)	1/2 cup (14.8)	3/4 cup (22.2)
—canned, whole	5 whole (5)	10 whole (10)	15 whole (15)	unlimited
Wax beans—canned, sliced	1/2 cup (4)	1 cup (8)	2 cups (16)	3 cups (24)
White beans—boiled	1/4 cup (4)	1/2 cup (8)	1 cup (15)	1 1/2 cups (24)
—canned	1/2 cup (4.5)	1 cup (9)	2 cups (18)	2 1/2 cups (22.5)
Yams—baked or boiled, pieces	*	1/4 cup (9.4)	1/3 cup (12.5)	2/3 cup (25)

Chapter 11

Motivation: Plan Your Work and Work Your Plan

I'll purge, and leave sack, and live cleanly, as a nobleman should do.

Falstaff, in *Henry IV, Part One,*
WILLIAM SHAKESPEARE

If only it were that simple, Falstaff's name might never have become eponymous for gluttony, hedonism, and corpulence. Unfortunately, as anyone who has tried it knows, changing your eating behavior is tough, hard work. An enormous reality gap exists between the ease of dieting as presented in most books and magazine articles on the subject and the actual day-to-day grind of a particular diet. What's advertised as a fast, easy, painless, you-won't-believe-how-quickly-your-fat-melts-away approach to weight loss and other benefits all too often becomes monotonous, restrictive, and ultimately abandoned. If it weren't so, the notorious 95 percent of people who always regain all their lost weight would still be thin.

So, how is this program different? In many ways it isn't—although unlike most other programs this one has a positive health approach that actually *will* heal you metabolically and make it easier to work your plan. Much as we'd like to tell you otherwise, the program we have outlined still requires discipline, self-denial, and just plain old hard work. But the reward for this effort is spectacular. In the course of our work with thousands of patients we have developed many techniques to make life easier for them, but it still isn't magic. Although it "fixes" your health problems quickly, it's not just a quick fix. We feel it's important to inform you in advance of the discipline required because the approach you take and the outlook you have at the beginning are of paramount importance.

214

The first decision you need to make is not that you need to lose weight or lower your cholesterol or reduce your high blood pressure or any or all of these. Your first decision must be to make these changes a *permanent* part of your life. That sounds simple, but in reality making that decision means that you are willing to abandon life (and all its dangerous goodies) as you know it today. It will be one of the best decisions you've ever made, but we want you to understand it for what it is—a major life-altering decision. Assuming you've made that decision, you've got to realize and accept the fact that the responsibility for this change is yours and yours alone. You have to do the work. We have provided all the information you need to be successful, but we can't do it for you. What we can do is give you some tips and tricks that have helped us and our patients achieve our goals.

The Worst Will Be Over Soon

In Phase I and Phase II, when it's so critical to follow the program to the letter, it helps to adopt a boot-camp attitude. Recruits go to boot camp knowing it's going to be strict, grueling, difficult, and probably not particularly pleasant. They also know it's going to be over. You need to think the same way. Compared to maintenance, these intervention phases are much more rigorous, but they will be over soon. Look upon it as a finite period of time you're spending to turn your health around and get on with it. When it's over, you can rejoice. As long as you stay on maintenance and don't eat unconsciously, you'll never have to go back to boot camp again.

Don't Get Hungry

Never let yourself get hungry. If you're not hungry, you will be much better able to avoid the temptation to eat those foods you know you shouldn't. The best approach is to stay ahead of the hunger curve. In other words, always try to eat before you get ravenously hungry—not after. Never skip breakfast. Keep a quantity of allowable snacks at the ready. You need to prepare these yourself and keep them handy because virtually all of the commercially manufactured snacks you'll find will be crawling with carbohydrates and despite their *no-fat* or *low-fat* labeling will sabotage you in a hurry.

Visualize Your Goals

A question we're often asked by weight-loss patients is: Since I have 220 pounds to lose, how can I stay motivated to stick to any diet long enough to lose all that weight? The answer is that you are *not* going on a diet of a predetermined length; you are adopting a new way of eating for the rest of your life, so it doesn't really matter how long it takes. Several years ago, when a twenty-two-year-old patient of ours, Michael, began our program weighing 420 pounds, he wondered if he would ever lose the 200-plus pounds that stood between him and his ideal body weight. When we told him to expect to lose at least 2 to 3 pounds a week, he grumbled that at that rate he would be twenty-five before he reached normal weight. Well, of course, in two years he was going to be twenty-five whether he lost the weight or not, so we said he might as well reach twenty-five thin instead of overweight. He started our program on August 13, 1993, and by June 17, 1994, four months short of his twenty-fourth birthday, he had lost 169 pounds. As Michael lost his excess body fat and developed a more positive self-image, he developed a social life for the first time in his life and sought and found a better job that required his moving out of the area. He has since become engaged and continues to do well. The results of the diet *became* the motivation. So take heart: no matter how much you have to lose, every pound lost takes you closer to your ultimate goal—becoming a leaner, fitter, healthier person. You've got the rest of your life to live healthy and fit—don't get caught up in the trap of deadlines.

Learn to set reasonable goals and use the power of visualization to achieve them. We're not New Age fans, but we can tell you that visualization works. Visualize clearly and vividly the changes you wish to take place and visualize them as if they had already taken place. You will set in motion all kinds of subconscious activity that will work behind the scenes to make your visual pictures a reality.[1] An excellent book on this subject that we find indispensable and can't recommend highly enough is *Maximum Achievement* by Brian Tracy (Simon and Schuster, 1993). As with all books we recommend, ignore any nutritional advice—we can never

---

[1] If it just seems completely unimaginable, you can send a current photo to Slim Photo (see appendix), and they'll send you back a slimmed-down photo, carefully to scale so you can see how you'll actually look at the end of all this—but of course you'll have better muscles in real life. Phone: (213) 964-1871.

understand why authors of books on nonnutritional subjects feel compelled to parrot the high-carbohydrate party line, but they do.

You're the Boss

It's astonishing that so many people fail at dieting. People who successfully overcome the uncontrollable vagaries of careers, higher education, marriage, and life in general succumb to the one, and maybe only, event over which they have total control—feeding themselves. We all seem to be about six years old when it comes to eating. But you need to realize that unless you are unconscious in a hospital bed undergoing tube feeding, *you, and only you, are in complete control over what you put in your mouth.* You may not be able to control the weather, the behavior of your children or your spouse, the intraoffice machinations at your workplace, the busybodies in your neighborhood, or the outcome of the Super Bowl, but you can take charge of the food you eat. We've all heard the excuse innumerable times from those who have been tempted from their diets by junk food of one sort or another: "I just couldn't resist it." As we say to our patients, "Yes, you *could* resist it; you just *chose* not to."

Temptation vs. You

It would be simplistic for us to act as though temptation doesn't exist or resisting it requires only a small effort of will. We love to eat, too (which is why we've built in occasional dietary vacations for maintenance). If it were easy, no one would be overweight. Although you can't make temptation go away, there are steps you can take to minimize its hold on you. In looking at these steps you'll get a better picture of how temptation actually works its wily magic on you and how you can turn the tables on it.

There are four components of any behavior—the physiological, the feeling, the thinking, and, finally, the doing. All behavior comprises some variation of these components in series. For example, let's say you suddenly find yourself in a threatening situation. The thinking component of behavior kicks in immediately with thoughts of all the potential harm you may be facing. Your adrenal glands begin pumping adrenaline—the physiological component. As a result you begin to feel the adrenaline rush we call *fear.* Finally, the doing component kicks in, and you remove yourself from the situation rapidly. These four behavioral components don't necessarily always proceed in this succession, but they are always there—some to a greater extent than others—driving all but unconscious activity. Although at first blush, especially in the situation we described, it appears that these progressions are beyond your control, in actuality by knowing what you're doing you can control them. How?

Of these four components you have total control over just one, the actual doing component, and partial control over one other, the thinking component. Over the other two, unfortunately, you have no *direct* control whatsoever, a fact not lost on your old adversary temptation, because these last two are its portals of entry into your behavior. If temptation can gain a foothold in your physiology and/or your feelings, it can often bend the other components to its will, resulting in self-destructive behavior. However, by controlling the doing portion of behavior you have the last say and can by force of your will drive the behavior the opposite way. You walk into the office break room to get your low-carb snack from the refrigerator and are overwhelmed by the fresh-baked aroma of still-warm doughnuts. There they are—at least a dozen fluffy, moist glazed ones in an open box with an attached note that says *help yourself!* Assuming you love doughnuts, what happens to you? You smell and see the doughnuts, which starts your physiology working. Your GI tract starts preparing for the incoming doughnuts, your pancreas actually releases a little squirt of insulin in preparation, and your whole being prepares for the consumption of the doughnuts—and all these changes are beyond your direct control. These physiological changes immediately cause you to feel consciously hungry and to crave the doughnuts. You begin thinking about how good the doughnuts would taste and how hungry you really are and how just one wouldn't hurt anything and how you could really buckle down to your diet tomorrow and . . . You break down and eat the doughnut, then another, then you say, "Oh, well, I've blown my diet. There's no sense in staying on it for the rest of the day. I'll start in earnest tomorrow. Now I think I'll have another doughnut." If someone who knows you're dieting walks in and discovers you in mid-debauch, you say, "I just couldn't resist." And temptation has played you like a violin. (If this happens in real life, jump right back into Phase I at the next meal.)

So you allowed the physiological and feeling components over which you have no control to run roughshod over your thinking and doing components. But you can drive the equation the other way. You walk into the break room, see and smell the doughnuts, and your physiology and feelings spring into action. Instead of allowing first your thinking and then your doing components to fall into line, reverse the order. Grab your low-carb snack and walk out. Get involved in some other activity. Think about something else. Make a phone call. Control the controllable components, and as you do your physiology will return to normal and your hunger will evaporate. By controlling the components you *can* control you end up indirectly controlling those you really have no direct control over. Take charge of your actions, and everything else will fall into line.

It sounds great in theory, you say, but it's difficult in real life. Sure it is, but so is getting up on Monday morning when the alarm goes off, which you do day after day. Why? Because you have a job you have to get to and you enjoy the house you live in, the car you drive, and the clothes you wear—all courtesy of the money you make from the job you have to get to. Your physiological component and your feeling component and especially your thinking component all want to stay in bed, but your doing component rousts them all up and into the shower, and your day begins. Muster the same force of will with your eating behavior, revel in your domination of temptation, and watch with delight as you begin to make a reality of your visualized image of a lean, strong, healthy you. Good luck!

Chapter 12

The Antiaging Formula: Exercise

Exercise is the goddamn key. The more I do, the better I get.

TED WILLIAMS

Here, more than elsewhere, I saw multitudes to every side of me; their howls were loud while, wheeling weights, they used their chests to push.

You stumbled into the fourth circle of Dante's hell? Nah, you just walked through the door of your local health club. Everywhere you look people are groaning, sweating, straining, flexing, posing, and pumping. You see fitness buffs of all descriptions from the archetypal 90-pound weaklings to guys who could give Arnold Schwarzenegger a run for his money. All these disparate people have their own pet theories on how to maximize their fitness gains from exercise, and they have their own ideas of the best nutritional strategy to help them along the way. The only unifying factor in all this chaos is that 99.9 percent of these nutritional ideas are incorrect. In this chapter you will learn the role proper nutrition plays in physical development. You will learn the best exercise for turning back the clock on aging while at the same time increasing your lean body mass and burning off your excess body fat.

Exercise is absolutely essential to milking all the pleasure you can from a long and healthy life. Sure it's hard, and sure it takes time and effort, and sure we often dread it ourselves. But when we don't want to get up off our duffs and go do it, we usually remind each other of one of our favorite quotes: "The only time you can coast in life is when you're going downhill" (A. Roger Merrill).

The goals of any physical exercise are to increase muscular strength and endurance and to enhance performance. Muscles increase strength by enlarging, becoming more dense, and more efficiently tapping into their fuel supply. They become more conditioned by increasing their blood supply so that they can better access oxygen to burn this fuel. And stronger, more conditioned muscles lead to better performance in all athletics and in most of life. To put the time spent in exercise to most efficient use in achieving these goals, the body's metabolic biochemistry has to do its part by creating the proper conditions for muscle growth and repair. Let's start by looking at a hormone we haven't yet discussed that comes closer to being an elixir of youth than anything known.

The Youth Hormone

Have you ever had this experience? You get up early and work out, go to your job and put in a full day, watch your diet and deny yourself virtually everything that sounds good to eat, then come home to find your teenager sprawled half asleep in front of the TV amid a jumble of empty pizza boxes, soft drink cans, and candy wrappers. As he (or she) comes to life and asks, "What's for supper?" you do a slow burn. You've worked hard all day, exercised, and dieted, and you still have a roll around your middle that you can't get rid of. Your kid, on the other hand, lies around all day, gets up only to eat, eats three times the calories you do, yet is slender, muscular, and, if forced, could run circles around you. What gives?

One of the major factors causing this unfair disparity between them and us is an almost magical substance called *human growth hormone.* They have a lot; we don't have much. And it makes an enormous difference. (Actually we have as much as they do, but sadly, we just can't get to it nearly as well.) Fortunately the nutritional program in this book helps you increase your growth hormone levels better than any way we know short of injecting it.

Human growth hormone is a profound anabolic, or tissue-building, hormone produced in the pituitary, a small gland located at the base of the skull, and secreted at intervals throughout the day. It causes growth, repairs tissue, mobilizes fat stores, and shifts the metabolism to the preferential use of fat. Like human insulin, human growth hormone is produced commercially by recombinant DNA, and doctors use it extensively to treat a variety of disorders. Severely burned patients and those with massive soft tissue injuries or those recovering from major surgery all benefit from growth hormone therapy. Children with growth hormone deficiency who would otherwise be doomed to a life of dwarfism achieve normal growth with the administration of recombinant growth hormone. In the July 5, 1990, issue of the *New England Journal of Medicine,* Daniel Rudman, M.D., and his research group at the Medical College of Wisconsin reported the results of their study on the effects of growth hormone administered to elderly males. Dr. Rudman's group showed that tiny amounts of growth hormone injected just beneath the skin of sixty-one- to eighty-one-year-old males produced almost unbelievable results in only six months: lean body mass increased by 8.8 percent, body fat decreased by 14.4 percent, bone density increased in the lumbar spinal bones, and skin thickness increased by 7.1 percent (thin, brittle skin is one of the consequences of aging). All these changes were a result of the growth hormone increase—the subjects didn't change their diet or exercise. After only six months' therapy with minuscule amounts of this extremely potent substance the more youthful changes these men exhibited were, in Dr. Rudman's words, "equivalent in magnitude to the changes incurred during 10 to 20 years of [reverse] aging." It's no wonder growth hormone clinics are popping up all over Mexico and other less medically regulated countries.

Another study, performed at the University of New Mexico, demonstrated that weight lifters injected with growth hormone for only six weeks lost four times more body fat and gained four times more lean body mass compared to those who received only placebo. These studies and others like them leave little doubt scientifically that growth hormone truly is the elixir of youth—it fosters a kind of regeneration of youth.

JUMP-STARTING YOUR YOUTH HORMONE

The growth hormone difference between adults and adolescents isn't a disparity in amount but in release. Teenagers are much more sensitive to all the factors that stimulate the release of growth hormone, whereas adults are less sensitive and become even less so with increasing age. In truth, teenagers typically have more stimulating factors present than do adults. So if you want more growth hormone—and who doesn't?—you need to increase and intensify those factors that stimulate its release from the pituitary gland.

Factors That Stimulate the Release of Growth Hormone[1]

Decreased blood glucose levels
Increased blood protein levels

---

[1] These are the factors stimulating growth hormone release that you can actually do something about; there are others, but they are predominantly drug-induced.

Carbohydrate-restricted diet
Fasting
Increased protein diet
Free fatty acid decrease
PGE$_1$ (a "good" eicosanoid)
Stage IV sleep
Exercise

Carbohydrate restriction, increased protein, good eicosanoids . . . hmmmm, sounds a lot like the nutritional regimen described in this book. That's not really so surprising, because if we've been programmed to perform optimally on this dietary structure by millions of years of evolution, it ought to exert positive effects throughout all parameters of our biochemistry.

Our nutritional plan will give you plenty of protein, keep your carbohydrates restricted, your blood glucose lowered, and your free fatty acids to a minimum and will induce the production of lots of good eicosanoids. As a result you should be stimulating the release of a fair amount of growth hormone. But you can get even more. Along with proper nutrition, sleep and exercise also stimulate the release of growth hormone—but not just any sleep and exercise; they must be the right kind.

It turns out Mom was right all those times she urged you to get to sleep early so you'd grow. Growth hormone is secreted in a pulsatile surge in stage III and stage IV sleep, the first hour or two after reaching deep sleep. So to maximize growth hormone release you need to make certain that you get deep, sound sleep every night.

Exercise stimulates the release of a powerful surge of growth hormone, which promotes repair and rebuilding of the muscle broken down during the workout. But the exercise must be strenuous and done until muscle exhaustion almost to the point of failure for maximum results. A few jumping jacks or a brisk stroll around the block will provide some cardiac benefit, but it won't stimulate the release of growth hormone. Although all strenuous exercise stimulates the release of growth hormone, resistance training (weight lifting) seems to stimulate the most. As you lift weights, your straining muscle develops microscopic tears. These minuscule injuries apparently call forth the growth hormone that then repairs them and, in addition, actually stimulates the growth of new muscle fibers to augment those with the microscopic damage. All the while this repair and tissue building are going on the growth hormone converts the muscles into little fat-burning machines and promotes the release of fat from adipose tissue to ensure them a steady supply of fuel.

As with almost every system in the body, there are two sides to this equation. Just as a number of factors stimulate the pituitary to give up its growth hormone, other factors inhibit this process. Since our sensitivity to all those release-stimulating factors diminishes with age, it becomes critical that we not only do everything we can to stimulate growth hormone release but also work to avoid those things that inhibit it.

Factors That Inhibit the Release of Growth Hormone

> Increased blood glucose levels
> Increased blood free fatty acids
> Obesity
> Pregnancy

Once again our regimen comes up a winner, pregnancy excepted. A couple of important points need to be made, however. First, since increased glucose levels inhibit the release of growth hormone, it behooves us to avoid anything sweet, starchy, or otherwise carbohydrate laden before we go to bed. Any of these substances will give us an elevation of blood glucose that will inhibit the normal shot of growth hormone released an hour or so after our falling asleep. See what all those snacks of milk and cookies at bedtime have been doing to you!

Second, the pulse of growth hormone released by exercise generally hits the circulation toward the end of the workout and immediately after. If you want to inhibit this growth hormone surge, all you have to do is to eat a power bar or a candy bar or drink fruit juice, as trainers often advise you to do before, during, and right after workouts in the mistaken notion that you need "explosive, high-carbo energy" as one of these products advertises. What you're really getting is no growth hormone. Always work out on an empty stomach, don't consume anything except water during the workout, and don't eat until an hour or so after. Then make sure it's a protein-rich meal—you need plenty of amino acids for the growth hormone to use to repair and rebuild your muscles.

Now that you've been introduced to the wonders of growth hormone, let's see how you can put it to work.

The Path of Most Resistance

The single best exercise you can do to improve your health is to lift weights. Yes, aerobic exercise is good, but it won't deliver the extra benefits of resistance training. And lifting weights is the best resistance training of all. Every day it seems a new medical study surfaces showing the efficacy of resistance training in improving the health of seniors, juniors, and all those in between. Working out with weights strengthens joints, increases the density of your bones to prevent osteoporosis, increases your muscle mass, improves your endurance if done correctly, *decreases* your insulin levels, and, as we've already seen, stimulates the release of growth hormone, which improves just about everything.

Each pound of muscle mass you pack on becomes a fat-burning dynamo, allowing you to increase your food intake without fear of fat gain. As your muscle mass continues to build, your body will begin to resculpt itself. You will lose all the little handles and bulges of fat you could never get rid of before, no matter how hard you dieted. Best of all, once that new muscle is there, and as long as you continue to work it, your metabolic rate will increase, allowing you to eat more than you can imagine— even of carbohydrate foods—without negative consequences. No more working hard to lose your weight only to watch it balloon back up as soon as you start eating normally again. You will actually be able to eat more than when you started and continue to lose fat. Sounds impossible, but it works like a charm—if you do.

If you're female, you may be thinking that this sounds great, but you're really not all that keen to look like the Incredible Hulk. Not to worry. Your female hormones and lack of male hormones will keep you unhulklike even if you train extensively. The women you see in body-building magazines who *do* look like well-developed males usually have had a little help from their friends, the anabolic steroids. Your friends— work, sweat, and your own growth hormone—will slim you down by decreasing your body fat. The muscle growth you experience will be in the filling-out of muscle tissue in places it has atrophied from underuse and in increasing the density of the rest of your muscles. When you start, your muscles will look like a piece of choice steak with fat marbled throughout. As you work out and follow this nutritional plan you will quickly begin to replace this intramuscular fat with more muscle, making your muscle not necessarily larger but denser.

A word of caution: if you're trying to lose weight, you may be disappointed if you follow the scales too closely, because as your muscles become more dense, they become heavier. The new muscle you add weighs more than the fat it replaces, but its increased metabolic requirement that is stoked by the fat stored elsewhere on your body ends up making you much smaller, not to mention better proportioned, than before, regardless of what the scales say. It's much better to measure your progress by the way your clothing fits than by the bathroom scale.

HOW DO I START?

There are any number of good books available on weight training. Just remember when you get one of these manuals, read and follow only the instructions on the exercise part—ignore any nutritional advice. We recommend *Dr. Bob Arnot's Guide to Turning Back the Clock* (Little, Brown and Company) by Robert Arnot, M.D., which has an excellent section on weight training, especially for men. It's easy to read, has good illustrations showing the various exercises, and describes a number of different workouts designed to fit your time constraints while helping you achieve your particular fitness goals. Another option is a television program, *The Body Electric*, a half-hour show produced by WFSV-TV in Tallahassee, Florida. *The Body Electric* works several muscle groups on each program and uses weights. It's broadcast all over the country and in Canada.

When you begin your resistance training program, you need to follow a few basic guidelines:

1. Start with light weights first to strengthen the ligaments, tendons, and connective tissue around your joints, which are the weakest link when you begin and are the most prone to injury and discomfort. Only after your joints have been stabilized and strengthened with several weeks of light weights should you begin your serious muscle building.

2. To achieve the quickest results, work your biggest muscles first. Do pushups, for instance. You're looking for the increased metabolism and fat burning you get from increased muscle mass, and working your biggest muscle groups—thighs, shoulders, butt, and chest—gives you more growth faster. A 5 percent increase in size and density of large muscle groups provides a lot more metabolic firepower than the same percentage increase in small muscle groups or individual muscles. Work on the size and definition of these smaller muscle groups later.

3. Use perfect form. The idea is to work and strengthen the particular muscle groups you are working on, not to lift a specific amount of weight. If you have to arch your back and change your position to complete your sets, go to a lesser amount of weight. As long as you keep your back straight, you will go a long, long way toward avoiding injury.

4. Don't forget to recalculate and increase your protein intake if you originally determined it based on a more sedentary level of activity. To make maximal gains and minimize the potential for injury, you must consume adequate protein, the stuff all that new muscle is made of.

5. To maximize growth hormone release, always perform your workouts on an empty stomach. Don't consume any carbohydrate snacks anywhere near the time of your workout, or you can kiss your growth hormone good-bye.

6. Work to increase *power*, not just strength. Strength is how much you can lift; power is how fast you can lift it. Power is strength divided by time and is a measure of what your muscles can do for you. Athletic performance and defensive living rely on power for optimal performance; whether you're trying to rifle a tennis serve or leap out of the way of an oncoming car, you depend on the power and quickness of your muscles, not just their strength. You develop power by increasing the speed with which you lift the weights first, then increase the weight. If, for instance, you are doing four sets of ten repetitions with a particular weight, perform them slowly and with perfect form. With subsequent workouts, increase your speed with the same weight until you are snapping that weight up briskly through all the sets—then move to a higher weight and start again slowly and perfectly, then work on increasing speed.

7. Make your workouts aerobic so that you get the benefit of both weight training and endurance exercise. You do this by following guideline 5 and by not slowing down and resting between sets. If you have to decrease your weights to keep from becoming exhausted, do so. As you follow your new diet, you will build endurance as quickly as you build strength and power, because the foods you eat will actually increase the amount of oxygen transported and released in your exercising muscles. How can your diet increase the amount of oxygen delivered to the tissues?

Oxygen is carried to the tissues in the red blood cells and released. To increase the delivery of oxygen, we need to get more red blood cells to the oxygen-deprived tissues—in this case our working muscles. We can do this in two ways: first by increasing the number of red blood cells, which our new diet does nicely thanks to its high content of readily absorbable iron, the element that drives the production of red blood cells; second by delivering more of these red blood cells to the meshwork of capillaries within the tissues, where the oxygen exchange actually takes place. The red blood cells are larger than the diameter of the capillaries, so they actually deform themselves as they snake their way through these tiny vessels. It's kind of like forcing a water balloon through a paper towel tube. The only way to get more of them through faster is to increase the diameter of the blood vessel and/or increase the deformability of the red blood cells so that more of them can work their way through more quickly. The good (series one) eicosanoids induced by our nutritional plan both dilate the blood vessels *and* increase the suppleness and deformability of the red blood cells, getting more of them to the working muscle faster.

8. Don't start your exercise program until at least a week after you start your new carbohydrate-restricted diet. We know you're fired up and ready to start pumping growth hormone today, but take our word for it and wait a week. When you change your diet from one of high carbohydrates to one of many fewer carbohydrates you are going to experience a few days of easy fatigability. You may even become a little short-winded just performing your normal daily tasks. After a few days, or maybe even a week, this breathlessness goes away and you will actually have more endurance. Why this phenomenon? Because of the enzymatic changing of the guard, as explained in the question-and-answer section at the end of Chapter 10.

What Will I Look Like?

You may be wondering what you'll end up looking like if you diligently follow all these instructions. For one thing, if you have a lot of weight to lose, you'll look great, not scrawny and wasted once you've come all the way down. And we can guarantee you'll feel better, look better, and enhance your performance in golf, tennis, squash, skiing, or whatever your activity of choice. If you don't have a sport you enjoy, find one. Athletics at any level improve your performance in life in general. No matter what you take up, you will find your coordination improved, your agility enhanced, your reflexes sharpened, and your outlook on life improved.

As the old saying goes, a picture is worth a thousand words, so take a look at the three photos in Figure 12.1. Amazingly, they are all of the same person, a 53-year-old printing supply salesman named Stan Kuter who lives in Little Rock. Let us give you a chronology of these truly astounding pictures. The first one (A) is Stan (with his daughter) when he was 43 years old and heavily into running and low-fat dieting. He appears kind of wasted and emaciated because . . . well, he was. The constant running—50 miles per week—was breaking down his muscles, and the inadequate protein component of his low-fat diet wasn't rebuilding them. To top things off, his carbo loading before his workouts ensured that he released no growth hormone to aid in the maintenance of his lean body mass. Because of his long-standing protein deficiency, he was immuno-suppressed—a fate common to many distance runners—and was chronically afflicted with colds, sore throats, and a host of other minor illnesses.

FIGURE 12.1

A

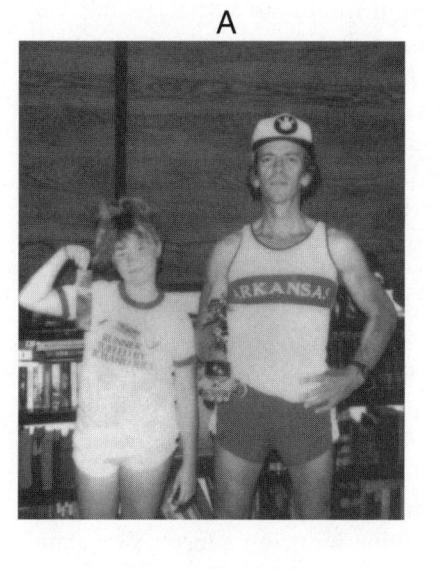

B

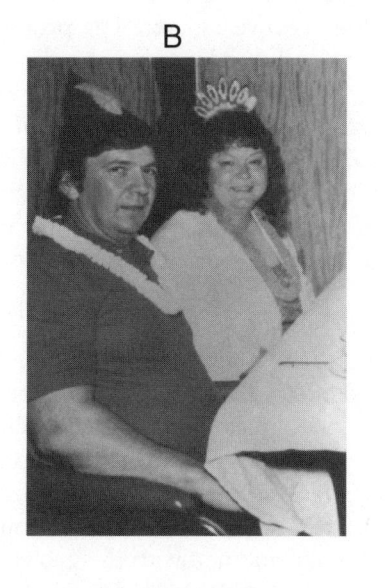

C

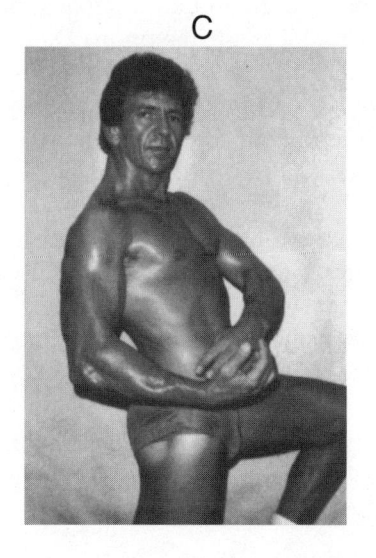

D

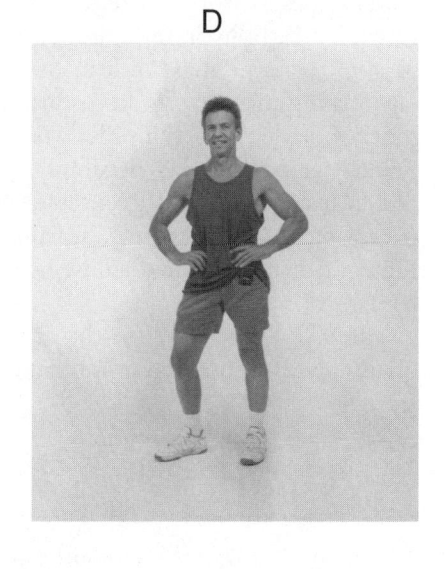

Stan finally had all the fun he could stand and decided to take a break from it all for a while, only to find himself in picture B (with his wife) a short two years later. The protein malnutrition Stan suffered while running and dieting reduced his muscle mass significantly and consequently reduced his metabolic rate as well. He had compensated for the decreased-lean-body-mass-induced metabolic burn by expending large amounts of energy running. When he quit running, however, the combination of reduced metabolic rate and no exercise opened the floodgates of body fat accumulation. This situation is one familiar to many who try to maintain their weight by running or other endurance exercises. They often find themselves in a trap. They can maintain their weight only as long as they continue to run. When they quit or even slow down, they find their weight increasing at a frightening rate.

Photo C shows Stan in his body-building phase. After tiring of being fat, Stan decided to take a different approach to conditioning. He got a copy of *Thin So Fast*, Mike's earlier book on the advantages of a restricted-carbohydrate nutritional program, followed it to the letter, and began a regimen of weight training. Only six months of adequate protein intake combined with the growth-hormone-inducing effects of resistance training transformed him from photo B to photo C.

Stan doesn't work out regularly anymore and doesn't always follow his restricted-carbohydrate regimen, but he still looks great—photo D. The reason: the large mass of lean tissue he built when he did work out is a fat-burning furnace that keeps his metabolic rate fired up, so he can have much more leeway on his diet without suffering the consequences. When he does gain a little fat, he simply cuts back on his carbohydrates slightly, and in just a few days the excess is gone. He works out with the weights occasionally, which keeps him from losing the muscle mass he has built. He isn't trying for new gains; he's simply maintaining what he already has.

The take-home lesson is that Ted Williams had it only half right: adequate dietary protein in combination with resistance training is the key.

The Bottom Line

Regular exercise plays an important role in helping you reclaim your health and vitality, not only in weight loss and maintenance but also in lowered blood pressure and improved lipid values. More important even than that, dedication to regular physical exercise helps you milk all the pleasure you can from a long and healthy life. The goals of exercise are simple: increased muscle strength and endurance. Stronger, better-conditioned muscles lead to improved physical performance—not just in sporting endeavors but in everyday activities. And best of all, exercise keeps you young! Although that may seem impossible, it's true: the right kind of exercise, coupled with the proper nutritional structure, will increase your release of growth hormone, that magic elixir of youth.

Our *Protein Power* program provides the proper nutritional framework to enhance release of growth hormone—the miraculous substance of youth that allows adolescents to escape the consequences of profound dietary abuse and sloth and still appear thin and fit. Or to withstand hours of exhausting physical activity and bounce up the next morning rested, raring to go, and none the worse for wear.

Growth hormone encourages growth and repair of body tissues, helps build lean body mass, mobilizes your fat stores, and shifts your metabolism into fat burning as a fuel source. Adults have more than adequate amounts of growth hormone locked away in the brain—we just have trouble getting to it, whereas teens release it easily. The chief time of release is about an hour or so after you fall deeply asleep. A number of factors help stimulate growth hormone release: stable low blood sugar, increased protein intake, a diet low in carbohydrate, fasting, deep sleep, a "good" eicosanoid balance, and exercise. Our nutritional regimen brings about all these positives except exercise—and we're adding that now. Other factors reduce growth hormone release: elevated blood sugar levels, obesity, and pregnancy. Again, our regimen comes up a winner (except for pregnancy, of course).

Although aerobic or endurance exercise is great for improving cardiovascular fitness, the best exercise to encourage release of growth hormone is the resistance kind—working your muscles against a resistance (a weight) to the point of near exhaustion. Weight training builds muscle (every pound of which burns calories and keeps you thin), strengthens joints, and increases bone strength. And done properly, it helps reduce elevated insulin levels and promote the release of growth hormone—both essential to your physical and metabolic rehabilitation.

Although good books detailing weight training exercise abound, they're usually filled with nutritional misinformation and constant reminders to load up on pasta and power bars and the like for their "explosive high-carbo energy." You must ignore their nutritional advice, because that high-carbo explosion will ensure you release little or no growth hormone. It's essential to your physical rehabilitation that you eat no carbohydrate foods before bedtime or your exercise regimen and drink only water to hydrate yourself while you exercise. One book we can recommend is *Dr. Bob Arnot's Guide to Turning Back the Clock* (Little, Brown and Company) by Robert Arnot, M.D.

Your exercise guidelines should be:

1. Start with light weights first and work up slowly.

2. Work your biggest muscles first—thighs, shoulders, buttocks, and chest—because you get bigger lean mass gains quicker.

3. Use perfect form during the exercise—if you have to twist and arch your back to lift a weight, it's too heavy. Lighten it.

4. As you increase the frequency or intensity of your workouts, don't forget to recalculate your protein requirements.

5. Always work out on an empty stomach.

6. Perform all exercises slowly and perfectly, then build speed—don't increase weight until you can smoothly, quickly, and perfectly perform the exercise at the current weight. This builds power and density of the muscle, not just strength.

7. Work aerobically during your weight training by moving quickly from one set to the next without long rest periods between.

8. Don't begin to exercise until you've been on your new nutritional regimen for at least a week. First set the stage and get stable nutritionally, then take off with your workouts.

If you bypassed the main body of the chapter in favor of this summary, you might want to back up for a moment to read the diet and exercise story of our patient Stan Kuter (page 228). As he has done for many of our other patients, Stan will amaze and inspire you. He's living proof that the right nutrition and resistance training are indeed the key to reclaiming your youth.

Chapter 13

Recipes

Protein is just as important as carbohydrates in meal planning. Our protein calculations, unless otherwise specified, are based on a 3-ounce portion in these recipes. You can adjust to your protein needs for an average of 7 grams protein per ounce of lean meat, fish, or fowl.

What's for Breakfast?

The fastest answer is cottage cheese, our Breakfast Fruit Smoothie, or hard boiled eggs. But here are some more interesting ideas. To pack in enough protein, breakfast should include eggs, cheese or cottage cheese, meat, chicken, or fish (well, maybe). On the carb front, don't forget that milk contains 6 carbohydrate grams per half cup, so in your coffee count .75 carbohydrate grams per tablespoon—half-and-half is .6. If you'd like fruit, choose a 5-carbohydrate-gram portion from pages 203–205 and be sure to add it into your total meal count. When you have time to sit down and really enjoy breakfast, try one of the breakfast dishes in the main recipe section.

HAM AND EGGS ON TOAST

Make a chunky salad mixture with finely chopped hard-cooked eggs, using 1 yolk to 2 whites, (2 ounces) slivered ham, minced scallions, salt, and pepper and just enough yogurt or sour cream to bind it. Mound the mixture on toast or crackers (maximum count 6 grams).

PER SERVING: 8 GRAMS CARBOHYDRATE, 16 GRAMS PROTEIN

FRIZZLED ORANGE BEEF WITH POACHED EGG

Sauté 2 ounces slivered dried beef (still sold in jars in the canned-meat section) in a little butter along with several wire-thin strands of orange zest, a generous sprinkle of chives, and some freshly ground black pepper. Poach an egg in the microwave (40 seconds on medium). Stir a rounded tablespoon of crème fraîche (or cream cheese) into the beef and let it melt but not boil. Pour the beef over a Jaret toast and top with the poached egg.

PER SERVING: 7 GRAMS CARBOHYDRATE, 22 GRAMS PROTEIN

SMOKED SALMON AND FRUIT

Spread cream cheese and smoked salmon on 4 grams of bread or crackers (page 205) and enjoy with $^1/_2$ cup of melon balls—these come frozen.

PER SERVING: 11.5 GRAMS CARBOHYDRATE, 10 GRAMS PROTEIN

ORANGE FRENCH TOAST WITH STRAWBERRIES

Soak a slice of Pepperidge Farm sandwich bread in 1 egg whisked with 1 tablespoon heavy cream. Sauté in a nonstick pan in $^1/_2$ pat of butter and a little grated orange zest until golden on both sides. Put $^1/_4$ cup sliced berries in the microwave with NutraSweet or Equal to sweeten and cook for a few seconds until you have a chunky sauce. Pour over the hot French toast.

PER SERVING: 12 GRAMS CARBOHYDRATE, 8 GRAMS PROTEIN

BREAD PUDDING WITH HAM AND CHEESE

Soak 2 Jaret toasts in 1 egg beaten with 2 tablespoons heavy cream until almost all the egg is absorbed. Lift one toast into a flat-rimmed soup plate with a spatula, fold over a slice of Black Forest ham (or Canadian bacon) on top, cover it with 2 tablespoons grated cheddar, and sandwich it with the second toast. Pour any remaining egg mixture over the top and sprinkle with a little more cheese. Microwave on high for $1^1/_2$ minutes.

PER SERVING: 13 GRAMS CARBOHYDRATE, 23 GRAMS PROTEIN

NOTE: Make this recipe open-faced with 1 Jaret toast and save 6 grams of carbs.

BLUEBERRIES AND CHEESE WITH COCONUT-CINNAMON TOAST

Mix $^1/_4$ cup fresh blueberries with $^1/_2$ cup cottage cheese and sweeten it to taste with NutraSweet or Equal. Toast 1 slice Pepperidge Farm Very Thin bread on one side only. Spread the other side with soft butter mixed with $^1/_2$ teaspoon brown sugar, a sprinkle of cinnamon, and 1 heaped teaspoon of unsweetened grated coconut (at the health food store or the freezer case of some supermarkets). Broil until bubbly and golden brown. Serve toast with the cottage cheese and berries.

PER SERVING: 11 GRAMS CARBOHYDRATE, 16 GRAMS PROTEIN

STEAK AND EGGS WITH MANGO

Sauté a $^1/_2$-inch-thick beef tenderloin (or ham) steak in butter, with or without a minced fresh jalapeño chili, top with a boiled egg, and surround with $^1/_3$ cup diced ripe mango. Add salt and freshly ground pepper.

PER SERVING: 11 GRAMS CARBOHYDRATE, 27 GRAMS PROTEIN

BREAKFAST BURRITO

Moisten 1 small flour tortilla on both sides with lightly dampened hands and soften it by holding it briefly over a gas flame or brushing it across a medium-high electric burner. Spread the center of the tortilla with 1 tablespoon drained and rinsed canned beans mashed to a paste with a little sour cream. Sprinkle it with a tablespoon of Mexican salsa verde and $^1/_4$ cup (not packed) of grated Monterey Jack or cheddar cheese. Very lightly scramble 2 eggs and spoon them across the center of the tortilla. Roll up the burrito like an egg roll, tucking in the ends. Heat it in the microwave for about 20 seconds, just long enough to melt the cheese.

PER SERVING: 15 GRAMS CARBOHYDRATE, 21 GRAMS PROTEIN

Fluffy Pancakes

SERVES 2

    2 extra-large eggs
 $^1/_3$ cup cottage cheese
    2 tablespoons cream cheese
       pinch of NutraSweet or Equal or to taste
    3 tablespoons wheat germ
    1 tablespoon rice flour or Wondra
    1 teaspoon baking powder
       pinch of baking soda

Whip the eggs in a food processor or by hand until frothy. Add the cheeses and beat until smooth. Add a little artificial sweetener. Add the rest of the ingredients and pulse to blend. Gently scrape the batter into a small bowl. Heat a nonstick skillet or griddle with a little butter as needed and when it's hot spoon the batter onto the griddle—about 10 pancakes. Cook over medium heat until the edges of the cakes are set and

Berry Syrups

· In lieu of syrup, make up a little fresh berry puree by pulsing
$^1/_2$ cup chopped fresh strawberries with 2 tablespoons orange juice
and a pinch of artificial sweetener. Microwave the mixture to a simmer and then let it cool down to warm before using. Leftover puree
will keep in the refrigerator for several days. Rhubarb is delicious in
this mix too. Microwave it in a little water and add the sweetener
after it's cooked.

Fresh raspberry puree is also wonderful with these pancakes. Use
Raspberry Crystal Light to liquefy the berries in the food processor. If the Crystal Light doesn't sweeten them enough, add a little
Equal or NutraSweet. After microwaving the berries, push them
through a strainer with the back of a spoon to remove the seeds.

PER 2-TABLESPOON SERVING: 2 GRAMS CARBOHYDRATE

---

large bubbles appear across the surface, about 1 minute. Carefully flip
them and cook for half as long as on the first side or until golden. Serve
on heated plates, with a drizzle of dietetic maple syrup or berry syrup
(above) and a couple of breakfast link sausages or crisp bacon (about 2
grams protein each).

PER SERVING: 10 GRAMS CARBOHYDRATE, 13 GRAMS PROTEIN

· Rice flour is available at most health food stores and Asian markets.
It's recommended for these pancakes because it results in a lighter texture.

· These pancakes don't keep particularly well, so just cut the recipe in
half if you're cooking them for yourself.

· Because this batter is very delicate, it's important that the baking
powder be fresh, not more than 2 months old, so it will puff up properly.

Rain Forest Pancakes:

Add $1^1/_2$ tablespoons finely chopped unsalted macadamia nuts, 1 tablespoon toasted unsweetened coconut, and a few drops of coconut extract to the batter.

PER SERVING: AN EXTRA 3 GRAMS CARBOHYDRATE, 2 GRAMS PROTEIN

If you're on maintenance, serve these little delectables with alternating *thin* slices of banana and kiwifruit between the pancakes, adding 5 carbohydrate grams to each portion.

Pecan Maple Pancakes:

Add 2 tablespoons finely chopped toasted pecans and a few drops of maple extract to the batter. Use dietetic maple syrup as a topping.

PER SERVING: AN EXTRA 2 GRAMS CARBOHYDRATE, 1 GRAM PROTEIN

Breakfast Fruit Smoothie

SERVES 1

   $^1/_2$ cup sliced strawberries, raspberries, or peaches, fresh or
       frozen
   $^1/_2$ cup cottage cheese
   $^1/_4$ cup plain yogurt
       Sugar free Tang or Crystal Light to taste (enough to cover
       everything else in the blender jar)

Mix in the blender. You can add ice if you're using fresh fruit.

PER SERVING: 17 GRAMS PROTEIN
              9 GRAMS CARBOHYDRATE (ALL STRAWBERRIES)
             11 GRAMS CARBOHYDRATE (ALL RASPBERRIES)
             14 GRAMS CARBOHYDRATE (ALL PEACHES)

Strawberry Jam

MAKES 2 8-OUNCE JARS, 32 TABLESPOONS

   1 pint fresh ripe strawberries
     juice of $^1/_2$ lemon
 $^1/_4$ cup water
   1 $^1/_4$-ounce envelope of unflavored gelatin
   5 teaspoons NutraSweet or 5 packets of Equal or less to taste

Wash, stem, and quarter the berries. In a medium saucepan, heat the berries with the lemon juice, covered, and simmer until the berries soften and give up their juice, about 3 minutes.

In a mixing bowl, pour the water over the gelatin and allow to soften for 1 minute. Add this to the berries and remove from the heat.

Mix in the NutraSweet and store covered in the refrigerator. Keeps for several weeks.

PER 1-TABLESPOON SERVING: 1 GRAM CARBOHYDRATE

Blender Hollandaise Sauce

SERVES 6

Great over cooked vegetables—especially asparagus and broccoli—or for eggs Benedict.

1 stick of butter
3 egg yolks (reserve whites for another use)
2 tablespoons fresh lemon juice
    dash of cayenne pepper

Melt the butter in a saucepan over low heat or in the microwave. In a blender or food processor, mix the egg yolks, lemon juice, and cayenne. With the motor running, add the melted butter in a slow stream. Blend for 30 seconds or until thick.

PER SERVING: 0.5 GRAM CARBOHYDRATE, 1.2 GRAMS PROTEIN

Light and Speedy Meals

Here are some ideas for lunches and dinners to put together when you're too rushed to focus on real recipes. Some are familiar dishes, and you may have your own favorite way of preparing them, in which case these notes will serve as reminders that they're permissible on this diet. Where quantities are necessary, they're for one serving, but everything is easily multiplied.

QUICK SALADS

Egg Salad

Chopped hard-cooked eggs with minced celery, scallions, and fresh dill, salt and pepper, and mayonnaise seasoned with Dijon mustard and lightened with yogurt two to one.

PER SERVING: LESS THAN 1 GRAM CARBOHYDRATE, 6 GRAMS PROTEIN PER EGG USED.

Stuff a medium tomato with it for another 4.1 grams carbohydrate.

Greek Salad

Cut up $^1/_2$ medium ripe seeded tomato, $^1/_2$ medium green pepper, and $^1/_2$ peeled and seeded cucumber and toss into a salad bowl. Add a slice of sweet onion separated into rings, a minced garlic clove, some chopped fresh dill, and lots of chopped parsley. Drizzle olive oil and red wine vinegar over the salad and top it with an ounce of crumbled feta cheese.

PER SERVING: 8 GRAMS CARBOHYDRATE, 8 GRAMS PROTEIN

Ham and Cheese Salad

Sliver a $^1/_4$-inch-thick slice of deli baked (or Black Forest) ham along with an ounce of Jarlsberg or Gruyère cheese. Mix with $^1/_2$ cup sliced raw mushrooms, a little chopped celery, minced parsley, and a couple of tablespoons of freshly grated Parmesan cheese. Shake up the dressing in a screw-top jar: 1 tablespoon olive oil, 1 teaspoon rice or white wine vinegar, $^1/_4$ teaspoon Dijon green peppercorn mustard, salt, and a tablespoon of heavy cream.

PER SERVING: 3 GRAMS CARBOHYDRATE, 19 GRAMS PROTEIN

Chicken Salad

Pull the meat from a carryout rotisserie chicken and mix with minced scallions, parsley, celery, and capers (or chopped stuffed green olives) and light mayonnaise mixed half and half with sour cream.

PER SERVING: 3 GRAMS CARBOHYDRATE, 21 GRAMS PROTEIN

Or mix the chicken with curried mayonnaise, grated orange zest, and yogurt. Add slivered jícama or water chestnuts for crunch and minced cilantro for sparkle. Serve with a couple slices of fresh ripe mango or papaya and $^1/_2$ diced avocado.

PER SERVING: 10 GRAMS ADDITIONAL CARBOHYDRATE, 2 GRAMS PROTEIN

Tuna Salad

Flake the tuna and mix with minced scallions, parsley, and grated lemon zest. Press a clove of garlic into the mayonnaise and add a squeeze of fresh lemon juice.

PER SERVING: 2 GRAMS CARBOHYDRATE, 24 GRAMS PROTEIN

Cottage Cheese and Tomato

Mix $^1/_3$ cup cottage cheese with lots of minced parsley and a minced clove of garlic. Stuff a medium tomato and serve over a big mixed green salad.

PER SERVING: 6.5 GRAMS CARBOHYDRATE, 14 GRAMS PROTEIN

Parsley Salad

This salad tastes wonderful with grilled lamb or roast chicken. Pull the leaves off a bunch of parsley and measure out 1 cup. Dress the parsley leaves with fresh lemon juice and freshly grated Parmesan cheese, salt, and pepper. You don't really need oil, but you can add a little olive oil if you like. Sliver 1 sun-dried tomato and toss it in.

PER SERVING: 6.5 GRAMS CARBOHYDRATE

Melon and Prosciutto

Slice $^1/_4$ 5-inch cantaloupe and wrap each slice in thin prosciutto slices. Arrange the wrapped melon slices on a plate and add a couple of wedges of lime to squeeze over them. Pass the peppermill.

PER SERVING: 10 GRAMS CARBOHYDRATE, 4 GRAMS PROTEIN

CREAMED CHIPPED BEEF WITH MUSHROOMS

Stouffer's creamed chipped beef has 5 grams carbohydrate per $^1/_2$ cup. Add $^1/_4$ cup sautéed mushrooms, 1 tablespoon minced scallions, and a dash of Tabasco. (Serve it over 10 steamed spears of fresh asparagus for an extra 5 grams carbohydrate.)

PER SERVING: 7 GRAMS CARBOHYDRATE, 9 GRAMS PROTEIN

Barbecue Sauce

Commercial BBQ sauces run between 5 and 14 grams carbohydrate per *tablespoon*. This one has only 2 grams per tablespoon (8.25 per $^1/_4$ cup). Mix together 2 tablespoons Heinz Light ketchup, 1 tablespoon Worcestershire sauce, 1 tablespoon Dijon honey mustard, 1 tablespoon minced shallot, 2 pressed garlic cloves, Tabasco sauce to taste, $^1/_4$ cup full-bodied red wine, a dash of liquid mesquite smoke, and a small pinch of NutraSweet or Equal.

SAUSAGE AND PEPPERS WITH ZUCCHINI

Sauté 3 ounces of your favorite sausage, links or patties, with $^1/_2$ cup chopped red or green bell pepper, $^1/_4$ cup chopped onion, and $^1/_2$ cup chopped zucchini.

PER SERVING: 7.5 GRAMS CARBOHYDRATE, 21 GRAMS PROTEIN

DILLED PANCAKES WITH SMOKED SALMON

Make the pancakes on page 235, adding minced fresh dill and minced scallions to the batter and leaving out the sweetener. Stack 5 of the pancakes with a teaspoon of sour cream and a thin slice of smoked salmon on top of each one.

PER SERVING: 13 GRAMS CARBOHYDRATE, 28 GRAMS PROTEIN

HAM STEAK WITH BEET SALAD

Roast 2 medium beets at 375° for about 40 minutes or until a knife tip easily pierces the beet. Cool the beets and slip off the skins. Sliver the beets and dress them with 2 tablespoons minced scallion and $^1/_4$ cup heavy cream mixed with a scant teaspoon horseradish mustard (or mix your own), salt and pepper, and a few drops of fresh lemon juice. Serve with a grilled 3-ounce ham steak.

PER SERVING: 13 GRAMS CARBOHYDRATE, 22 GRAMS PROTEIN

STIR-FRY DISHES

Simple vegetable stir-fries with the addition of thinly sliced beef, chicken, pork, tofu, or whole shrimp are perfect hurry-up, low-carb meals. Look up the carbohydrate gram counts of the vegetables you want to use in Chapter 10. Choose from mushrooms, green beans, eggplant, red pepper, bok choy, asparagus, scallions, baby corn, carrots, spinach, snow peas or sugar snaps, celery, bamboo shoots, and water chestnuts. Heat the wok until it's hot and add peanut oil, minced garlic, a slivered coin of ginger, and a dried hot chili or two if you like your stir-fries spicy. Briefly cook the meat first, remove it (and chilies) to a side bowl, and then briefly toss and cook the vegetables. Add the meat back in and season with soy sauce, tamari, oyster sauce, or one of the many good liquid stir-fry seasonings available at gourmet stores. Check labels; some of these are loaded with carbs.

PER SERVING: Carbohydrate gram counts will vary according to the vegetables chosen. Watch the quantities!

GARLIC SHRIMP WITH SALSA

Sauté jumbo shrimp in garlic oil and add a tablespoon of hot Mexican salsa to each serving. Serve with a mixed green salad with $1/2$ sliced avocado and 4 or 5 strips of jícama.

PER SERVING: 5 GRAMS CARBOHYDRATE, 21 GRAMS PROTEIN

SALMON OLIVADA

Smear olivada paste over a thick salmon fillet or steak and broil it. A 6-ounce salmon steak provides 42 grams protein.

CHEESE TOAST WITH TOMATO, BACON, AND AVOCADO

Melt 1 ounce grated cheese on 1 Jaret toast with a thin slice of tomato on the bottom. Top with 2 slices of crisp bacon and a slice of avocado.

PER SERVING: 7 GRAMS CARBOHYDRATE, 11 GRAMS PROTEIN

Snacks: 5 Carbohydrate Grams or Less

Remember: subtract your snack carbohydrates from your meal allowance.

- $1/4$ cup Planter's mixed salted nuts with peanuts (3 grams)
- 1 Swedish ginger snap with a thin slice of natural cheddar (4 grams)
- 2 celery ribs filled with 1 tablespoon of chunky natural peanut butter or cream cheese with scallions (5 grams)
- 4 slices of hard salami (or cervelat with garlic and pepper-corns) spread lightly with cream cheese and rolled around a thin scallion or half of a larger one (2 grams)
- 2 thin slices of boiled or baked ham spread with cream cheese and chives, rolled (1 gram)
- 2 thin slices of ham spread with spicy mustard and rolled up with thin slices of Gruyère (1 gram)
- 1 Wasa sesame cracker with 1 tablespoon of any cheese spread of your choice (3 grams)
- 2 slices of rare deli roast beef spread lightly with 1 table-spoon cream-style horseradish, rolled (1 gram)
- 5 pieces Talk o' Texas Okra Pickles—hot or mild (5 grams)
- $1/4$ cup roasted and salted sunflower seeds (4 grams)
- 5 Wheat Thins (5 grams)
- 2 ounces string cheese or mozzarella with 2 cherry tomatoes (3 grams)
- 1 deviled egg (1 gram)

COD WITH TOMATO SHRIMP SAUCE

Mix 2 tablespoons crème fraîche or sour cream with minced chives, a squeeze of sun-dried tomato paste from a tube, a pinch of cayenne, and a squeeze of lemon. Fold in 1 ounce chopped cooked shrimp and serve the sauce over a *thick* 4-ounce fillet of cod steamed in the microwave.

PER SERVING: 3 GRAMS CARBOHYDRATE, 36 GRAMS PROTEIN

HUEVOS CARACAS

Frizzle some dried beef in butter with a little chili powder. Add $^1/_2$ seeded and chopped tomato and a dash of hot sauce. Cook for about 2 minutes. Add a tablespoon of grated Parmesan cheese and then fold in 2 beaten eggs. Lift and turn until the eggs are firm.

PER SERVING: 2.5 GRAMS CARBOHYDRATE, 21 GRAMS PROTEIN

GRUYÈRE AND ZUCCHINI FRITTATA WITH SAUSAGE

In a nonstick omelet pan, melt butter and sauté $^1/_2$ cup matchstick-cut zucchini with salt and pepper until it's tender. Pour in 3 beaten eggs and a handful of grated Gruyère cheese. Cook over low heat, continually lifting this flat omelet to let the uncooked portion flow to the bottom of the pan. Serve with a couple of small grilled sausages.

PER SERVING: 3.1 GRAMS CARBOHYDRATE, 31 GRAMS PROTEIN

Soups

Spicy Tomato and Celeriac Soup

MAKES 1 QUART; 4 SERVINGS

   2 cups canned Italian plum tomatoes, drained
   2 cups beef broth
$^3/_4$ cup grated celery root
   2 garlic cloves, minced
   1 tablespoon minced flat-leaf parsley
   1 teaspoon fresh thyme leaves or $^1/_4$ teaspoon dried
$^1/_4$ teaspoon Tabasco sauce or to taste
     pinch of NutraSweet or Equal
     salt to taste

Put everything but the NutraSweet and salt in a saucepan and cook over low heat until the celeriac and garlic are soft. Add a small pinch of sweetener and some salt. Puree the soup in a food processor or blender.

PER 1-CUP SERVING: 7 GRAMS CARBOHYDRATE

• To serve this soup for a full meal, mix $^1/_2$ pound ground chicken with 6 minced scallions, $^1/_4$ teaspoon dried oregano, salt and pepper, and an egg yolk mixed with a bit of heavy cream. Form into little meatballs and sauté them quickly in olive oil. Put a few of them in the bottom of the soup bowls and freeze the rest for another use. Slices of cooked sausage would also be good. Additional protein grams: 16.

• Try replacing the beef broth with 1¹/₂ cups clam broth and simmer chunks of sea bass or cod in the soup. Additional protein grams: 16.

Kind-of-Mexican Chicken and Vegetable Soup

MAKES 2 QUARTS; 5 SERVINGS

  2 tablespoons olive oil
¹/₂ cup chopped scallion
  1 garlic clove, minced
  1 tablespoon minced canned chipotle chili or canned green
      chili plus a shake of liquid smoke and hot sauce
  1 quart chicken broth
  2 celery ribs, chopped
  1 carrot, sliced
¹/₂ cup cut green beans
¹/₂ cup diced zucchini
  1 cup diced Muir Glen organic canned tomatoes
¹/₂ cup canned hominy, rinsed
  1 cup shredded cooked chicken
      salt and pepper to taste
¹/₄ avocado, diced, per serving
  1 thin slice of lime per serving

Heat the oil in a soup pot, then sauté the scallion, garlic, and chili in the hot oil over medium heat until the garlic is soft, about 2 minutes. Add the broth and all of the vegetables and simmer uncovered until the vegetables are soft. Add the hominy, chicken, salt, and pepper and heat for 2 minutes. Add more chipotle or some Tabasco sauce if you like the soup spicier. Garnish each portion with avocado and lime.

PER 1¹/₂-CUP SERVING: 10 GRAMS CARBOHYDRATE, 12 GRAMS PROTEIN

Spinach, Leek, and Bacon Soup with Scallops

SERVES 2

> 4 strips of smoked bacon
> 3 leeks, trimmed, cleaned, and minced
>   salt and pepper to taste
> 1 cup cooked frozen whole-leaf spinach, chopped
> 3 cups chicken broth
> 2 egg yolks mixed with $1/4$ cup heavy cream
>   pinch of cayenne pepper
> 10 ounces bay scallops
> 2 lemon wedges for garnish

Crisp-cook the bacon and crumble it for garnish; set aside. Reserve 2 tablespoons of the bacon fat and sauté the minced leeks in it over medium heat until soft. Add salt and pepper. Add the spinach and broth and puree in a food processor or blender. Return to the stove over medium-low heat. Ladle a little hot broth into the yolk mixture and whisk, then whisk the mixture into the rest of the broth, stirring until the soup is thickened. Taste for salt and add the cayenne. Add the scallops and cook for a minute or two to heat through. Serve with the bacon bits on top and garnish with a lemon wedge.

PER SERVING: 9 GRAMS CARBOHYDRATE, 25 GRAMS PROTEIN

Double-Mushroom Soup

MAKES 1 QUART; 4 SERVINGS

> 4 tablespoons ($1/2$ stick) butter
> 2 cups chopped mixed mushrooms
> $1/2$ cup minced scallion
> 2 garlic cloves, minced
>   salt and cayenne pepper to taste
> 1 teaspoon dry mustard
> 2 teaspoons wild mushroom powder (grind dried wild
>   mushrooms in a food processor)
> 3 cups chicken broth

2 tablespoons dry sherry
2 egg yolks mixed with $^1/_4$ cup heavy cream

Melt the butter in a large skillet over medium-low heat. Sauté the mushrooms, scallion, and garlic in the butter for about 30 minutes, until the mixture is thick. Add the salt and cayenne, dry mustard, and mushroom powder, mix well, and cook for 5 minutes. Pour in the chicken broth and sherry and bring the soup to a simmer. Whisk a little of the hot liquid into the yolk mixture and then whisk that mixture back into the soup, stirring until it thickens.

PER 1-CUP SERVING: 3 GRAMS CARBOHYDRATE, 5 GRAMS PROTEIN

• Serve before a roast chicken or a broiled fish fillet and add a big mixed green salad with lemon vinaigrette.

Gazpacho

SERVES 2

1 16-ounce can Muir Glen organic stewed tomatoes
2 garlic cloves, pressed
1 tablespoon mayonnaise
  pinch of cayenne pepper
1 teaspoon red wine vinegar
  salt and pepper to taste
$^1/_4$ cup minced scallion
$^1/_2$ medium cucumber, peeled if waxed, seeded and diced
$^1/_4$ cup diced green bell pepper

Puree half of the stewed tomatoes in a food processor or blender with the pressed garlic, mayonnaise, cayenne, and vinegar. Add salt and pepper. Add the rest of the tomatoes and pulse on and off to blend, preserving some texture. Mix the remaining vegetables together and refrigerate separately from the soup base until both are well chilled. Serve the soup very cold with the chopped vegetables stirred in.

PER SERVING: 10.5 GRAMS CARBOHYDRATE

Chilled Red Pepper Soup with Cilantro

SERVES 2

    ³/₄ cup drained canned roasted red peppers
    1 cup chicken broth
      salt to taste
    1 garlic clove, pressed or minced
      pinch of cayenne pepper
    2 tablespoons minced cilantro
    3 tablespoons sour cream
    1 tablespoon yogurt

Puree the red peppers with the chicken broth in a food processor or blender. Add the salt, garlic, and cayenne and pulse to blend. Chill for at least an hour. Whisk the cilantro into the sour cream and yogurt. Serve the soup with the herbed cream feathered into it with a fork.

PER SERVING: 6 GRAMS CARBOHYDRATE, 3.5 GRAMS PROTEIN

 • Serve this soup with a couple of broiled or grilled lamb chops and a mixed green salad, including some spinach.

Chilled Almond Avocado Soup

SERVES 2

    1 ripe Hass avocado, chopped
    ¹/₂ cup blanched almonds, toasted
    1 cup chicken broth
    ¹/₄ teaspoon fresh lime juice
      salt and pepper to taste
      pinch of nutmeg, preferably freshly ground
    ¹/₂ cup light cream
    1 tablespoon slivered almonds, toasted

Puree the avocado and blanched almonds in a food processor or blender until smooth. Pour the mixture into a small saucepan and add the chicken broth, lime juice, salt and pepper, and nutmeg. Bring to a boil, then lower the heat, and simmer uncovered for 5 minutes. Stir in the cream. Chill the soup for at least an hour. Serve with the slivered almonds sprinkled on top.

PER SERVING: 15 GRAMS CARBOHYDRATE, 15 GRAMS PROTEIN

• Serve with jumbo shrimp sautéed in garlic oil and red pepper flakes over spinach salad. (12 cooked shrimp have about 21 grams protein.)

Gingered Egg Drop Soup with Chicken

SERVES 2

2 chicken breast halves, skinned and boned
1 coin of fresh ginger
3 cups chicken broth, preferably homemade
  salt and Szechuan pepper to taste
4 scallions—the bulb, and 1 inch of the green parts, slivered
8 snow peas, trimmed and cut on the diagonal into thin strips
1 egg, beaten

Cut the chicken breasts lengthwise into 3 sections and then into diagonal strips. Simmer the chicken strips with the ginger coin in the chicken broth in a small saucepan until the chicken is opaque, about 6 minutes. When the chicken is cooked, remove and discard the ginger. Salt the broth and grind in some Szechuan pepper. Add the scallions and snow peas. Whisk the egg and drizzle it into the broth. Serve the soup immediately.

PER SERVING: 4 GRAMS CARBOHYDRATE, 36 GRAMS PROTEIN

• Serve with 3 Japanese sesame rice crackers for an extra 4.5 carbohydrate grams.

Salads

Indonesian Vegetable Salad with Peanut Sauce

SERVES 2

$^1/_2$ cup bean sprouts
1 cup very thinly sliced red cabbage
$^1/_2$ cup sliced young green beans

$^1/_2$ cup chopped zucchini
$^1/_4$ large red bell pepper, cut into thin strips
  2 tablespoons creamy natural peanut butter
$^1/_4$ cup Thai unsweetened coconut milk
  1 garlic clove, pressed
$^1/_2$ teaspoon Thai hot chili sauce or to taste
  1 tablespoon tamari or soy sauce
    pinch of NutraSweet or Equal
$^1/_6$ lime in a wedge
    water as needed
  8 scallions, trimmed and quartered
  2 tablespoons grated carrot
$^1/_2$ cucumber, peeled if waxed, sliced
  3 cups spinach, washed and dried
  2 hard-cooked eggs, sliced

Pour boiling water over the bean sprouts and let them sit for only a second. Strain and reserve. Steam the cabbage, beans, zucchini, and red pepper in the microwave together until crisp-tender, about 5 minutes. In a small bowl, mix the peanut butter, coconut milk, garlic, chili sauce, tamari, and NutraSweet into a sauce using the back of a spoon. Squeeze the lime wedge into the sauce. Add water to the sauce to bring it to the consistency of heavy cream. Adjust the seasoning. Arrange the cooked and raw vegetables around a bed of spinach, keeping each variety separate. Overlap the egg slices in the center and serve the salad with the peanut sauce on the side.

PER SERVING: 15 GRAMS CARBOHYDRATE, 8.5 GRAMS PROTEIN

 • Serve with broiled or charcoal-grilled pork baby back ribs rubbed with salt and cayenne pepper.

Caesar Salad with Shrimp

SERVES 2

  4 hearts of romaine, broken into bite-size pieces

Dressing:

  6 tablespoons olive oil
  2 tablespoons fresh lemon juice

salt and pepper to taste
pinch of dry mustard
dash of Worcestershire sauce
$^1/_2$ inch squeeze of anchovy paste from a tube (optional)
1 egg yolk

Topping:

2 tablespoons freshly grated Parmesan cheese
12 large shrimp, cooked and peeled
12 garlic croutons

Put the romaine into a salad bowl. Put the dressing ingredients in a screw-top jar and shake vigorously. Taste for seasoning and adjust—the dressing should be lemony and piquant. Toss the greens with enough dressing to coat the leaves, reserving a little. Sprinkle the leaves with the grated Parmesan. Dip the shrimp into the reserved dressing and place them on top of the salad along with the garlic croutons. (Make the croutons from diced rustic bread. Coat them with garlic olive oil and toast on a baking sheet in a 375° oven until golden and crisp.)

PER SERVING: 9 GRAMS CARBOHYDRATE, 13 GRAMS PROTEIN

Barbecued Pork, Zucchini, and Roasted Red Pepper Salad

SERVES 2

Dressing:

$^1/_4$ cup olive oil or avocado oil
2 tablespoons sherry vinegar
1 garlic clove, pressed
$^1/_4$ teaspoon ground cumin
salt and pepper to taste

Salad:

any amount of mixed salad greens
1 cup sliced mixed green and yellow summer squash

$^1/_4$ cup diced jícama
1 canned roasted red pepper, torn into strips
　any amount of barbecued pork tenderloin, sliced*

Shake the dressing in a screw-top jar. Toss the salad vegetables with the dressing and arrange the cold pork slices around the edge of the salad.

Per serving: 8 grams carbohydrate

Spinach, Avocado, Bacon, and Goat Cheese Salad

Serves 2

Salad:

　any amount of spinach leaves
3 celery ribs, cut into 2-inch sticks lengthwise
6 scallions, trimmed and quartered
2 ounces goat Gouda or any firm goat cheese, cut into thin
　　strips
1 medium Hass avocado, sliced

Dressing:

$^1/_4$ cup sunflower or light olive oil
2 tablespoons fresh lemon juice
1 teaspoon Dijon honey mustard
2 teaspoons minced fresh dill
　salt and pepper to taste

Toppings:

4 strips of smoked bacon, cooked and crumbled
2 tablespoons roasted sunflower seeds

---

* To barbecue the pork, rub a pork tenderloin all over with 1 tablespoon olive oil mixed with a minced garlic clove, $^1/_4$ teaspoon oregano, $^1/_8$ teaspoon ground cumin, and a jolt of liquid smoke and Tabasco. Massage the seasonings into the meat. Broil the pork 4 inches from the heat for 6 minutes on each side.

Toss the salad ingredients with the blended salad dressing and add the toppings.

PER SERVING: 9 GRAMS CARBOHYDRATE, 12 GRAMS PROTEIN

GOING FOR THE CRUNCH

You'll quickly notice that the low-carb kitchen is short on crunch—no rice cakes, no pretzels, no buckets of popcorn. But here are some ideas for snacks that offer a little crunch for very few carbs.

- unlimited pork rinds—zero carbohydrate
- 2 Wasa Sesame Rye crackers—4 grams carbohydrate
- 5 Wheat Thins—5 grams
- 1 cup Cape Cod cheddar cheese popcorn—5 grams
- 2 breadsticks—5 grams (check labels)
- $^1/_2$ cup Planter's mixed salted nuts with peanuts—7 grams
- 1 Jaret (melba) toast—6 grams

Main Dishes

Antipasto Supper

SERVES 2

This long list of ingredients shouldn't intimidate you since there's no cooking involved. A great antipasto can be put together in minutes.

    arugula or other flat salad greens
3 tablespoons Hellmann's Light mayonnaise
2 large garlic cloves, pressed
1 tablespoon fresh lemon juice
1 $6^1/_2$-ounce can white tuna, packed in oil
1 teaspoon tiny capers or minced large capers

$^1/_2$ cup Progresso or Giovanni's eggplant caponata
$^1/_4$ cup oil-packed artichoke hearts
   red wine vinegar
   salt and pepper to taste
4 slices of imported prosciutto
1 tablespoon whipped cream cheese with minced onion
8 slices of Italian hard salami
4 scallions, split lengthwise
2 red hot cherry peppers or pickled okra
8 mushrooms, thinly sliced
   oil and vinegar
   fresh thyme leaves
8 cherry tomatoes
8 Italian or Greek black olives
2 ounces ricotta salata or fresh mozzarella, cut into strips

Line a round serving platter with arugula leaves. Mix the mayonnaise, garlic, and lemon juice in a small dish. Turn out the tuna onto paper towels to drain, keeping the fish in the round compressed shape. Blot the top and sides and set the round of tuna in the center of the platter. Spread with the garlic mayonnaise and dot with capers. Set all the other components around the tuna like the spokes of a wheel: First the canned caponata. Drain the artichoke hearts and drizzle some red wine vinegar over them. Add salt and pepper. Next, ruffle the prosciutto. Then place a dot of the cream cheese in the center of each slice of salami. Place the white end of a scallion half on the dot and gather the salami up around it, using the cream cheese as the "glue." Next lay out the cherry peppers or okra. Dress the sliced mushrooms with oil and vinegar and the leaves from a couple of stems of fresh thyme. Arrange the tomatoes, the olives, and finally some fingers of cheese.

PER SERVING: 12 GRAMS CARBOHYDRATE, 31.5 GRAMS PROTEIN

Tex-Mex Cheese Flan with Chunky Salsa

SERVES 2

These puffy little flans are not only versatile and ready in a flash but are perfect for company, as either an accompaniment or a first course.

   vegetable or olive oil spray
1 jumbo egg

$^1/_4$ cup nonfat ricotta or large-curd cottage cheese
$^1/_4$ cup grated Monterey Jack cheese, lightly packed
   2 tablespoons light sour cream
   1 tablespoon minced cilantro (optional)
      salt and pepper to taste
   2 tablespoons chunky Mexican salsa
   2 cilantro sprigs for garnish

Preheat the oven to 350°. Lightly spray two $^1/_2$-cup soufflé ramekins or custard cups. Put all the ingredients except the salsa and cilantro sprigs in a blender or food processor. Blend or process until very smooth and creamy. Divide the mixture between the ramekins—they should be about two-thirds full. Bake for 20 minutes or until nicely domed and puffed. Run a sharp knife around the edge of the ramekins and turn the flans out onto serving plates. Top with a tablespoon of salsa, garnish with cilantro, and serve immediately.

PER SERVING: 4 GRAMS CARBOHYDRATE, 12 GRAMS PROTEIN

   • Serve the flan with chicken sausage and a large mixed green salad with $^1/_2$ avocado, sliced.

PER SERVING: AN ADDITIONAL 7 GRAMS CARBOHYDRATE, 24 GRAMS PROTEIN

Italian Flan:

Use grated fontina cheese or half fontina and half fresh mozzarella—try smoked mozzarella. Arrange a couple of basil leaves or one large one on the bottom of the ramekin before filling it. Top the finished flan with a tablespoon of hot marinara sauce (additional 1 gram carbohydrate).

Feta-Dill Flan with Shrimp:

Use cottage cheese, crumbled feta, minced dill, and 2 minced scallions in the flans. Serve with 6 large shrimp, tails on, sautéed in olive oil with minced garlic and a sprinkle of hot red pepper flakes. Just before serving, toss a large handful of baby spinach leaves into the shrimp and toss until the spinach wilts but remains bright green.

PER SERVING: AN ADDITIONAL 5.5 GRAMS CARBOHYDRATE, 11 GRAMS PROTEIN

Nutty Chicken Thighs

SERVES 2

These crunchy baked chicken thighs are close cousins to southern fried chicken.

    4 tablespoons (^{1}/$_2$ stick) butter, melted
^{1}/$_4$ cup peanut oil
    1 egg, lightly beaten with 3 tablespoons buttermilk
^{1}/$_4$ cup ground raw peanuts
    1 tablespoon sesame seeds
    2 tablespoons flour
      salt and pepper to taste
    4 chicken thighs

Preheat the oven to 350°. Mix the melted butter with the oil and pour it into a shallow ovenproof pan. Slide the pan into the oven while you dip the chicken. Whisk the buttermilk and egg together in a flat soup bowl and mix the ground peanuts, seeds, flour, and seasoning in another. Dip the chicken pieces into the buttermilk/egg and then coat completely with the dry mixture. Place the chicken in the hot pan, spooning up the butter and oil to completely moisten the coating. Bake for 30 to 40 minutes or until the chicken is well browned and crisp.

PER SERVING: 10 GRAMS CARBOHYDRATE, 40 GRAMS PROTEIN

• Serve the chicken with a large green salad, including some spinach, a few thinly sliced red onion rings, and 4 halved cherry tomatoes. Dress the salad with olive oil, red wine vinegar, and a dash of balsamic vinegar.

PER SERVING: AN EXTRA 3 GRAMS CARBOHYDRATE

Maintenance Additions:

Serve each portion of chicken with ^{1}/$_2$ cup steamed whole skinny green beans and coleslaw. To make the coleslaw, mix ^{1}/$_2$ cup shredded raw cabbage with 2 tablespoons grated carrot, ^{1}/$_4$ minced sweet red pepper, and a scant tablespoon of Hellmann's Light mayonnaise with a splash of apple cider vinegar.

PER SERVING: AN EXTRA 9 GRAMS CARBOHYDRATE, 2 GRAMS PROTEIN

Chicken with Chèvre, Smoked Bacon, and Pepper Salsa

SERVES 2

4 single chicken breasts, pounded thin
$^1/_4$ cup soft goat cheese
2 thick slices of smoked bacon, diced
2 garlic cloves, minced
$^1/_2$ cup chopped onion
$^1/_2$ cup chopped mixed peppers (red, green, yellow, and jalapeño)
2 tablespoons minced cilantro

Spread 2 of the pounded chicken breasts with the cheese. Cover them with the remaining chicken breasts and sandwich them together, securing them with toothpicks. Fry the diced bacon in a skillet large enough to hold the chicken breasts. Remove the crisp bacon and set aside. Pour off all but 2 tablespoons of the bacon fat. Sauté the chicken on both sides over medium heat until lightly golden. Remove them to a microwave-safe dish and cover with plastic wrap. Sauté the garlic, onion, and mixed pepper salsa until limp but not soft. Toss in the cilantro. When you're ready to serve, cook the chicken in the microwave for about 5–6 minutes. Top the chicken with the salsa and bacon.

PER SERVING: 6 GRAMS CARBOHYDRATE, 35 GRAMS PROTEIN

• Serve with a mixed green salad with slices of $^1/_2$ avocado, 3 to 4 cherry tomatoes, and a lime vinaigrette.

PER SERVING: AN EXTRA 8 GRAMS CARBOHYDRATE, 2 GRAMS PROTEIN

Turkey Burgers with Red Wine Sauce

SERVES 2

3 tablespoons olive oil or butter
2 tablespoons chopped shallot
2 garlic cloves, minced
   pinch of dried thyme

pinch of dried rosemary
pinch of dried oregano
1 teaspoon mustard with green peppercorns
1 cup Zinfandel or other fruity red wine
$^3/_4$ pound ground turkey or mixed chicken and turkey

Heat the oil in a small skillet and sauté the shallot and garlic over medium heat until wilted but not brown, about 2 minutes. Add the dried herbs and mustard and mix well. Add the red wine and reduce by half over high heat. Loosely form the meat into 2 patties and fry them over medium heat in another small skillet. Cook the burgers about 6 minutes on each side. Pour the sauce over the burgers.

PER SERVING: 8 GRAMS CARBOHYDRATE, 36 GRAMS PROTEIN

• Serve with $^1/_2$ cup chopped mushrooms sautéed with $^1/_2$ cup chopped green and yellow summer squash.

PER SERVING: AN EXTRA 3 GRAMS CARBOHYDRATE

Lemon Chicken with Choron Sauce

SERVES 2

This sauce is a French classic, named after the chef who invented it.

1 roasting chicken or carryout rotisserie chicken
  salt and pepper to taste
3 lemons
6 garlic cloves, peeled
$^1/_2$ medium onion
  olive oil

Choron Sauce:

3 egg yolks
2 tablespoons fresh lemon juice
$^1/_2$ teaspoon salt
  pinch of cayenne pepper
$3^1/_2$ tablespoons butter
$^1/_4$ cup tomato puree

If you're roasting your own chicken, preheat the oven to 375°. Rinse the chicken inside and out and pat dry. Salt and pepper the cavity. Pierce the lemons all over with a fork and stuff them into the chicken along with the garlic and the half onion cut in two. Skewer the cavity closed (using meat skewers or wooden kebab sticks) and tie the legs together. Rub the chicken with olive oil and roast for 1 to $1^{1}/_{2}$ hours, depending on its size. Remove the chicken from the oven, discard the stuffing, and let the bird sit while you make the sauce.

Beat the yolks in a blender until thick and yellow. Add the lemon juice, $^{1}/_{2}$ teaspoon salt, and the cayenne. Melt the butter in the microwave and, while still hot, drizzle it slowly into the yolks with the blender running. The sauce will thicken quickly. Add the tomato puree and pour the warm sauce over the carved chicken.

PER SERVING: 4 GRAMS CARBOHYDRATE, 45 GRAMS PROTEIN (PER 6-OUNCE PORTION)

✓ Serve with 1 cup buttered steamed broccoli with toasted pine nuts.

PER SERVING: AN EXTRA 3 GRAMS CARBOHYDRATE, 2 GRAMS PROTEIN

Chicken Breasts Stuffed with Prosciutto and Mozzarella

SERVES 2

    2 whole chicken breasts, boned and split
    4 paper-thin slices of prosciutto
    4 thin slices of mozzarella
    1 tablespoon Pillsbury Shake & Blend flour
    3 tablespoons olive oil
$^{2}/_{3}$ cup dry white wine
$^{1}/_{2}$ cup tomato sauce
$^{1}/_{4}$ teaspoon dried oregano
       salt and pepper to taste
       minced parsley for garnish

Pound the chicken breasts between 2 pieces of wax paper until very thin. Put a slice of prosciutto and a slice of cheese on top of each. Roll the breasts up, tucking in the sides and securing the ends with toothpicks. Sprinkle each breast very lightly with the instant flour. Brown the rolls in the olive oil in a sauté pan over medium-high heat and transfer them to a microwave-safe covered dish. Pour the wine into the sauté pan and simmer vigorously, scraping up any browned bits and reducing the wine by half. Add the remaining ingredients and simmer for another minute or two. Pour over the chicken rolls and microwave on high for 3 to 4 minutes. Garnish with minced parsley.

PER SERVING: 10 GRAMS CARBOHYDRATE, 42 GRAMS PROTEIN

• Serve with a mixed green salad with arugula and bitter greens or spinach. Add $^1/_4$ cup canned marinated artichoke hearts to each serving.

PER SERVING: AN EXTRA 3.5 GRAMS CARBOHYDRATE, 1 GRAM PROTEIN

Chicken Chile Verde with Pepitas

SERVES 4

   3 tablespoons peanut oil
   4 chicken thighs and 4 breasts, boned
   4 garlic cloves, minced
$^1/_2$ cup chopped onion
    salt and pepper to taste
   2 teaspoons ground cumin
   4 tomatillos, husked and finely chopped
   1 cup chopped canned mild green chilies
   2 to 3 canned jalapeños to taste, minced
$^1/_2$ cup chicken broth
$^1/_4$ cup minced cilantro
   1 tablespoon per serving roasted, shelled pumpkin seeds
   2 tablespoons sour cream

Heat the oil in a large skillet over medium heat. Sauté the chicken in the oil until golden, about 4 minutes on each side. Add the garlic and onion, reduce the heat, and cook until the garlic is soft, about 3 minutes. Add salt and pepper and sprinkle in the cumin. Add the tomatillos, chilies, and broth. Cover and simmer until the chicken is tender and the sauce thickened, about 30 minutes. Add the cilantro and serve the chicken sprinkled with the pumpkin seeds and a dollop of sour cream.

PER SERVING: 7.5 GRAMS CARBOHYDRATE, 46 GRAMS PROTEIN

• Serve with $^1/_2$ sliced avocado on Caesar salad (page 250).

PER SERVING: AN EXTRA 3.7 GRAMS CARBOHYDRATE, 2 GRAMS PROTEIN

Barbecued Chicken Wings

SERVES 10

Our friend Bill Parker developed this wonderful recipe, which has become a family favorite. The secret is to cook the wings long and slowly, then dunk them in the sauce just before serving. Be careful not to burn the wings—if you don't have a cover on your grill, just use a big piece of foil.

The sauce:

    1 cup water
  1/2 cup olive oil
  1/2 cup vinegar, white or apple cider
    2 tablespoons chili powder
  1/2 teaspoon cayenne pepper

Mix the sauce ingredients together in a saucepan and bring to a boil over high heat. Boil 5 minutes, then set aside.

The wings:

    5 pounds chicken wings
      salt and pepper

Prepare a grill for barbecuing. Snip the wing tips off and sprinkle the wings with salt and pepper. Arrange the wings on the grill when the coals are glowing red and covered with white ash or set the grill for medium-hot. Cook the wings covered for 1 to 1 1/2 hours, turning frequently, until the wings seem a bit dry.

Remove the wings from the grill and immediately dunk them in the sauce. Arrange on a platter and serve.

PER SERVING: 1.4 GRAMS CARBOHYDRATE, 38 GRAMS PROTEIN

Baked Grouper with Parsley and Lemon

SERVES 2

$^3/_4$ to 1 pound grouper, flounder, or any firm white fish fillet
1 egg beaten with 1 tablespoon milk
3 tablespoons wheat germ
2 tablespoons freshly grated Parmesan cheese
1 tablespoon almond or olive oil
1 tablespoon butter
2 tablespoons minced parsley
1 teaspoon grated lemon zest

Soak the fish in the egg wash for 30 minutes. Mix the wheat germ with the Parmesan and dip the fish into it on both sides to form a light coating—no more than needed. Preheat the oven to 375°. Heat the oil and butter together in a nonstick skillet with an ovenproof handle and lightly brown the fillet on both sides over medium heat. Remove the skillet to the oven and bake for 15 minutes or until the fish is firm. Garnish with parsley and lemon zest.

PER SERVING: 4.5 GRAMS CARBOHYDRATE, 47 GRAMS PROTEIN

• Serve with $^1/_2$ cup peeled, seeded, and chopped cucumber sautéed in butter with 1 tablespoon grated carrot.

PER SERVING: AN EXTRA 4 GRAMS CARBOHYDRATE

Coconut Salmon

SERVES 2

$^1/_4$ cup peanut oil
2 large shallots, thinly sliced
1 tablespoon turmeric
   pinch of cayenne pepper
   pinch of ground mace
$^3/_4$ pound salmon fillet, cut into 2 servings
$^1/_2$ cup Thai unsweetened coconut milk
   cilantro sprigs for garnish

In a small skillet, heat the peanut oil over medium-high heat. When it's very hot, add the shallots and fry until deep brown, about 5 minutes. Strain them out onto a folded paper towel to crisp—set aside. Mix the spices in a small saucer and dip the salmon into them, rubbing the fillets all over to coat them lightly. Put the salmon into a covered microwave-safe dish and pour in the coconut milk. Microwave on high for about 3 minutes or until the salmon is opaque and just firm to the touch. Serve with the crispy shallots on top and a sprig of cilantro.

PER SERVING: 3 GRAMS CARBOHYDRATE, 36 GRAMS PROTEIN

• Serve with 1 cup sautéed fresh or cooked frozen spinach. Sauté the fresh spinach in a tablespoon or more of olive oil and a minced garlic clove or lightly butter the cooked frozen spinach. Add salt and pepper.

PER SERVING: AN EXTRA 3 GRAMS CARBOHYDRATE, 5.4 GRAMS PROTEIN

Portobello Mushrooms Stuffed with Salmon and Spinach

SERVES 2

    2 large portobello mushrooms, stemmed
    3 teaspoons sunflower oil or light olive oil
      salt and pepper to taste
    2 tablespoons minced scallion
  $^1/_2$ pound salmon fillet, skinned and chopped
    1 10-ounce package frozen whole-leaf spinach, thawed
    3 tablespoons cream cheese

Brush the mushrooms with the oil, and salt and pepper them. Broil them upside down for 3 minutes. Preheat the oven to 375°. Sprinkle a tablespoon of minced scallion on each mushroom and divide the chopped salmon between them. Cook the spinach according to the microwave instructions and drain well. Blot out most of the water and chop it coarsely. Put 1 cup of the spinach back in the microwave with the cream cheese just to melt the cheese. Mix it well with a fork. Add salt and pepper. Pile the spinach over the salmon and bake the stuffed mushrooms for 20 minutes.

PER SERVING: 4 GRAMS CARBOHYDRATE, 29 GRAMS PROTEIN

• Serve with a lettuce and tomato salad.

PER SERVING: AN EXTRA 4 GRAMS CARBOHYDRATE

Grilled Tuna Steak with Gingered Slaw

SERVES 2

  2 tablespoons avocado or light olive oil
  1/4 teaspoon Sriracha Thai chili sauce or other hot sauce
  2 tuna steaks, 1 inch thick

Gingered Slaw:

  2 cups very thinly sliced red cabbage
  2 cups very thinly sliced Napa cabbage
  6 scallions, trimmed and slivered lengthwise
  1/2 cup skinny green beans, slivered lengthwise
  1/4 large yellow bell pepper, cut into thin strips
    salt and pepper to taste

Dressing:

  1/2 teaspoon toasted sesame oil (Asian)
  3 additional tablespoons avocado or sunflower oil
  1 tablespoon rice wine vinegar
  1 teaspoon soy sauce
  1 tablespoon sesame seeds
  2 teaspoons minced pickled ginger
    small pinch of NutraSweet or Equal or a couple of drops of
      Sweet 10

Mix the oil and chili sauce and rub it into the tuna steaks on both sides. Combine all of the prepared vegetables in a large bowl. Lightly salt and pepper them. Whisk together the dressing ingredients. Grill the steaks over white ash–coated coals, or sauté them for about 1 minute on each side. Toss the salad and serve.

PER SERVING: 10 GRAMS CARBOHYDRATE, 29 GRAMS PROTEIN

• Tuna cooks particularly fast because of its oil content, so be sure not to overcook it or it will be very dry. As soon as the steak hits the heat you can actually monitor the cooking process by watching the edge of the meat. The opaque gray color will rise like a thermometer. Turn the steak before the color line reaches the center and remove it from the heat while the center is still red.

Crab Cakes

SERVES 2

1/2 pound lump or backfin crabmeat
2 tablespoons Hellmann's mayonnaise
1 tablespoon sour cream
  Tabasco sauce to taste
3 scallions, both white and green parts, minced
2 tablespoons minced parsley
1 teaspoon capers, chopped, or 1/4 teaspoon lemon zest
6 Sunshine oyster crackers, finely crushed
2 teaspoons Wondra flour
2 tablespoons butter

Pick over the crabmeat to remove any cartilage without breaking up the lumps. Mix together the next 6 ingredients and fold carefully into the crabmeat. Add the crushed oyster crackers and lightly form the meat into 4 round cakes without compressing it. Refrigerate the cakes for 1 hour. Lightly dust both sides with presifted flour. Melt the butter in a skillet large enough to hold the crab cakes. Sauté them in the melted butter over medium-low heat until golden brown and heated through, about 4 minutes on each side.

PER SERVING: 5 GRAMS CARBOHYDRATE, 28 GRAMS PROTEIN

• Serve with 1/2 avocado stuffed with radish salad: mix finely slivered red and white radishes with salt and pepper, then drizzle with a little balsamic vinegar.

PER SERVING: AN EXTRA 4 GRAMS CARBOHYDRATE, 2 GRAMS PROTEIN

Scallops and Ham with Honey Mustard Sauce

SERVES 2

  2 scallions, minced
  3 thin slices of domestic prosciutto or Black Forest ham
  1 tablespoon safflower or light olive oil
12 large sea scallops
  2 tablespoons Dijon honey mustard
  1 teaspoon grated fresh ginger with juice
  2 teaspoons Chinese oyster sauce

In a nonstick pan, sauté the scallions and ham in the oil over medium heat until the ham is lightly frizzled and the scallions soft, about 3 minutes. Blot the scallops dry on paper towels. Push the ham and scallions to the side of the pan and sauté the scallops over medium-high heat, turning them frequently. When the scallops have patches of golden brown, reduce the heat and add the mustard, ginger, and oyster sauce. Toss all the ingredients together and simmer until the scallops are cooked through.

PER SERVING: 4 GRAMS CARBOHYDRATE, 12 GRAMS PROTEIN

• Serve the scallops with $1/2$ cup sugar snap peas or snow peas stir-fried with 2 sliced water chestnuts and mushrooms.

PER SERVING: AN EXTRA 6.5 GRAMS CARBOHYDRATE, 1 GRAM PROTEIN

Greek Shrimp with Feta Cheese

SERVES 2

   3 tablespoons olive oil
   2 garlic cloves, minced
     hot red pepper flakes to taste
$1/2$ teaspoon crushed dried oregano
$1/2$ cup strips of drained canned Italian plum tomatoes
   3 tablespoons bottled clam juice
   2 tablespoons chopped fresh dill
   1 tablespoon drained capers

    salt and pepper to taste
1¹/₂ tablespoons butter
 12 to 16 large shrimp, peeled but tails left on
  3 tablespoons crumbled feta cheese

In a small skillet over medium heat, sauté the garlic, pepper flakes, and oregano in the olive oil until the garlic is soft and golden, about 2 minutes. Add the tomatoes and clam juice and simmer until most of the liquid evaporates, about 3 minutes. Add the dill, capers, and salt and pepper. Preheat the oven to 400°. Pour the sauce into a bowl and wipe out the skillet. Heat the butter over medium-high heat until it starts to brown. Toss and sauté the shrimp very briefly—just sealing and glazing the exterior and not cooking them through. Divide the shrimp between 2 ovenproof gratin dishes, arranging the tails up. Spoon the sauce over the shrimp and sprinkle the cheese on top. Bake for 15 minutes.

PER SERVING: 4.5 GRAMS CARBOHYDRATE, 15 GRAMS PROTEIN

• Serve with a big green salad.

Beef Provençal

SERVES 4

Make this dish the day before you plan to serve it to give the flavors a chance to develop fully.

 ¹/₄ pound sliced slab bacon
  2 pounds boneless chuck or rump roast, cut into 2-inch cubes
  2 medium onions, quartered
    salt and pepper to taste
  1 small fennel bulb, trimmed and thinly sliced
  1 head of garlic, separated into cloves and peeled
  6 large strips of orange zest
  1 bay leaf
    pinch of dried thyme
  1 cup full-bodied, fruity red wine
  1 cup canned beef broth
 12 Mediterranean black olives, pitted

Use a 12-inch sauté pan with a tight lid. Sauté the bacon over medium heat until crisp and set it aside. Leave the bacon fat in the pan. Brown the meat and glaze the onions in the bacon fat. When they're golden, salt and pepper the meat and onions and add the rest of the ingredients except the olives, barely covering them with the liquid. Cover the pan and simmer the stew over very low heat for a couple of hours. Let it cool with the cover on, then refrigerate. Before reheating the next day, skim off any solidified fat that's risen to the surface. Serve the stew garnished with the crumbled bacon and the black olives along with a large green salad vinaigrette sprinkled with grated Parmesan.

PER SERVING: 8 GRAMS CARBOHYDRATE, 60 GRAMS PROTEIN

Zesty Beef Sangria

SERVES 4

Since leftovers of this dish are delicious, this recipe makes enough for 2 meals for 2 people.

> 2 pounds rump roast, chuck, or brisket
> 2 tablespoons chili powder
>   salt to taste
> $^1/_4$ pound smoked slab bacon, diced
> $^1/_4$ cup chopped onion
> 4 garlic cloves, minced
> 2 canned chipotle chilies, minced (optional)
> 1 cup Zinfandel or Spanish Rioja
> 2 tablespoons Triple Sec
>   zest of $^1/_2$ medium orange

Rub the meat well with the chili powder and salt. Let it sit until it comes to room temperature. Cut it into $1^1/_2$-inch cubes. In a large skillet with a tight cover, sauté the diced bacon over medium-high heat until most of the fat is rendered. Pour off all but about 3 tablespoons of bacon fat. Sauté the beef in the skillet with the bacon until it's well browned on all sides. Add the onion, garlic, and minced chipotle. Stir and toss until the onion and garlic softens and browns lightly. Add the wine, Triple Sec, and orange zest, cover the pan, and simmer over very low heat until the meat is fork-tender, about 1 hour, or longer, depending on the cut of beef selected.

PER SERVING: 4 GRAMS CARBOHYDRATE, 56 GRAMS PROTEIN

• Serve with $^3/_4$ cup baked acorn squash, buttered and sprinkled with a little cinnamon. Or serve it over $^3/_4$ cup spaghetti squash.

PER SERVING: AN EXTRA 8 GRAMS CARBOHYDRATE, 1 GRAM PROTEIN

Bulgogi

SERVES 2

This is an indoor version of the classic Korean beef barbecue. Actually you'll end up eating less than the 5 grams of carbohydrate listed here, since most of the marinade stays behind.

1 pound flank steak, rib-eye, or tenderloin

Marinade:

  $^1/_4$ cup chopped scallion
   2 garlic cloves, minced
  $^1/_2$ teaspoon grated fresh ginger
   2 tablespoons soy sauce
   1 tablespoon toasted sesame seeds, crushed
    pinch of NutraSweet or Equal
   2 teaspoons freshly ground black pepper
$1^1/_2$ tablespoons sake or dry sherry

   3 tablespoons peanut oil
   6 scallions, sliced diagonally, for garnish
   1 teaspoon toasted sesame seeds for garnish

Slice the meat across the grain into very thin slices about 3/8 inch thick. Combine the marinade ingredients and rub into the beef with your hands. Place in a covered dish or plastic bag and leave it to develop flavor for 2 hours in the refrigerator.

Drain the meat and sear in the hot peanut oil in a nonstick skillet or a wok over high heat for 1 minute. Do not overcook. Serve garnished with the sliced scallions and a sprinkling of sesame seeds.

PER SERVING: 5 GRAMS CARBOHYDRATE, 57 GRAMS PROTEIN

• Serve with 1 cup steamed broccoli pieces tossed with 2 sliced water chestnuts for an extra 4 grams carbohydrate and 2 grams protein.

• You can also omit the peanut oil and simply add the meat, marinade and all, to the hot skillet.

Chili-Stuffed Peppers

SERVES 2

   2 large red or green bell peppers
$^3/_4$ pound ground chuck
   2 garlic cloves, minced
   1 small red onion, minced
   1 canned chipotle chili in adobo or 1 canned jalapeño plus a
      dash of liquid smoke
    salt and pepper to taste
   1 teaspoon ground cumin
   1 teaspoon dried oregano
$^1/_2$ cup grated cheddar or Monterey Jack cheese

Grill the peppers over an open flame or directly under the broiler, turning often, until the skin is totally charred. Watch them closely so the peppers don't collapse. As soon as they are blackened, put them into a plastic bag and let them sit for a few minutes until they're just cool enough to handle. (Don't let them sit too long, or the steam in the bag will soften the peppers too much.) Rub off all the skin. Carefully cut around the stem and pull it out. Carefully scoop out the seeds with a teaspoon. If you mistakenly tear a pepper, don't despair; they'll taste good anyway. Preheat the oven to 350°.

Mix the meat well with the remaining ingredients except the cheese. Stuff the peppers and stand them up or sit them down on a pie plate or shallow oven pan. Bake them for about 20 minutes and then remove them from the oven to mound the cheese on top. Return the peppers to the oven to melt the cheese and ensure that the meat is cooked.

PER SERVING: 8.5 GRAMS CARBOHYDRATE, 32 GRAMS PROTEIN

• Serve with an avocado salsa made with $^1/_2$ cubed avocado tossed with a couple of slivered cherry tomatoes, minced scallion, and cilantro. Add salt and pepper to taste.

PER SERVING: AN EXTRA 6 GRAMS CARBOHYDRATE, 2 GRAMS PROTEIN

Microwaved Stuffed Peppers:

Slice the stem end from the peppers at the point where the edge is straight. Shake and pull out the seeds and stand the peppers up in a small microwave-safe dish. Stuff them with the meat mixture and pour $1/2$ inch beef broth in the bottom of the dish. Cover the dish with plastic wrap and microwave for 6 to 8 minutes on high. Remove the plastic wrap, pile the cheese on top, and put them back in the microwave for 20 seconds.

Italian Stuffed Peppers:

Using green bell peppers and the same procedure, stuff them with $3/4$ pound of ground veal or mixed ground chicken and turkey. Season the meat with 3 slivered slices of prosciutto, 2 pressed garlic cloves, 3 tablespoons minced parsley, 1 teaspoon lemon zest, and salt and pepper to taste. Mix in 1 egg whisked with 2 tablespoons of crème fraîche or sour cream, a pinch of freshly grated nutmeg, and $1/4$ cup of grated Parmesan cheese. Top off each cooked pepper with a little dollop of crème fraîche or sour cream.

Cabbage Lasagne

SERVES 8

The "noodles" here are cabbage leaves. You can use Swiss chard the same way.

> 1 medium to large head of cabbage
> 1 tablespoon olive oil
> 2 garlic cloves, minced or pressed
> 1 medium onion, chopped
> 1 green bell pepper, chopped
> $3/4$ pound ground beef
> 1 6-ounce can Hunt's tomato paste
> 1 8-ounce can Hunt's tomato sauce
> 1 teaspoon dried oregano

2 teaspoons salt
1 teaspoon black pepper
1 cup grated mozzarella cheese
$^1/_2$ cup ricotta or cottage cheese
$^1/_2$ cup freshly grated Parmesan cheese

Preheat the oven to 350°. Wash the cabbage and remove the tough outer leaves. Cut the head in half. Carefully peel back the leaves, trying to keep them intact; these will serve as the lasagne noodles. Arrange the individual leaves on a steamer basket or tray and steam until nearly tender, about 3 to 5 minutes. (You can also do this in the microwave.) Set aside.

Put the olive oil in a large skillet over medium-high heat. Sauté the garlic, onion, and green pepper until the onion is translucent. Add the ground beef and brown thoroughly. Drain or skim the accumulated fat and water. Add the tomato paste, tomato sauce, and seasonings to the mixture and combine well.

Coat a 9- by 13- by 2-inch baking pan with a little olive oil. Line the bottom with a layer of cabbage leaves. Top with half of the meat mixture. Add a third of the mozzarella and half of the ricotta cheese. Add another layer of cabbage leaves, the remaining half of the meat mixture, another third of the mozzarella, and the remaining half of the ricotta. Top with the remaining mozzarella and finish by scattering the Parmesan on top.

Bake, covered, for about 20 minutes. Uncover and bake for 5 minutes more.

PER SERVING: 9 GRAMS CARBOHYDRATE, 20 GRAMS PROTEIN

• This dish freezes well. Cool, then cut into 8 servings. Wrap individually in freezer wrap. To reheat, thaw and heat in the microwave for approximately 4 minutes on high.

• Serve the lasagne with a big green salad tossed with a red wine vinegar and olive oil dressing.

Finnish Meat Loaf

SERVES 6

This typical Finnish meat loaf is traditionally wrapped with sour cream pastry and taken along on cross-country skiing picnics. It's delicious either hot or cold and should be served with a big dollop of sour cream.

    1 cup chopped mushrooms
 $^1/_2$ cup chopped onion
    4 tablespoons ($^1/_2$ stick) butter
    3 pounds ground meat: $1^1/_2$ pounds beef and $^1/_2$ pound each
        pork, ham, and veal
 $^1/_4$ cup minced parsley
      freshly ground pepper to taste
    1 cup grated Gruyère cheese
 $^1/_2$ cup heavy cream

Preheat the oven to 350°. Sauté the chopped mushrooms and onion in the butter over medium heat until the onion is soft, about 5 minutes. Add the cooked mixture to the ground meat and remaining ingredients, reserving $^1/_4$ cup of the cheese for the top. Mix it all together with your fingers and press the mixture into a loaf pan. Sprinkle the top with cheese and bake the meat loaf for an hour.

• If you don't use the ham, add a teaspoon of salt to the mixture.

PER SERVING: 2.5 GRAMS CARBOHYDRATE, 66 GRAMS PROTEIN, PLUS SOUR CREAM GARNISH AT .5 GRAM CARBOHYDRATE AND 1 GRAM PROTEIN PER TABLESPOON

• Serve with $^1/_2$ cup sliced roasted beets seasoned with olive oil, salt and pepper, and a splash of balsamic vinegar. (Roast whole unpeeled beets in a 375° oven for about 1 hour or until the tip of a knife pierces them easily. When cool enough to handle, slip the skins off with your fingers. These beets reheat well in the microwave.) Add a spinach salad with slivered scallions.

PER SERVING: AN EXTRA 6 GRAMS CARBOHYDRATE, 38 GRAMS PROTEIN

Veal Scaloppine with Ricotta and Swiss Chard

SERVES 2

 $^3/_4$ pound veal scaloppine
    2 eggs, beaten with a pinch of salt and pepper
    1 bunch of Swiss chard, stemmed
    2 garlic cloves, minced
    2 tablespoons butter
 $^1/_2$ cup ricotta cheese
    3 tablespoons sour cream

nutmeg, preferably freshly grated
salt and pepper to taste
1 **tablespoon freshly grated Parmesan cheese**

Soak the veal in the beaten egg for 30 minutes. Meanwhile, stack and roll up the Swiss chard leaves, then slice across the roll into 1-inch ribbons. Sauté the chard with the garlic in the butter over medium-high heat for 10 minutes. Remove and reserve 1 cup.

Preheat the oven to 375°. In the same skillet, over low heat, add half the veal slices one at a time and cook just long enough to set the egg coating on both sides. Remove the slices as they're cooked to an ovenproof gratin dish. Put the ricotta and sour cream in the processor or blender with a pinch of nutmeg, salt and pepper, and the grated Parmesan. Blend until smooth. Spread half the cheese mixture over the veal with the back of a spoon. Layer $^1/_2$ cup Swiss chard on top. Cook the rest of the scaloppine and cover the first batch. Layer on the other $^1/_2$ cup Swiss chard and then spread the rest of the cheese on top. Bake for about 30 minutes or until the cheese topping is set.

PER SERVING: 9.5 GRAMS CARBOHYDRATE, 46 GRAMS PROTEIN

• Serve with a mixed green salad vinaigrette.

Grilled Lamb Burgers with Roasted Eggplant Puree

SERVES 2

The spicy eggplant puree transforms simple ground lamb patties into something special. The leftover puree will keep for several days in the refrigerator and is equally good as a vegetable dip or an accompaniment to a cold roast chicken.

1 **medium eggplant**
2 **tablespoons roasted garlic paste, Consorzio brand or**
    homemade
$^1/_2$ **teaspoon harissa (Moroccan hot sauce), available at specialty**
    food stores and some supermarkets, or other hot sauce
$^1/_4$ **cup minced cilantro**
3 **tablespoons minced scallion**

1 tablespoon fresh lemon juice
3 tablespoons olive oil
   salt to taste
   grilled lamb burgers

Pierce the eggplant skin in a few places and roast it in a 400° oven un-til it's soft all the way through, about 30 minutes. Slit it lengthwise and let it cool. Meanwhile, mix together everything else but the olive oil, salt, and lamb into a thick paste, then slowly whisk in the olive oil. Spoon out the eggplant flesh into a food processor and add the seasoning paste. Blend until smooth but not soupy. Add salt to taste. Add more harissa if you like things spicier. Add more oil if necessary. Grill the lamb burgers and top with a spoonful of eggplant.

PER SERVING: 3 TO 5 GRAMS CARBOHYDRATE, DEPENDING ON HOW MUCH EGGPLANT YOU DEVOUR, 28 GRAMS PROTEIN

• Serve with $1/2$ cup baby carrots, blanched in the microwave and then sautéed in butter until lightly brown.

PER SERVING: AN EXTRA 3 GRAMS CARBOHYDRATE

Cold Lamb with Raw Vegetable Salad

SERVES 2

This is not only a great way to make a meal from leftover roast lamb or any roast meat or poultry, but it's delicious enough not to seem like left-overs at all.

      sliced roast lamb, turkey, chicken, or ham, about 6 ounces
$1/4$ pound cream cheese, softened in the microwave
$1/4$ teaspoon paprika
$1/4$ teaspoon salt
  2 tablespoons fresh lemon juice
  2 tablespoons minced parsley
  2 tablespoons minced fresh dill
$1/4$ cup olive oil
$1/2$ cup sliced firm white mushrooms
$1/2$ cup red bell pepper strips
  1 cup thin slices of zucchini
  8 cherry tomatoes, cut in half
  6 scallions, both white and green parts, minced
     pepper to taste

Use a food processor to blend the cream cheese with the next 5 ingredients. When it's smooth, drizzle in the olive oil a little at a time until the seasoned cheese absorbs it all and the sauce is thick but pourable. Taste for salt, pour over the mixed vegetables, and give the salad a few grinds of fresh pepper. Serve alongside the cold sliced meat.

PER SERVING: 11 GRAMS CARBOHYDRATE, 26 GRAMS PROTEIN

Butterflied Pork Chops with Bourbon Mustard Sauce

SERVES 2

> salt and pepper to taste
> 2 butterflied pork chops, ³/₄ inch thick
> 3 tablespoons butter, preferably clarified
> 1 tablespoon olive oil
> 3 tablespoons bourbon
> 2 tablespoons minced shallot
> 1 cup thinly sliced mushrooms
> ¹/₈ teaspoon dried thyme
> 1 tablespoon Dijon mustard
> ¹/₄ cup heavy cream
> 1 tablespoon minced parsley

Salt and pepper the chops. In a skillet large enough to hold the chops, sauté them in 2 tablespoons of the butter and the olive oil over medium-high heat until nicely browned on both sides. Pour in the bourbon and swirl it around in the pan over medium-high heat until it reduces to a thin syrupy glaze. Add the shallot and mushrooms, cover the pan, and cook for 5 minutes. Crush the thyme between your fingers and sprinkle over the chops. Add the mustard and cream, cover the pan, and simmer for 25 minutes. Remove the chops to serving plates, add the remaining butter to the pan, and swirl it into the mustard sauce. Pour the sauce and mushrooms over the chops and sprinkle with the parsley.

PER SERVING: 3 GRAMS CARBOHYDRATE, 21 GRAMS PROTEIN

• Serve with 1 cup steamed spinach.

PER SERVING: AN EXTRA 3.1 GRAMS CARBOHYDRATE, 5.4 GRAMS PROTEIN

Ranch Chili with Cheese

SERVES 2

    3 tablespoons peanut oil
    1 pound beef chuck, minced or ground once
  $1/2$ cup chopped onion
    2 garlic cloves, minced
    2 tablespoons chili powder
  $1/2$ teaspoon crushed dried oregano
  $1/2$ teaspoon paprika
  $1/2$ teaspoon ground cumin
  $1/4$ teaspoon cayenne pepper
  $1/2$ cup Contadina tomato puree
  $1/2$ cup strong leftover black coffee or canned beef broth
    1 tablespoon masa harina or cornmeal, optional
    3 tablespoons grated cheddar cheese

Heat the oil in a large skillet over medium-high heat. Add the beef and brown it, then add the onion, garlic, and all the seasonings. Stir and cook until well mixed and the onions are limp. Transfer to a covered saucepan and add the tomato puree and coffee. Cover and simmer the chili for an hour, adding a little water if it becomes dry. The chili should be thick and soupy. Add the masa and simmer for 10 more minutes. Serve in bowls, sprinkled with cheddar.

PER SERVING: 10 GRAMS CARBOHYDRATE, 56 GRAMS PROTEIN

• You can add chopped green bell peppers to this chili—1 medium pepper, added along with the onions, will contribute a little less than 2 additional grams carbohydrate. You may want to delete the cornmeal in that case to keep the dish under 10 grams.

Desserts

Chocolate Chip Cheesecakes

SERVES 12

You don't have to use ersatz sugar for these little tarts, but each cheese-cake is only 2 grams carbohydrate if you use NutraSweet instead.

> 12 1³/₄-inch fluted paper cups
>   12-cup mini-muffin tin
> 1 large graham cracker, finely crushed
> 1 extra-large egg
> ¹/₄ cup sugar or NutraSweet Spoonful
> ¹/₄ teaspoon vanilla extract
> 1 8-ounce package Philadelphia cream cheese, softened
> 2 tablespoons semisweet mini chocolate chips

Preheat the oven to 350°. Place the paper cups in the muffin tin and distribute the crushed graham cracker among the cups. Put all the ingredients except the chocolate chips into a food processor and blend thoroughly—or beat the egg, sugar, and vanilla together well with a whisk and then incorporate the cheese. Fold in the chocolate chips and then spoon the blended mixture into the cups. Bake for 15 minutes or until the edges are set and the center is still moist. Remove the cheesecakes from the muffin tin and let them cool. Refrigerate for at least an hour before serving.

PER SERVING: 5 GRAMS CARBOHYDRATE (MADE WITH SUGAR), 2 GRAMS CARBOHYDRATE (NUTRASWEET), 3 GRAMS PROTEIN

• Use different flavorings to change these little treats. Substitute a couple of teaspoons of instant espresso coffee powder for the chocolate chips or leave in the chips for a mocha cheesecake. Use lemon extract or a tablespoon of fresh lemon juice instead of the vanilla and add some grated lemon or lime zest. Sprinkle the tops of the cheesecakes with toasted unsweetened coconut for a little crunch—or bury a single whole toasted almond in each cake and flavor with almond extract. Remove the paper and serve two on a plate with a drizzle of fresh raspberry puree (page 236) for an extra 1 gram carbohydrate.

Meringue Tart Shells

SERVES 6

These elegant little company dessert jewels can be filled with berries and whipped cream. It may take you a few trial runs to get them crispy. Don't open the oven door too soon.

    3 egg whites
  $^1/_4$ teaspoon salt
    3 teaspoons NutraSweet Spoonful or 3 packets of Equal
    1 teaspoon almond extract
  $^1/_2$ cup grated almonds
  $^1/_2$ cup shredded unsweetened coconut (optional)

Preheat the oven to 250°.

In a bowl, combine the egg whites, salt, NutraSweet, and almond extract. Beat until stiff. Add the almonds and coconut.

Drop by large spoonfuls onto a buttered cookie sheet. Create a depression in each mound with the bottom of a glass. Bake for 30 minutes. Then turn off heat—*don't* open the oven door. Leave the meringues in the oven for another 30 minutes.

PER SERVING: 3.5 GRAMS CARBOHYDRATE, 5.5 GRAMS PROTEIN

Coconut Flan

SERVES 6

    1 cup unsweetened coconut milk
    1 cup light cream
  $^1/_4$ cup sugar or NutraSweet Spoonful
    4 extra-large eggs
    1 teaspoon vanilla or coconut extract
       nutmeg, preferably freshly grated

Preheat the oven to 325°. Heat the coconut milk, cream, and sugar in a glass pitcher in the microwave for 5 minutes on high or in a saucepan over medium heat until a skin begins to form on the surface. In a heat-proof bowl, whisk together the eggs and extract and, continuing to whisk, add the hot cream in a thin stream. Divide the mixture evenly among six $^1/_2$-cup custard or soufflé cups. Dust the tops with nutmeg. Space the cups apart in a shallow pan—or a glass or ceramic casserole for the microwave—and pour water into the pan about a third of the way up to the top of the cups. Bake for 30 minutes or cook on high for about 6 minutes. Do not overcook; the centers should wiggle slightly. After cooling them completely, refrigerate for at least 4 hours before serving.

PER SERVING: 9.5 GRAMS CARBOHYDRATE (NUTRASWEET), 16.5 GRAMS CARBOHYDRATE (SUGAR), 6 GRAMS PROTEIN

• Try adding a little rum extract or Myers's dark rum. Decorate with a slice or two of kiwifruit or a strip of ripe mango.

• If you're not fond of coconut, leave the coconut milk out and make this flan with 2 cups light cream.

Irish Lace Cookies

MAKES 2 DOZEN COOKIES

$^1/_2$ cup boiling water
2 cups rolled oats
1 tablespoon unsalted butter
4 teaspoons NutraSweet or 4 packets of Equal
2 extra-large eggs
1 teaspoon vanilla extract
2 teaspoons baking powder
$^1/_2$ teaspoon salt

Preheat the oven to 375°.

Pour boiling water over the oats, mix, cover, and set aside to soak. Meanwhile, beat the butter, NutraSweet, eggs, and vanilla together until fluffy and smooth. Add the baking powder and salt to the oats, then pour the oats into the creamed mixture and combine well.

Drop teaspoonsful 2 to 3 inches apart on a lightly greased cookie sheet. Bake for 12 to 15 minutes. Cool completely on a rack. Store in an airtight container in layers separated with wax paper or paper towels.

PER COOKIE: ABOUT 4 GRAMS CARBOHYDRATE, LESS THAN 1 GRAM PROTEIN

Sweets If You Must

Unfortunately, one sweet treat usually begs another, and the unhealthy devotion to sugar can last a lifetime. The good part is that the craving quickly disappears if the temptation is just ignored. Try it—wait ten minutes and reconsider. Once you're into the dynamic phase of weight loss, your cravings will virtually disappear. But we recognize that this is a particularly tough habit to break, so here are a few mini-desserts for when your chin starts to wobble. Since the insulin rush of sugar is lessened if it's consumed or digested with protein, having a sweet with your after-dinner coffee is the best time to sin. If you must indulge between meals, precede it with $1/2$ cup of cottage cheese or other available protein. The suggested candy on this list is individually wrapped to make it easier not to exceed the calculated portions.

GRAMS	CANDY
5	1 Hershey's Nugget with Almonds
6	1 Milky Way Miniature
5.5	1 Chocolate Parfait Nips
4.2	1 tablespoon (12) Nestlé's Goobers (chocolate-covered peanuts)
5	8 Starbucks chocolate-covered espresso beans
5	2 Andes chocolate crème de menthe thins
2	1 Life Savers sugar-free popsicle
4.5	2 Hershey's Kisses with Almonds
4	1 Irish Lace Cookie (page 280)

Warm Brie with Chutney and Almonds

SERVES 4

This makes an unusual dessert served with the apple slices—or an interesting hors d'oeuvre, for that matter.

1$1/4$ pound wedge of Brie cheese or a mini Brie wheel with the rind
2 tablespoons Major Grey chutney, finely chopped
1 to 2 tablespoons sliced blanched almonds to taste

Preheat the oven to 350°. Put the cheese on a piece of aluminum foil on a baking sheet. Spread the chutney over the top of the cheese. Sprinkle with sliced almonds and bake for 5 to 7 minutes or until the cheese is slightly runny. Using a wide spatula, transfer the cheese to a serving plate. Serve with crackers or thinly sliced apples dipped in lemon juice for an additional 1–2 grams of carbohydrate per cracker or apple slice.

PER SERVING: 6 GRAMS CARBOHYDRATE, 7 GRAMS PROTEIN

Espresso Ice Cream with Cinnamon

SERVES 5

¹/₃ cup Italian espresso powder
 1 quart light cream or 2 cups heavy cream plus 2 cups milk or half-and-half
¹/₂ teaspoon ground cinnamon
¹/₂ cup NutraSweet Spoonful to taste

Put the coffee powder, cinnamon, and cream in a microwave-safe bowl and bring it to the brink of a boil in the microwave. Or heat the mixture in a saucepan on top of the stove. Remove from the heat, stir well, and let the coffee and cream steep for at least 30 minutes. Strain it if there are any lumps. Add NutraSweet. Freeze in an ice cream maker according to the manufacturer's directions.

PER SERVING: 9 GRAMS CARBOHYDRATE, 8 GRAMS PROTEIN

Appendix

Sources and Resources

Purveyors of Wild Game

Denver Buffalo Company
1120 Lincoln Street
Denver, CO 80203-9790
Phone: (800) BUY-BUFF; (800) 289-2833
Fax: (303) 831-1292
catalog available

Game Exchange/Polarica
105 Quint Street
San Francisco, CA 94124
Phone: (800) 426-3872
catalog available
    or
73 Hudson Street
New York, NY 10013
Phone: (800) 426-3487
catalog available

Prepackaged Nutritional Meal Replacement Products

If you would like more information about some of the high-quality-protein meal replacement products we use in our practice and how to incorporate them into your new nutritional strategy, call (800) 925-1373.

Other Food Sources

Soya Bluebook
P.O. Box 84
Bar Harbor, ME 04609
Resource guide to manufacturers and distributors of soy products worldwide.

Newsletter

We are in the process of preparing a newsletter for our patients. For subscription information, send your name and address to:
Newsletter
Eades Medical Clinic
11025 Anderson Rd., Suite 130
Little Rock, AR 72212

Pertinent Worthwhile Reading

Neanderthin: A Cave Man's Guide to Nutrition
Ray Audette, Ph.D., Paleolithic Press
This interesting and well-written book adopts a true caveman and almost mystical approach to nutrition: if a caveman could hunt it or gather it to eat it, so can you. An approach more restrictive than we think necessary, but an interesting perspective from a bright and creative writer. Available for $12.00 plus $3.00 shipping and handling from:
Paleolithic Press
6009 Laurel Oaks
Dallas, TX 75248

Diabetes Type II
Richard K. Bernstein, M.D.
Prentice-Hall Press, 1990
Currently out of print, but the best treatise on this disease around. If you have diabetes, make the acquisition of this book a priority. You may find it in the library, through interlibrary loan services, used-book stores, or a book search service. Dr. Bernstein is in the process of revising and updating a new edition of this work, which Little, Brown and Company is slated to publish in 1997.

The Zone
Barry Sears, Ph.D.
HarperCollins, 1995
Currently available in bookstores and written by a close friend of ours, this book looks at nutrition from an eicosanoid-modulating perspective. Although Dr. Sears takes a somewhat different approach from ours, the underlying science is fundamentally the same, and his book has great chapters on nutrition and chronic fatigue syndrome, cancer, heart disease and other chronic illnesses, and sports performance.

Motivational Tool

For $39.95, you can have an anatomically correct photograph of yourself at your ideal weight. If you have trouble imagining yourself thin, this photo on your refrigerator may be a powerful totem. Send a front-on whole-body shot plus a check to Slim Photo, 7616 Lindley Avenue, Reseda, CA 91335. Call (213) 964-1871 for an order form.

INDEX

DATE DUE